Outdoor Envii
for People with Dementia

Outdoor Environments for People with Dementia has been co-published simultaneously as *Journal of Housing for the Elderly*, Volume 21, Numbers 1/2 and 3/4 2007.

Outdoor Environments for People with Dementia

Susan Rodiek, PhD, NCARB
Benyamin Schwarz, PhD
Editors

Outdoor Environments for People with Dementia has been co-published simultaneously as *Journal of Housing for the Elderly*, Volume 21, Numbers 1/2 and 3/4 2007.

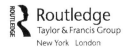

Routledge
Taylor & Francis Group
New York London

First published by

The Haworth Press, 10 Alice Street, Binghamton, NY 13904-1580 USA

This edition published 2012 by Routledge

Routledge
Taylor & Francis Group
711 Third Avenue
New York, NY 10017

Routledge
Taylor & Francis Group
2 Park Square, Milton Park
Abingdon, Oxon OX14 4RN

Outdoor Environments for People with Dementia has been co-published simultaneously as *Journal of Housing for the Elderly*, Volume 21, Numbers 1/2 and 3/4 2007.

Library of Congress Cataloging-in-Publication Data

Outdoor environments for people with dementia / Susan Rodiek, Benyamin Schwarz, editors.
        p. ; cm.
        "Co-published simultaneously as Journal of Housing for the Elderly, Volume 21, Numbers 1/2 and 3/4 2007."
        Includes bibliographical references and index.
        ISBN 978-0-7890-3804-3 (hard cover : alk. paper) – ISBN 978-0-7890-3805-0 (soft cover : alk. paper)
        1. Dementia–Patients–Care–Psychological aspects. 2. Dementia–Patients–Long-term care–Psychological aspects. 3. Long-term care facilities–Landscape architecture–Psychological aspects. 4. Long-term care facilities–Design and construction–Environmental aspects. 5. Dementia–Patients–Recreation. 6. Outdoor recreation–Therapeutic use. 7. Outdoor recreation–Psychological aspects. 8. Gardens–Therapeutic use. 9. Gardens–Psychological aspects. 10. Nature, Healing power of. I. Rodiek, Susan. II. Schwarz, Benyamin. III. Journal of housing for the elderly.
        [DNLM: 1. Dementia–psychology. 2. Dementia–therapy. 3. Environment Design. 4. Aged–psychology. 5. Gardening. 6. Homes for the Aged. 7. Nature. WT 155 O945 2007]
RC521.O94 2007
362.196'83–dc22

                                                                        2007043815

Outdoor Environments for People with Dementia

CONTENTS

ABOUT THE EDITORS

Susan Rodiek, PhD, NCARB, teaches architectural design at Texas A&M University, where she holds the Ronald L. Skaggs Endowed Professorship in Health Facilities Design, and is also Associate Director of the Center for Health Systems & Design. Her work applies professional practice and environment-behavior expertise to healthcare and long-term care facilities.

Her recent research has focused on the benefits of outdoor access for both residents and staff in assisted living facilities. Currently Dr. Rodiek is developing a multimedia educational series to translate evidence-based design principles into practical solutions to improve the quality of outdoor space for older adults. Funded by SBIR grants R43 AG024786 and R44AG024786 from the National Institute on Aging (NIA), this award-winning educational tool targets a broad range of industry professionals, including architects, landscape architects, long term care providers, policy planners, and consumer advocates.

Dr. Rodiek is Coordinator of the combined Environment-Gerontology Network of the Environmental Design Research Association (EDRA), and the International Association of Person-Environment Studies (IAPS). She is an Advisory member of the Texas Healthy Aging Network and the Program on Health Promotion and Aging, School of Rural Public Health of the Texas A&M University System Health Science Center. Dr. Rodiek holds a doctorate in Architecture from Cardiff University, and is a nationally-registered architect with more than twenty years' experience in both landscape and architectural projects. She publishes in the areas of environmental gerontology, healthcare and therapeutic garden environments.

Benyamin Schwarz, PhD, is a Professor in the Department of Architectural Studies at the University of Missouri-Columbia. His teaching specialty areas include design fundamentals, environmental analysis, housing concepts and issues, design studio, architectural programming, and environmental design for aging. He received his bachelor's degree in Architecture and Urban Planning from the Technion, the Institute of Technology of Israel, and his Ph.D. in Architecture from The University of Michigan with an emphasis on Environmental Gerontology. He designed numerous facilities for the elderly in Israel and in the U.S. His research addresses issues of long-term care settings in the United States and abroad, environmental attributes of dementia special care units, assisted living arrangements, and international housing concepts and issues. Dr. Schwarz has been the editor of the *Journal of Housing for the Elderly* since 2000. He is the author of *Nursing Home Design: Consequences of Employing the Medical Model.* His co-edited books with Leon A. Pastalan, include *University-Linked Retirement Communities: Student Visions of Eldercare* and *Housing choices and well-being of older adults: Proper Fit.* He co-edited with Ruth Brent the books, *Popular American Housing: A Reference Guide* and *Aging Autonomy and Architecture: Advances in Assisted-Living.* Dr. Schwarz co-edited with Susan Rodiek *The Role of the Outdoors in Residential Environments for Aging.* His other publications include *Assisted Living: Sobering Realities* and numerous articles in various academic and professional venues.

About the Contributors

Stacey Biddle, COTA/L, has combined her creative talents with degrees in Art Therapy and Occupational Therapy by providing direct service for 15 years to seniors in long term, sub-acute, and home health care. She has extensive experience adapting and modifying the environment to enhance the quality of life of older adults. Ms. Biddle has applied her expertise through project management of research on HIV, dementia, adapted wardrobe systems and incontinence studies.

Elizabeth C. Brawley is a senior interior designer who specializes in supportive, therapeutic environments for aging and Alzheimer's special care. She is the author of the newly released *Design Innovations for Aging and Alzheimer's–Creating Caring Environments*, a detailed guide for a broad range of design issues essential to maintaining independence and functional abilities. She was awarded the 1998 Polsky Prize for her landmark book *Designing for Alzheimer's Disease: Strategies for Creating Better Care Environments*. Ms. Brawley has gained national and international recognition as an expert and industry leader in the area of environmental design for aging.

Margaret Calkins, PhD, is widely recognized as an expert in the creation and evaluation of long-term care settings, particularly for people with dementia. She is President of I.D.E.A.S., Inc., and Chair of the Board of the IDEAS Institute, both of which seek to improve environments for elders through the conduct of rigorous, applied research, dissemination of evidence-based information and resources, and individual partnering with designers and care providers. She is a frequent keynote speaker at conferences in the US and abroad, making over 20 presentations annually.

Garuth Eliot Chalfont, PhD, has designed therapeutic landscapes in the UK and the US for 15 years, and now integrates architecture, landscape and care practice in the design of total living environments for people with mental health needs (www.chalfontdesign.com). He aims to improve the lived experience of people in care environments by evolving how research, design and care are taught and practiced, with particular emphasis on connection to the natural world for ecological and spiritual sustainability. His new book entitled *Design for Nature in Dementia Care* is a Bradford Good Practice Guide, published by Jessica Kingsley, London, UK. He currently researches enabling environments in the School of Architecture at the University of Sheffield.

Nancy J. Chapman, PhD, is Professor Emerita in the Nohad Toulan School of Urban Studies and Planning at Portland State University. She received her PhD in environmental and social psychology from the University of California, Berkeley. Among her research and teaching interests is a focus on housing and environments for the elderly. In this field, she has publications on gardens, urban form and physical activity, accessory apartments, and privacy issues for families visiting dementia facilities.

Pamela D. Clarke, MSc, is a researcher in Primary Care at the University of Liverpool. A qualified social worker and health psychologist, she has extensive experience of teaching, research and practice in a range of health, welfare and higher education settings. Pamela's particular interests are in psycho-social health, human rights and equality.

Jiska Cohen-Mansfield, PhD, is a Professor at the Sackler Faculty of Medicine at Tel-Aviv University, director of the Research Institute on Aging of the CES Life Communities, and a professor of Health Care Sciences and of Prevention and Community Health at the George Washington University Medical Center and School of Public Health. Her research has included two main tracks: understanding persons with dementia, and health promotion in community-dwelling older persons. Dr. Cohen-Mansfield has served as Principal Investigator on studies funded by the Alzheimer's Association, the National Institute of Aging, the National Institute of Mental Health, the Agency for Healthcare Research and Quality, and other funding agencies. She has authored over 200 articles. She is a Diplomat in Behavioral Psychology from the American Board of Professional Psychology (ABPP), a fellow of the Gerontological Society of America and of the American Psychological

Association, and a member of several other associations including the American Geriatrics Society, and the International Psychogeriatric Association. She serves on the editorial and advisory boards of several gerontological journals. Dr. Cohen-Mansfield has received several awards, including the Outstanding Service Award from the Alzheimer's Association (1999), Recognition Award for Outstanding Contributions in Gerontological Research from the Maryland Gerontological Association (1994), and the Busse Research Award for Social/Behavioral Sciences (1993), and the Barry Reisberg Award for Alzheimer's Research (2003). She is a Highly Cited Researcher as listed by ISI.

Bettye Rose Connell, PhD, is a Health Research Scientist at the Atlanta VA's Rehab Research and Development Center and an Assistant Professor in the Division of Geriatric Medicine and Gerontology at Emory University. She has 20 years experience investigating the effect of physical and social environments of care on functioning, behavior, and quality of life of persons with dementia. Her research includes evaluating the efficacy of outdoor activity programming combined with bright light exposure, nighttime noise reduction, and sleep hygiene interventions on improving sleep in nursing home residents.

Clare Cooper Marcus is Professor Emerita in the Departments of Architecture and Landscape Architecture at the University of California, Berkeley, and Principal of Healing Landscapes, Berkeley, CA. She is the author/co-author/editor of several books including *Housing as if People Mattered, People Places, House as a Mirror of Self,* and *Healing Gardens*. She speaks internationally on the topic of outdoor space in healthcare facilities.

Keith Diaz Moore, PhD, is associate professor and Chair of the Architecture program at the University of Kansas. Dr. Diaz Moore's research into the design and performance of care settings for the elderly has been funded by numerous foundations, including the Alzheimer's Association and the Helen Bader Foundation, and has been published in numerous journals and book chapters. His co-authored book *Designing a Better Day: Guidelines for Adult and Dementia Day Services Centers* was recently published by the Johns Hopkins University Press. Keith currently serves as Chair of the Environmental Design Research Association, and just completed a term as a Trustee for the National Adult Day Services Association Foundation.

Grant Gibson, MA, is a Research Assistant in the Division of Psychiatry, at the University of Liverpool, United Kingdom. His research interests focus on the relationship between older people and the physical environment, and interactions between older people and technology.

Charlotte F. Grant, PhD, presently owns a landscape design business called MAKING PLANS based in the Lake Oconee area of Georgia and in Chattanooga, TN. She utilizes over 15 years of research experience in the fields of environment-behavior and therapeutic gardens in her residential and health care design projects as well as speaking engagements.

Teresia Hazen, MEd, is a registered horticultural therapist and coordinator of six Legacy Health System Therapeutic gardens on two campuses in Portland, Oregon. Two of the gardens, the Legacy Emanuel Children's Hospital Garden and the Legacy Good Samaritan Hospital garden, received the Therapeutic Garden Award from the American Horticultural Therapy Association in 1998 and 2000 respectively. She holds a BA in Education from the University of Washington, a school administration credential from Central Washington University and MEd from the University of Portland, and is actively involved in training horticultural therapists in Portland and healthcare garden design nationally.

Donna Lewis, RN, is a gerontological nurse practitioner in the Atlanta VAMC Geriatric Research, Education, and Clinical Care Center and serves as an adjunct faculty at Emory University's Nell Hodgson School of Nursing. She has worked directly with elderly patients for over 20 years in inpatient psychiatric, intensive care and long-term care settings. Ms. Lewis's areas of interest include interdisciplinary approaches to common geriatric problems in long-term care.

Eunice Noell-Waggoner, BS, is president of the Center of Design for an Aging Society, a not-for-profit organization, dedicated to improving homes, public buildings, and public outdoor spaces to support dignity, independence, health and safety of our aging population. She served as the Project Coordinator for the Portland Memory Garden. Ms. Noell-Waggoner has a strong interest in the photobiological affects of light as well as appropriate light to maximize aging vision.

Rebecca Ory Hernandez, MS, has a degree in Environmental Design with an emphasis in Gerontology from the University of Missouri-Columbia. She is an interior and garden designer who has worked as a consultant in the areas of commercial and residential design. Rebecca resides and gardens in Ogden, Utah and is employed at Weber State University as a Development Director for the *Dumke College of Health Professions.*

Erja Rappe, PhD, is Planning Officer, Department of Applied Biology, at the University of Helsinki where she works. Rappe has been involved in research projects concerning health related effects of green environments. Her main research area is the use of horticulture in health promotion, especially among elderly and individuals recovering from mental disorders. She is interested in finding out the mechanisms how green environment and plant related activities are associated with human well-being.

Jon A. Sanford, MArch, is a Research Architect at the Rehab R&D Center, Atlanta VA and a Senior Research Scientist and Adjunct Associate Professor of Architecture at Center for Assistive Technology and Environmental Access at Georgia Tech. He has been actively engaged in housing for older adults for the past 25 years and is well recognized for his expertise in universal design and home modifications. Mr. Sanford has been the Principal Investigator on numerous projects and is widely published on issues related to accessibility codes and design of environments to meet the needs of older adults.

Andrew Sixsmith, PhD, is Director of the Gerontology Research Center at Simon Fraser University in Vancouver, British Columbia, Canada. His current interests focus on factors that influence the quality of life of older people. He has a particular interest in how new technologies can facilitate the delivery of community health and welfare services. Formerly teaching in Social Gerontology in the Department of Primary Care at the University of Liverpool, he has been a member of the British Society of Gerontology Executive Committee and has been UK representative on the EU's COST-A5 Committee on Ageing and Technology. Dr. Sixsmith has directed a number of European and UK funded projects in recent years. The ENABLE-AGE project funded by the EU Quality of Life programme examined the home environment as a determinant for autonomy, participation, health and well-being in very old age. As part of the EU-funded CareKeys project he has been looking at the relationship between quality of life and quality of care of frail older people in long term care. As director of the INDEPENDENT consortium, he has been developing and evaluating technologies for people with dementia, funded by the UK Engineering and Physical Sciences Research Council

Joseph G. Szmerekovsky, PhD, is an Assistant Professor of Management, Marketing and Finance at North Dakota State University. His research interests are in project management, complex systems, supply chain management, and RFID systems. He has published papers in top journals such as *Management Science, Naval Research Logistics* and *European Journal of Operational Research.* He currently has several working papers under development. Joseph received his PhD in Operations Research, his MS in Management Science, and his BS in Applied Mathematics from Case Western Reserve University in Cleveland, Ohio.

Päivi Topo, PhD, is Adjunct Professor of Sociology of Medicine at the University of Helsinki, Department of Public Health. She is Research Director of the National Research and Development Centre for Welfare and Health in Helsinki, Finland, and is Academy Research Fellow at the Academy of Finland. She has published several papers related to women's ageing, disability, enabling technology for people with dementia, ethics of care and assessment of the quality of dementia care from the clients' point of view.

Judith M. Torrington, BArch, RIBA, is an architect and researcher with extensive experience in designing buildings for older people. Now Reader in Architecture at the University of Sheffield her research focus is on the impact architecture can make on well-being, both positively and negatively.

Jean Wineman, DArch, is Professor of Architecture, Associate Dean and Chair Doctoral Program in Architecture at the Taubman College of Architecture & Urban Planning, University of Michigan. Her research interests focus on the links between visual and spatial properties of architecture and behavioral and educational outcomes. Her recent research and scholarship examine application of spatial design measures in predicting residential satisfaction/behavior, in exploring the effects of spatial layout on educational outcomes in zoos and museums, and in facility design to support work performance.

John Zeisel, PhD, co-founded Hearthstone Alzheimer Care & the Hearthstone Alzheimer's Family Foundation in the early 1990s. Hearthstone manages small-scale assisted living residences for people with Alzheimer's employing innovative non-pharmacologic treatments, including explicit evidence-based therapeutic environmental design and gardens. John lectures widely and has served on the faculty at Harvard University, Yale, McGill, the University of Minnesota, and Salford University in the UK. The Hearthstone Foundation's Artists for Alzheimer's™ program is a leader in linking artists and cultural institutions to those living with Alzheimer's–among these are guided programs for people with Alzheimer's at the National Gallery of Australia in Canberra, and the Museum of Modern Art in New York. John's work focuses on the neuroscience aspects of design programming, design projects, and evaluation–namely, the ways in which physical environment supports brain development and function and how environments reduce symptoms of aggression, agitation, social-withdrawal, and delusions. In this connection he serves on the Board of the Academy of Neuroscience for Architecture. His revised classic text *Inquiry by Design: Environment/ Behavior/Neuroscience in Architecture, Interiors, Landscape, & Planning,* linking research, neuroscience, and design was published by W. W. Norton in 2006.

PART I

Introduction:
Outdoor Environments
for People with Dementia

Benyamin Schwarz
Susan Rodiek

This volume is about people who are afflicted with dementia, about nature and outdoor environments, and about the relationship between them. There are special problems associated with providing care for cognitively impaired persons and support to their families; these problems are recognized by researchers, funding agencies and care providers. We view this collection of articles as a contribution to the task of expanding the knowledge base for the design of outdoor environments for people with Alzheimer's disease and other kinds of dementia. While we consider the outdoors to be essential component in the intervention efforts in dementia care, we have a complementary task to set limits on what are believed to be achievable goals in the care for this population. As Lawton and Rubinstein have cautioned us: "For a condition whose biological substratum is irreversible, it is tempting to foster unrealistic hope that is good for neither science nor families with an impaired person" (2000, p. xiv).

The first objective of the volume is to maintain the position in which empirical studies and direct observations constitute the foundation on which hope is kept alive. A second objective is to provide a basis for hope that recognizes the significance of connection to nature in any stage of dementia, and looks for fa-

[Haworth co-indexing entry note]: "Introduction: Outdoor Environments for People with Dementia." Schwarz, Benyamin, and Susan Rodiek. Co-published simultaneously in *Journal of Housing for the Elderly* (The Haworth Press, Inc.) Vol. 21, No. 1/2, 2007. pp. 3-11; and: *Outdoor Environments for People with Dementia* (ed: Susan Rodiek and Benyamin Schwarz) The Haworth Press, Inc., 2007, pp. 3-11. Single or multiple copies of this article are available for a fee from The Haworth Document Delivery Service [1-800-HAWORTH, 9:00 a.m. - 5:00 p.m. (EST). E-mail address: docdelivery@haworthpress.com].

Available online at http://jhe.haworthpress.com
doi:10.1300/J081v21n01_02

3

vorable outcomes of intervention in the interactions between people with dementia and their outdoor environments.

ABOUT PEOPLE WITH DEMENTIA

According to a report released in March 2007 by the Alzheimer's Association, there has been a 10 percent increase in the number of people afflicted with dementia since 2002. The number of Americans with Alzheimer's disease is now more than 5 million, which supports the long-forecast dementia epidemic as the American population ages. One in eight people 65 and older have this mind-devastating disease, and nearly one in two people over 85 has it. Unless scientists discover a way to delay the onset of the illness, some 7.7 million people are expected to have the disease by 2030, the report says. By 2050, that toll could reach 16 million.

"The fundamental pathology of Alzheimer's disease is the progressive degeneration and loss of vast numbers of nerve cells in those portions of the brain's cortex that are associated with the so-called higher functions, such as memory, learning and judgment. The severity and nature of the patient's dementia at any given time are proportional to the number and location of cells that have been affected." At the same time there is "a marked decrease in acetylcholine, the chemical used by these cells to transmit messages" (Nuland, 1993, p. 91). Patients with Alzheimer's disease experience high rates of non-cognitive, behavioral, and psychiatric symptoms that may include hallucinations, delusions, depression, physical aggression, pacing, wandering, and sleep disorders. The cause of the disease is still unknown and there is no known cure for it. Today's available pharmacological treatments alleviate symptoms only temporarily, and there is no evidence that non-pharmacological therapies can improve cognitive performance. At this point there are nine drugs in late-stage clinical trials, including a few that aim to slow Alzheimer's worsening (Associated Press, 2007).

Central to the ethics of dementia care is enhancing well-being and making the most of the strengths that are still present within the person. Stephen G. Post has suggested that "above all, we must recognize that the quality of life for the person with dementia is always partly subjective and is somewhat a matter of emotional adjustment facilitated by interactions and environment" (Post, 2000, p. 94). Compelling advice to caregivers was presented by Nancy L. Mace and Peter V. Rabins: "Since dementing illnesses develop slowly, they often leave intact the impaired person's ability to enjoy life and to enjoy other people. When things go badly, remind yourself that, no matter how bad the other person's memory is or how strange his behavior, he is still a unique and special human being. We can continue to love a person even after he changed drastically, even when we are deeply troubled by his present state" (1999, p. 12).

Lawton (1983) described four components of quality of life: perceived quality of life, behavioral competence, objective environment, and psychological well being. Two of these components, perceived quality of life and behavioral competence, are crippled by Alzheimer's progressive brain degeneration. However, caregivers may impact the two remaining components of quality of life: appropriate physical and social environment; and accommodating conditions for psychological well being (Volicer, 2000). Clearly in addition to the physical needs such as safety, nutrition, and good health, people with dementia have the same psychosocial needs as other individuals. They need to feel secure, they need stimulation and companionship, and they need to be valued as unique individuals. Consequently the main caregiving goals for residents with advanced dementia are maintenance of quality of life and the preservation of dignity and comfort. *Thus the experience of nature, which is perceived as a vital part of subjective quality of life, should be central to intervention programs for people with dementia.* Because by eliminating interaction with natural elements from their daily lives, we "exclude people with dementia from the pleasurable sensory experiences most of us enjoy every day" (MacDonald, 2002).

ABOUT NATURE AND OUTDOOR ENVIRONMENTS

Human relationships with nature are a fundamental genetically based need. According to Wilson (1984) who coined the word *Biophilia* to describe the need, this instinct emerges unconsciously in human cognition and emotions, and is revealed "in the predictable fantasies and responses of individuals from early childhood onwards" (p. 85). Studies have shown that direct contact with nature benefits a wide range of people across cultures. In addition it can benefit prisoners, hospital patients, and autistic children, as well as adults with Alzheimer's disease (Kaplan & Kaplan, 1989; Tyson, 1998; Carstens, 1998; Marcus & Barnes, 1999; Ulrich, 1999; Kahn, 1999; Rodiek & Schwarz, 2005).

Kaplan and Kaplan (1989) noted that the "immediate outcomes of contacts with nearby nature include enjoyment, relaxation, and lowered stress levels. In addition, the research results indicate that physical well-being is affected by such contacts. People with access to nearby natural settings have been found to be healthier than other individuals. The long-term, indirect impacts also include increased levels of satisfaction with one's home, one's job, and with life in general" (p.173). At the end of their book Kaplan and Kaplan (1989) reiterate their point: "Viewed as an amenity, nature may be readily replaced by some great technological achievements. Viewed as an essential bond between humans and other living things, the natural environment has no substitutions" (pp. 203-204).

If this essential cross-cultural human need has merit, it helps to form some normative principles such as "If you want to support your physical and psychological health, then affiliate with nature." Or, in the context of this volume, "If we want to provide holistic care for people who suffer from dementia we need to maintain their affiliation with nature".

ABOUT OUTDOOR ENVIRONMENTS
FOR PEOPLE WITH DEMENTIA

In recent years, there has been a growing awareness that persons with dementia should have the necessary environmental support and freedom to access the outdoors, and a substantial crop of 'wandering parks,' 'healing gardens,' 'treatment gardens,' and 'restorative gardens' has sprung up as a result. However, even with wide scale endorsement of this concept, relatively little is known about how persons with dementia respond to specific environmental features, and how planned activities and environmental conditions can encourage usage and/or benefit residents. Even fewer studies have explored what beneficial health-related and behavior-related outcomes may result from having access to the outdoors, partly due to the complexity of measuring physical environment interventions, and partly due to the difficulty of obtaining reliable and valid data on dementia resident outcomes.

Some of the potentially beneficial health outcomes for older persons with dementia may be similar to the potential benefits for older adults without a diagnosis of dementia: multiple physical and psychological benefits associated with increased physical activity; the hormonal balance associated with exposure to bright outdoor light; and psychological benefits from contact with nature elements. In addition to benefits that may be derived from actual usage of outdoor space, it is theorized that *merely having access to the outdoors* may in itself have substantial positive benefits, especially for persons with dementia, because of the potential impact on autonomy, independence, sense of freedom, and self-esteem.

The E-B inventory for dementia environments developed by Zeisel, Hyde and Levkoff (1994) used the term "outdoor freedom" to describe the benefits to residents. Their model attempts to support individual treatment goals with measurable positive outcomes on resident behavior, mood, social interaction, and active engagement in activities. This emphasis on the freedom engendered by nature contact is echoed by Tyson, who said the "ultimate goal of treatment gardens is to facilitate self-initiated and independent engagement in ordinary outdoor activities by providing residents access to supportive environment and the freedom to do so" (2002, p. 55).

Integrating insights from the nursing profession and landscape architecture, Randall and her colleagues (1990) proposed design solutions in the outdoor environment to specifically address symptoms of Alzheimer's disease such memory loss; apraxia (inability to perform motor acts); agnosia (the inability to understand or use sensory information); frailty; wandering; disorientation; plant ingestion; sundowning; and delusions and hallucinations. The authors caution that the proposed design solutions were not the only approaches to mitigate the symptoms of dementia but they tried to carefully address the issues necessary to achieve the goal of comfortable and secure outdoor environments for the patients.

ORIENTATION TO THE BOOK

In the opening chapter of this volume, John Zeisel explores the issue of therapeutic gardens for people with dementia. Drawing on the growing field of neuroscience and design, Zeisel (2006) describes the design process and links it to the specially designed therapeutic gardens. In the last section of his chapter the author provides eight basic design criteria for the review of these gardens. Zeisel stresses the synergy that can come from the holistic design approach to the indoor and the outdoor space of special care environments for people with dementia.

In the second chapter, Jiska Cohen-Mansfield provides a broad picture of the field of *Outdoor Wandering Parks for Persons with Dementia*. The article is based on a national survey of 672 long-term care facilities with outdoor gardens. The purpose of the survey was to identify features of outdoor areas and clarify the relationship between design attributes and utilization and satisfaction with these areas in nursing home with dementia special care units. The results indicate that most outdoor spaces are used by residents for whom they were originally intended (cognitively impaired residents and wanderers) but also by other residents, family members, staff members and volunteers. The author points out that "outdoor areas were reported to have a positive impact on all users, as well as on public relations and marketability of the facilities."

The next paper is based on findings from the first phase of the INDE-PENDENT Project in the United Kingdom that investigates enabling environments for people with dementia. The authors, Gibson, Chalfont, Clarke, Torrington, and Sixsmith, discuss their findings from interviews with people who suffer from the disease, as well as from focus groups with family and professional caregivers regarding nature based activities. Participants in the study included both people living in their homes and residents of long term care facilities. The findings from the study indicate that access and participation in nature-related activities can benefit people with dementia, as long as their real needs are understood and addressed.

Keith Diaz Moore's chapter deals specifically with what he coins *Restorative Dementia Gardens*. The term is anchored in Kaplan's Attention Restoration Theory (2001) and aims at interventions to restore people with dementia having directed-attention fatigue. The author describes the Exemplary Dementia Garden Project that came into existence following a symposium in Oregon in 2005, in which twelve recognized experts in the field identified several Dementia Gardens in the US. This expert panel developed a survey protocol which was sent out to individuals associated with the gardens and a rich data based was developed. The article focuses on data from five therapeutic gardens designed for people experiencing dementia.

The next three chapters discuss various evaluation tools developed by the authors for gardens for people with dementia. Charlotte F. Grant and Jean D. Wineman review results from a study conducted in five outdoor environments in long-term care facilities designed for people with dementia. The authors discuss the *Garden-Use Model,* which serves as a theoretical base grounded in the rich data collected in their research. They recommend this model as an evaluation instrument for gardens in long-term care facilities and outdoor environments for people with dementia. Garuth Eliot Chalfont addresses the problems of dementia patients who are often deprived of opportunities to venture outdoors. Because of these limitations, the author claims, residents of facilities for dementia care may be excluded from a wide range of natural and sensory experiences. To that end the author proposes "a comprehensive checklist for investigating the potential for connection to nature for people living in dementia care environments." The PLANET tool evolved as a response to observational studies in the US, the UK, and Scandinavia. Clare Cooper Marcus provides another assessment tool for evaluating gardens for dementia care. The rationale for the Alzheimer's Garden Audit Tool (AGAT) is explained in the article and its use is discussed.

The chapter written by Rebecca Ory Hernandez is a report about research conducted in two gardens in assisted living facilities for people with dementia in the Midwest. The author used several methods in her post occupancy evaluation of the sites: interviews with family members, staff, administrators and design professionals, behavioral mapping, and other forms of observation. The findings of the study lead to several design recommendations for future gardens.

The next two chapters address two separate studies regarding the connection between outdoor activities and sleep patterns of residents who suffer from dementia. Bettye Rose Connell, Jon A. Sanford, and Donna Lewis discuss their one-year pilot study of the effects of an outdoor activity program on sleep patterns and behaviors of nursing home residents with dementia. The authors found that the group of residents who were engaged in outdoor activities experienced better sleep duration and reduced verbal agitation, compared with a control group engaged in indoor activities. In another study of nursing home residents, Margaret Calkins, Joseph Szmerekovsky, and Stacey Biddle found that "increased time spent outdoors resulted in a modest improvement in sleep, and mixed or immeasurable impact on agitation."

In a paper from Finland, Erja Rappe and Päivi Topo discuss theories and empirical studies about healing gardens. In the second part of their chapter, the authors report findings from their study of the impact of plants and outdoor activities on people with dementia in day care and residential care homes. Obviously, the weather patterns in Finland are one of the hindrances for outdoor activities. The outside temperatures for nine months of the year prevent residents from going outside and deter staff from changing their clothes in order to go out. Despite these severe conditions, the researchers stress the significance of gardens for people with dementia, particularly because of the outdoor capability to stimulate residents' "all senses".

Nancy J. Chapman, Teresia Hazen, and Eunice Noell-Waggoner discuss their program for training staff in long-term care facilities to increase their knowledge about horticulture and encourage them to involve residents in outdoor activities. The authors point out that following the training sessions, staff members were able to improve activity programs as well as recommend modifications to design attributes of outdoor environments in their facilities.

Written by Elizabeth C. Brawley, the next chapter takes a different format. It is a set of general guidelines for developing an outdoor space for people with dementia. The author reviews issues such as the overall layout, safety and security, visibility of garden areas from inside the special care unit, visible connections to destination in the garden, walking paths, places to sit, activities, opportunities for social engagement, and transition spaces.

In the final chapter, Clare Cooper Marcus discusses an exemplary outdoor space in Grand Rapids, Michigan. Designed by landscape architects Martha Tyson, Elizabeth Dunn and Jeanne Senis, the garden serves the clients and meets many of therapeutic needs of the residents, family members and staff. Although this chapter is not a rigorous post-occupancy evaluation of the garden, the author analyzes the attributes of the garden, and provides design recommendations for future outdoor environments for people with dementia

"Dementia," writes Steven Post, "is both a decline from previous mental state and a terrible breaking off from the values of the dominant culture. The moral task is always to enhance the person with AD. What cues seem to elicit memory? What music or activity seems to add to well being? How can capacities that are still intact be creatively drawn out? How can modalities of touch and voice convey love to the person? Rather than thinking of people with dementia as out of reach because of forgetfulness or as unworthy because cognitive disability, the moral task is to bring them into discourse in creative ways" (2000, p. 94). We believe that maintaining connections to the outdoors is one of the manifestations of this discourse. It is our hope that this volume serves as a small step towards creating better outdoor environments that may enhance dementia victims' quality of life.

REFERENCES

Associated Press. 2007. "Report: Over 5M Living With Alzheimer's." *The Associated Press*, March 20th 2007.

Carstens, D. Y. 1989. Outdoor spaces in housing for the elderly. In C.C. Marcus and C. Francis (eds.) *People places: Design guidelines for urban open space*. New York: Van Nostrand Reinhold.

Kahn, Jr. P.H. 1999. *The human relationship with nature*. Cambridge, MA: The MIT Press.

Kaplan, R., and Kaplan, S. 1989. *The experience of nature: A psychological perspective*. Cambridge: Cambridge University Press.

Kaplan, S. 2001. Meditation, restoration, and management of mental fatigue. *Environment and Behavior*, 33 (4): 480-506.

Lawton, M. P. 1983. The varieties of wellbeing. *Exper Aging Res* 9:65-72.

Lawton, M. P. and Rubinstein R.L. (eds.) 2000. *Interventions in dementia care: Toward improving quality of life*. New York: Springer Publishing.

MacDonald, C. 2002. "Back to the real sensory world our 'care' has taken away." *Journal of Dementia Care*: 10 (1) 33-36.

Mace, N.L., and Rabins, P.V. 1999. *The 36-hour day*, 3rd ed. Baltimore, MD: The Johns Hopkins University Press.

Marcus, C. C., and Barnes, M. (eds.). 1999. *Healing Gardens: Therapeutic benefits and design recommendations*. New York: John Wiley & Sons.

Nuland, S. B. 1994. *How we die: Reflections on life's final chapter*. New York: Alfred A. Knopf.

Post, S. G. 2000. *The moral challenge of Alzheimer disease*. Baltimore, MD: The Johns Hopkins University Press.

Randall, P., Burkahrdt, S.S.J., and Kutcher, J. 1990. Exterior space for patients with Alzheimer's disease and related disorders. *The American Journal of Alzheimer's Care and Related Disorders& Research*, July/August, pp. 31-37.

Rodiek, S., and Schwarz, B. (Eds.) 2005. *The role of the outdoors in residential environments for aging.* New York: The Haworth Press.

Tyson, M. M. 1998. *The healing landscape: Therapeutic outdoor environments.* New York: McGraw-Hill.

Tyson, M. M. 2002. Treatment gardens: Naturally mapped environments and independence. *Alzheimer's Care Quarterly,* 3(1): 55-60.

Ulrich, R. S. 1999. Effects of gardens on health outcomes: Theory and research. In C.C. Marcus, and M. Barnes, (eds.) *Healing Gardens: Therapeutic benefits and design recommendations.* New York: John Wiley & Sons.

Volicer, L. 2000. Goals of dementia special care units. *Research & Practice in Alzheimer's Disease (RPAD) Volume 4, Special care Units. Paris:* Serdi Publisher.

Wilson, E. O. 1984. *Biophilia.* Cambridge, MA: Harvard University Press.

Zeisel, J., Hyde, J., and Levkoff, S. 1994. Best practices: An environment-behavior (E-B) model for Alzheimer's special care units. *American Journal of Alzheimer's Care and Related Disorders and Research,* vol. 9, no. 2 (March/April) pp.4-21.

doi:10.1300/J081v21n01_01

Creating a Therapeutic Garden That Works for People Living with Alzheimer's

John Zeisel

SUMMARY. Therapeutic gardens specially designed for people living with Alzheimer's disease can improve the quality of life of those who use them, and can be helpful in reducing what are called "problem behaviors." This article explores this statement and describes how the design process can best achieve a garden that is truly therapeutic. The article is in three parts, each of which represents a critical step in design: image, present, test. The last section presents eight basic design criteria to apply in therapeutic garden design review. The article is intended to leave the reader with the big idea that inside and outside environments must be designed as one to respond to the needs of the Alzheimer's mind. doi:10.1300/J081v21n01_02 *[Article copies available for a fee from The Haworth Document Delivery Service: 1-800-HAWORTH. E-mail address: <docdelivery@haworthpress.com> Website: <http://www.HaworthPress.com> © 2007 by The Haworth Press, Inc. All rights reserved.]*

KEYWORDS. Alzheimer's, nonpharmacologic, treatment, therapeutic, garden, design

John Zeisel, PhD, is Founder & President, Hearthstone Alzheimer Care & the Hearthstone Alzheimer's Family Foundation, 23 Warren Avenue, Suite 140, Woburn, MA 10280 (E-mail: zeisel@TheHearth.org).

[Haworth co-indexing entry note]: "Creating a Therapeutic Garden That Works for People Living with Alzheimer's." Zeisel. John. Co-published simultaneously in *Journal of Housing for the Elderly* (The Haworth Press, Inc.) Vol. 21, No. 1/2, 2007, pp. 13-33; and: *Outdoor Environments for People with Dementia* (ed: Susan Rodiek and Benyamin Schwarz) The Haworth Press, Inc., 2007, pp. 13-33. Single or multiple copies of this article are available for a fee from The Haworth Document Delivery Service [1-800-HAWORTH, 9:00 a.m. - 5:00 p.m. (EST). E-mail address: docdelivery@haworthpress.com].

INTRODUCTION

Therapeutic gardens specially designed for people living with Alzheimer's disease can improve the quality of life of those who use them, and can be helpful in reducing what are called "problem behaviors." This article explores this statement and describes how the design process can best achieve a garden that is truly therapeutic. The article is in three parts, each of which represents a critical step in design: image, present, test. *Image:* To design effectively for a specific group, designers start with a picture in their minds of how the users–in this case people living with Alzheimer's disease–see the world. Neuroscience has provided us with insights into this, some of which are presented below. Broad imageable design concepts, such as natural mapping and landmarking, are also described in this section. *Present:* In sketching the first concept, or in schematic design, straightforward design rules of thumb can keep the design process on track. The rules of thumb presented here can serve as the basis for therapeutic garden designs that respond to basic needs. *Test:* Continual improvement through repeated design review is critical to achieving a successful buildable garden. The last section presents eight basic design criteria to apply in therapeutic garden design review. The article leaves the reader with the big idea that inside and outside environments must be designed as one to respond to the needs of the Alzheimer's mind.

This approach to design for Alzheimer's draws heavily on the growing field of neuroscience and design, a focus of the Academy of Neuroscience for Design (www.ANFArch.org)–particularly the brain's "environment system" as it is described in the author's recently revised *Inquiry by Design: environment / behavior / neuroscience for architecture, interiors, landscape and planning.*

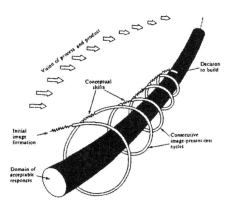

Design development spiral

LINKING THERAPEUTIC GARDEN DESIGN
INTO THE DESIGN PROCESS

The design process comprises cycles of three activities repeated several times, each time with increasing specificity and focus.

These three activities are imaging, presenting, and testing.

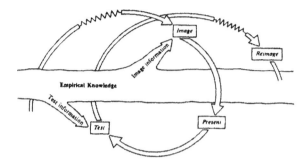

The resource for making appropriate design decisions–empirical knowledge–lies at the center of this process. Personal experience, research data, evidence-based guidelines, and best practices in design and operations all inform design. While the term "empirical" tends commonly to be used to describe objective, usually rigorous and research-based, knowledge, its dictionary meaning focuses on the fact that it is knowledge based on experience (from the bottom up) rather than knowledge that some theory tells us is the knowledge to employ (top down.)

The goal of this ever tightening design spiral is an environment that meets the needs of direct users, the organization for which the environment is being planned, and the physical environment context in which it sits. (Zeisel, 2006)

In designing environments to be used primarily by people living with Alzheimer's or another dementia, having access to information organized according to how it feeds the design process, can be most useful. My own experience described in this article is organized into image, presentation, and test information.

One result of organizing information in this way is that a single powerful message about the design process emerges for therapeutic gardens meant for people living with Alzheimer's. In fact the design process used in every living environment for these individuals and groups of people living with this illness would do well to follow this dictum: *Always include both inside and outside spaces linked into a single environment throughout the entire design process for any environment which will be used for people living with Alzheimer's–from the first conceptual sketch until construction documents.*

The following is not an exhaustive set of design guidelines or a thorough review of the field of designing for dementia. Rather what follows are somewhat idiosyncratic heuristic keys I employ in my own work with designers to guide the process of therapeutic garden design to a fruitful end.

IMAGE INFORMATION

Image information is empirical knowledge that can be used to "picture in the mind" the person who might use an environment, the way such a person thinks, and the environment that will emerge through the design process. In the first set of image information presented here, we are talking about the image the designer holds in his or her mind–the picture in the designer's mind of how potential users think, behave, and see the world We might call the object of the designer's first image, the user's image. The second set of image information, presented below, relates to environmental design constructs, such as indoor/outdoor unity and temporal supports. Image information is employed to create an initial picture in the mind of the designer of the final project that is "right" enough, so that the ever-tightening design spiral will lead to an environment that eventually "works" well.

Image information #1: How the deficits of the Alzheimer's brain influence the way people living with this illness interact with their environment. There are six important physiological changes that take place that can help designers gain imaging insight into the users of therapeutic gardens.

Loss of "complex sequencing" executive function. Executive function in the brain is the process that takes place in the frontal lobe whereby each of us first identifies the myriad micro-activities that make up larger actions, and then organizes these into a coherent sequence to a single end. On the simplest level, without a fully operational executive function area in the brain and without help from others, we could not brush our teeth, get dressed, or eat a meal successfully. Designers would not be able to organize the tools they need to draw a sketch, or operate a computer.

In using an everyday environment, unless continuous use has embedded knowledge of that environment in the person's long term memory, a person living with Alzheimer's would encounter difficulty making the connections and sequencing steps needed to get outdoors:

- Deciding that the garden that she sees out one window is the garden that she can get to out the door in another room.

- Figuring out how to operate a complex door lock system to open an exterior door.
- Deciding where to go once in the garden.

Difficulty creating and embedding new "wayfinding" cognitive maps. The parts of the brain used to remember places and sequences of places is also compromised. As the illness progresses, it is increasingly difficult to "remember" a new environment one experiences. This is not simply a matter of bad memory. Rather it comes about because those brain elements employed in creating a cognitive map, made up mostly of remembered landmarks and their associate meaning, is compromised. The clearer garden access is, and the more self-evident the organization of the garden and its implied uses, the less burdensome that environment is for its intended users.

Damaged supra-chiasmatic "timekeeping" nuclei. The timekeepers in the brain, linked to the physiological timekeepers throughout our bodies, are damaged in those with Alzheimer's disease. When gardens and interior environments for these users include clear and evident "zeitgebers," users are more oriented to time and place. Zeitgebers, the term taken from German meaning "time givers," can be natural elements like the sun, the moon, and the light or darkness of the day, as well as constructed elements like clocks or even signs on which the time of day and the day of the week are written. Windows located where people living there can have a view out into a garden whatever room they are in can be effective zeitgebers, if appropriately located and designed.

Compromised hippocampal "event tagging": The hippocampus, a small seahorse-shaped element in the brain's limbic system, tags experiences we have and events we engage in with a virtual "time and place stamp" that enables people with fully functional brains to remember events clearly. This tagging device is damaged by Alzheimer's disease, just as it is compromised when a person has had too much to drink, been given certain medications and drugs, and under certain emotionally stressful situations. The hippocampus seems to do a better job of time and place stamping, when the events themselves have greater meaning to the person, and when strong emotions are attached to the experience. Garden design that maximizes environmental zeitgebers–when a person is in the garden or when a person is inside a setting looking out–will be effective in overcoming some of the event tagging deficits a person living with Alzheimer's experience.

Limited thalamus, orbito-frontal cortex, and hippocampal "impulse control": When most of us face stressful events, aggressive people, or sexually loaded situations, no matter what we may feel at the moment, we hold back any urge we might have to fight back, run away, or behave inappropriately. With damage to the impulse control system in the brain, people who live with

Alzheimer's increasingly lose their ability to control such impulses. Even when there is no increase in aggression or sexuality, such behaviors are more prevalent. One thing one can do to help a person in such a situation, is decrease the contextual threats that elicit strong, often negative, reactions. Gardens, with their soothing colors, temperature, sensory inputs, and familiar natural elements can serve this purpose.

Healthy "emotional expression" amygdala: The amygdala, a small almond shaped organ in the brain's limbic system ("amygdala" means almond, in Greek) is the center of emotions and feelings. This system operates successfully long into Alzheimer's disease, and can thus be accessed in communication, relationship, and through design. Therapeutic garden elements that elicit positive emotion, such as intimate seating areas, comfortable benches surrounded by flowering bushes, and planting areas for vegetables all build on the health of the amygdala in Alzheimer's disease.

Active "procedural learning" systems: The complex damage to the brain that is called Alzheimer's disease, makes it difficult for people living with the illness to learn new things the way most people learn in school–lists of names of people and places, mathematical and chemical formulae, words in another language. This type of learning is called *declarative* learning, and the systems that enable it are increasingly impaired during the progress of Alzheimer's. However, there is another learning system that is less impaired–the brain's *procedural* learning system. This is the system that embeds new skills and abilities through a mix of cognitive and body repetition. Riding a bicycle, eating with chopsticks, and instinctively knowing the way home, are skills that are procedurally learned. Gardens with embedded routines, repetition, familiarity, and sequences can contribute to the ability of people with Alzheimer's to learn in this way.

Garden and landscape designers who develop a coherent image of the users of their gardens as people with more or less of these deficits and abilities, will design better therapeutic gardens.

Image information #2: Another set of imaging concepts helpful in designing therapeutic gardens are environmental design constructs that relate to the unique way people living with Alzheimer's are likely to conceptualize the world. These include:

- Indoor/outdoor unity
- Natural mapping
- Temporal support
- Learning support, and
- Landmarking.

Indoor/outdoor unity: For most people the building they work in, their home, and their school represent holistic environments that they comprehend and to which they relate. Outside such settings is another conceptual whole comprising streets, parks, shops, and transportation–the larger public world. Out of doors includes in-between places such as front porches, lawns, back patios, and front and back yards which–while out of doors–are actually extensions of indoors. The boundary between such in-between places and the more public world of streets, parks, and sidewalks is usually as symbolic as they are physical barriers–a low fence indicating that the lawn is private property, or a planted hedge indicating that the public is only allowed there if they have business with those living in the house. This complex interrelated set of constructs may be confusing to people living with Alzheimer's as they increasingly cope with the changes in their brains.

For them, a simple distinction between indoors and outdoors suffices. In fact it not only is sufficient to orient such a person and keep them safe, it is necessary. The question raised, then, is where to draw the line between inside and out.

My experience tells me that the line is best drawn not at the juncture between interior and exterior–between the front or back door and the porch, patio, or lawn–but around these indoor extension areas, separating both interior and them clearly from the often dangerous more public sidewalks, streets, parks, woods, and roads. The garden or front yard fence demarcates that boundary inside of which everything must be safe and Alzheimer's-friendly, and outside of which is out of bounds.

The unified concept of what's mine, what's safe, and what's accessible includes not only interior areas, but therapeutic gardens as well.

Natural mapping: Another central imaging concept when designing gardens for people living with Alzheimer's is natural mapping. Originally formulated to describe small objects that contain all the information needed to let an uninitiated user know how to use and manipulate that object, (Norman, 1990) I have found it is equally helpful to describe the best environments for people with Alzheimer's. Appliances like most toasters and tools like hammers and screwdrivers, don't need written instructions to let users know what to do with them. A toaster is naturally mapped because the openings on the top are shaped like a slice of bread, the plunger clearly drops the toast in and simultaneously turns the toaster on, and either a 1-5 scale or a light-to-darker visual scale clearly indicates that the purpose of the adjacent knob is to indicate whether the toast should be more or less toasted–left in longer or shorter time. The same cannot be said for television remote controls–especially those that also control DVD machines, VCR machines, and possibly a cable or satellite subscription with hundreds of stations. For this small instrument an instruction booklet is definitely needed.

Well-designed therapeutic gardens for people living with Alzheimer's are naturally mapped. A single pathway moves from near the garden entrance on one side to near it on the other. There are a series of clearly understood small and large destinations along the pathway–landmarks by which users orient themselves. These might include park benches, flowering trees, a mailbox, a car, a laundry drying rack, and planter boxes. There are also areas with clear meaning in the context of home: front porch, back patio, back yard, and front yard. There are no hidden areas that might confuse users, and any minor pathways–short cuts–intersect the main path, at a 90° angle so that the intersection provides an evident choice between main and side pathway–not a confusing fork in the path. This self-evident character in the design must be part of the initial image the designer begins her work with.

Temporal Support: People living with Alzheimer's disease may develop difficulty knowing the time–hours, days, and seasons–without external cues.

FIGURE 1. Naturally Mapped Walking Path

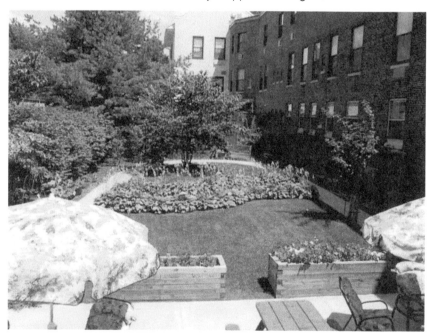

All photographs are from gardens at Hearthstone Alzheimer Care treatment residences in Palisades and White Plains, NY, and Marlborough, and Woburn, MA

Gardens are simple ways of offsetting this particular disability. The degree to which the garden can be seen from interior spaces provides one part of its ability to support its users temporally. The same is true for the ease with which users can find the garden, get into it, and leave when they want to–all encouragements to use the garden as often as possible. The more a garden can be used in all four seasons–to enjoy the out of doors, for horticultural therapy, to plant and harvest, to mow the lawn or shovel snow–the more it represents a temporal support.

Learning Support: We know that people living with Alzheimer's can learn using their procedural memory abilities. Procedural memory is reinforced through repetition and routine, among other characteristics of space. If a person repeats the same task or trip over and over in the same way, that person gets to know it–learns that skill of that behavior–in a deep way. Garden design supports procedural learning when the garden presents the same aspect to users each time they see it and use it, and if the image presented has strong emotional or symbolic content: a striking rose bush, a chicken coop, a bar-b-cue.

Landmarking: We all remember our way around indoor and outdoor places by recollecting the landmarks that indicate where we have to make a locational

FIGURE 2. Temporal Support Balcony

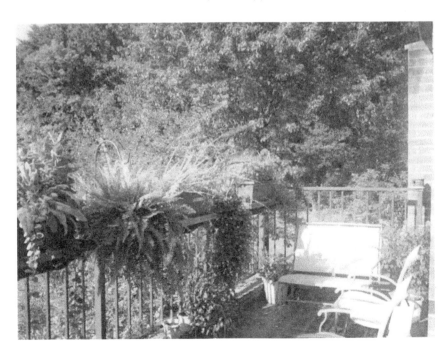

decision–turn, move into or out of a place, decide to act one way or another. This hardwired instinct to employ landmarks in wayfinding means that designers of gardens for people living with Alzheimer's must begin with an image of clear and evident landmarks connected by clear and evident pathways, without the whole garden becoming either trite or simplistic.

PRESENTING

Designs are presented in sketches, words, plans, section, and vignette. Most designs for living make a major distinction between the interior of a building–number of beds, width of hallways, size of common rooms–and the exterior–the garden. There are a few specific design rules of thumb that can help every garden designer achieve at least a good therapeutic garden when built, if not an exceptional one.

Rule of thumb #1: Always design inside and outside together. The principles of therapeutic garden design presentation begin with how the design process for such a project is organized. The first rule is to always think about and

FIGURE 3. Temporal Support Rooftop

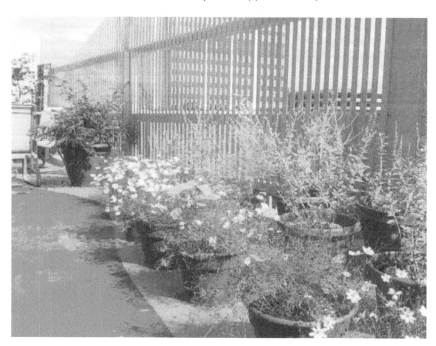

FIGURE 4. Landmarking

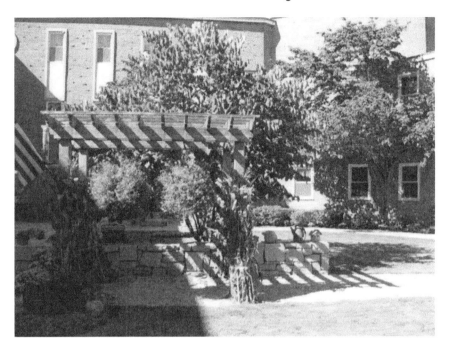

design the inside of a residence and the outside at the same time. As yin and yang dimensions of the same design event, a designer who designs them in sequence sacrifices benefits the garden might gain from proximity to the interior and the quality of interior spaces does not derive as much from being next to a garden. From the start of the first sketch, to working drawings, the building and the adjacent garden have to be thought of together, planned at the same scale, and detailed to the same degree. So often I have seen building plans for Alzheimer's residences, without a garden drawn in. When the garden is included in the drawing, often either the building or the garden is rendered in color and with furniture, seldom both at the same time and in the same drawing.

Rule of thumb #2: A park in the garden: Most therapeutic gardens will be enclosed and separate from public streets and parks. The front and back yard in the garden, and the porch and patio are by definition oriented outward, away from the residential building. Therefore, in an enclosed garden with only residential features, the exclusion of outsider public areas is evident to everyone in the garden. One way to reduce the impact of excluding public areas in the

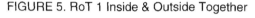

FIGURE 5. RoT 1 Inside & Outside Together

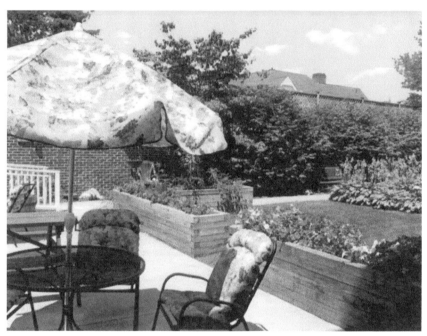

therapeutic garden is to include a "park" in the garden design. This can be a small area with different paving and planting, and it can include a park bench or two. The main design characteristics of the internal park is that it be located as far as possible from the garden entrance, has its back to the fence enclosure, and the benches faces back towards the garden itself. In this way, people sitting on the benches feel they are outside looking into the garden–as close to being in an outsider public area as possible in such a setting.

Rule of thumb #3: Continually visible re-entry: No matter how the garden path is laid out, and no matter what the design of the doorway, the place people come into and leave the garden needs to be visible from every spot in the garden–the path, the park bench, the front porch, the back patio, the planting gardens, the front lawn, and the back yard. The comings and going of residents, visitors, and staff re-enforce each person's procedural memory of place–each event of this sort saying to the person living with Alzheimer's–this is the way home.

Rule of thumb #4: Plan the entrance and exit to and from the garden as a landmark: Every garden has an entrance that is likely to be the major way into

FIGURE 6. RoT #2 View from the Park

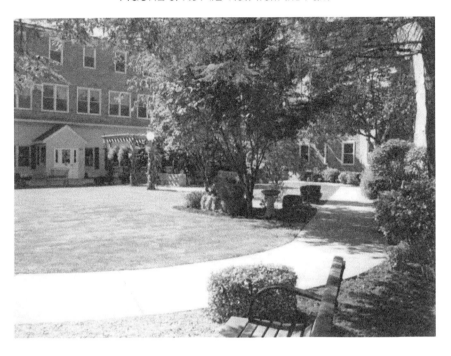

the garden for residents. The easier it is for residents to get outside to a safe therapeutic garden by themselves, and the easier it is for them to find their way back inside, the more they will use the garden on their own. By "easier" I mean both cognitive as well as physical ease. The simplest way to guarantee that this happens is to make the door itself a visual landmark. A bright color can do this; a typical doorway shape can work as well.

As Grant (2003) has shown in her research, this leads to residents being more independent in their decisions and actions. In 216 observed separate uses of the Hearthstone garden at Marlborough, Massachusetts, fully 61% of the trips into the garden were independent and self-initiated by residents, and this figure jumped to 75% of those re-entering the building through the iconic sloped roof front door—actually the door leading back into the safety of the residence living room. Because of the door's placement and design, three out of four residents who used the garden came back into the residence on their own initiative. Interesting as well, is that fully a third (36%) used the iconic and evident park bench to sit for a while on their trip around the garden.

FIGURE 7. RoT #3 Continually Visible Re-Entry

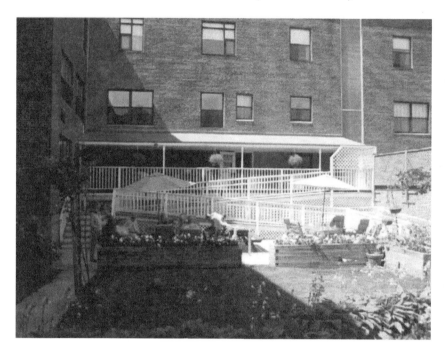

Rule of thumb #5: Absolute safety and security: There can be no compromises with treatment garden safety and security, not only because of resident safety, but also because of family member and staff behavior. For every treatment garden, there will be both a symbolic and actual *gatekeeper*. The administrative, symbolic gatekeeper makes decisions about hours of access, programs to be carried out there, whether or not family or paid partners must accompany users, and if so how many, who has control over access, and other such gate-keeping decisions. Actual gatekeepers lock and open the doors to the treatment garden, decide when to hold activities there, and whether the garden is an inviting active place, or one to which special visits are made.

Among every partner's major objectives is to be caring, thoughtful, and above all responsible. Responsible means keeping the person safe–and that means absolutely safe. No matter what the symbolic or administrative gatekeeper says, if the garden is not 100% secure, the actual gatekeeper will make 100% responsible decisions–keep the door locked most of the time, make certain there are always partners in the garden when people living with Alzhei-

FIGURE 8. RoT #4 Entrance as a Landmark

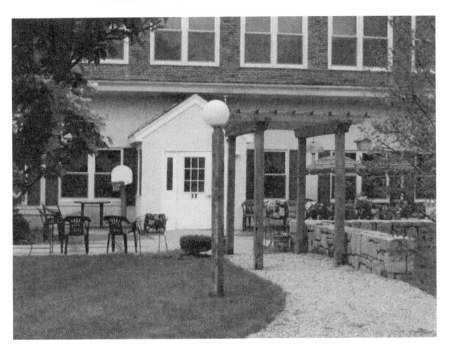

mer's are using it, and in other ways limit users independence. The person is not being mean or controlling, she is being responsible.

On the other hand, with a 100% secure garden gatekeepers can relax and provide a welcoming environment that fosters independence, a sense of self, and joy. Security can be achieved with a fence that is high enough to prevent climbing over, even if a bench or chair is moved close to the fence. An eight-foot fence (2.2 meters) is generally high enough. If a gate to the outside is necessary, it needs to be camouflaged with no visible lock or evident pathway leading to it. Enclosure should have no places for a resident to grab hold of and lift himself over. My own experience is that in active areas, for example when the garden is next to a parking area or an active street, it is better to use materials that prevent seeing through, so that even the idea of "getting out" does not occur to garden users. Although this principle may be less relevant in rural areas, or gardens next to fields, other gardens, and woods, I tend to feel it is a pretty good rule of thumb to keep in mind when presenting a 100% safe treatment garden.

FIGURE 9. RoT #5 Absolute Safety

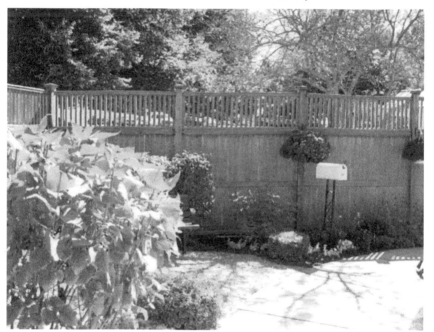

And remember, 100% safety is not an end in itself. It leads to gatekeeper generosity, greater access, greater independence, and thus greater sense of self and personhood.

Rule of thumb #6: The 90° shortcut: Intriguing forks in the road, enchanting secondary pathways, and mysterious hidden areas to be alone are all wonderful garden design concepts, but not for most people living with Alzheimer's. Each of these fantasies poses a challenge which may lead to joy and learning, but which also may lead to frustration and catastrophic reactions. Within the concept of natural mapping, there can be choices–as long as the choices are clear-cut. The idea is simple. If a major pathway leads in one direction to a destination, a secondary pathway cutting the trip shorter is a clear choice if it parts from the major pathway (or joins it) at a 90° angle. In addition, the greater the distinction between the two paths, and the greater the environmental announcement that the intersection of the two paths is, in Kevin Lynch's (1960) term, a "node," the greater will be the clarity of choice. Distinction can be achieved by specifying a different material for the short cut, or a different color, or a different planting scheme. A cluster of plants, a park bench, a bird

FIGURE 10. RoT #6 90 Degree Shortcut

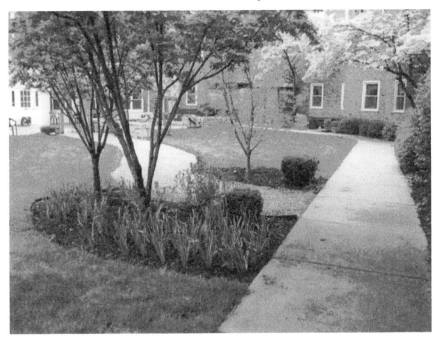

feeder, or a mailbox can announce a node. In every case a 90° angle is an integral part of the design equation.

There are more presentation rules of thumb, but this is not a design guideline article. This article aims to orient our design minds as best we can towards seeing the world the way someone living with Alzheimer's might, so that resulting treatment gardens have a chance of supporting their brains–giving them a chance for independence, control, understanding, low stress, access to memories related to nature, sense of self, and joy.

TESTING INFORMATION

Employing the design spiral as a guide, each concept sketch, bubble diagram, schematic design, and even construction document needs to be reviewed and tested against what we know about the environment being designed and its users–what the design ought to respond to–so that designs can be continually improved and eventually achieve their treatment goals. Because imaging, presenting, and testing in design all triangulate on the same issues in slightly different ways, and with emphasis on different dimensions of the same issue, it should not be surprising that issues such as security and landmarks appear again in this section.

One way to do this is to use a checklist of design objectives to determine at each stage how well the design meets those objectives. This is a rather dry way of testing designs, although effective in many instances.

Here I would like to suggest that eight to ten major principles underlie successful treatment gardens, and that if they are kept in mind and made explicit in the "test" phase of each design cycle, resulting environments will have a good chance of actually treating–reducing symptoms–of Alzheimer's disease. Some of these have been elaborated earlier in this article; others are new or have only been dealt with by implication.

Test information, is not based on new data in the design process; it draws on the same data as image and presentation information, presenting it in a form that can be used more easily in a rapid-fire test situation, sometimes with several people taking part. In a design review / test meeting there might be other similar designers, designers of different disciplines, paying clients, users living with Alzheimer's, family or paid partners including garden gatekeepers, horticultural therapists, and contractors. Test information has to be presented simply and straightforwardly with no confusing jargon.

Safety and security: To maximize usability and access to treatment gardens they need to be 100% safe and secure. Plan enclosures that are high enough and smooth enough to prevent climbing, yet still feel friendly and empowering–as if they are keeping dangers out, rather than restricting the person's freedom. Avoid hidden areas that cannot be easily seen from inside or other parts of the garden. Camouflage exits from the garden to unsafe areas.

Walking pathways: To give greatest respect and dignity to users, do not plan "wandering paths," rather plan all pathways to be "walking paths." People walk to destinations. People use landmarks to orient themselves when they walk. Check at each design stage to be sure that the walking paths are designed with visible destinations, evident landmarks, 90° angle shortcuts, and are clear enough that with repeated use, users living with Alzheimer's will eventually learn the garden's organization using their procedural memory.

Landmarks: Landmarks are the building blocks of place-knowing and way-finding. So that users know where they are and can find their way without too much trouble, be sure to pepper the environment with recognizable landmarks. Include familiar objects like birdfeeders and mailboxes, benches and stonewalls, beds of flowering shrubs, and vegetable plots–possibly raised beds. Make sure that the treatment garden does not look like an illustration in a design student's textbook. I said "pepper", not include every landmark you can think of. Subtlety and grace remain characteristics of good design, even for this population.

Territory: To be comfortable, everyone needs to be able to recognize and appropriate for herself some territory–even temporarily. Dynamic and comfortable gardens provide those opportunities. Test the designs to be sure that there are several small places that might be called "take over areas." The goal is to be sure that users with Alzheimer's can say, even for a short time, I like to sit on "my bench," plant in "my veggie garden," and rake "my lawn."

Shared places: One of the depressing side effects of living with Alzheimer's is social isolation and withdrawal. Friends and family may avoid the person. Strangers who do not know what "living with Alzheimer's" means, may turn away. Gardens can help people overcome their feelings of isolation by providing places that draw groups of people together, even just groups of two or three. Make sure that in addition to "take over" territories for individuals, there are also "together places" where users are likely to meet each other naturally. Raised planting bed with edges wide enough to sit on, invite users to come together. The same is true for a patio with round socio-petal tables each with its own sun umbrella, or a gently swinging bench with place for two or three people.

Sensory experiences: As people age, with or without Alzheimer's, and one or another sense becomes less sensitive–hearing, sight, smell–the more they can use several senses at the same time, the more they understand their environment, the more in control they feel, and the more empowered they are. There is no better place to provide such experiences than in a treatment garden. In reviewing plans, make sure that consideration is continually given to the colors of both person-made objects like benches, stonewalls, and fences, and also to planting schemes. Plantings can be organized to provide fragrant places, objects and plants can be planned to maximize the textures users come in contact with and touch, and all garden elements together can provide joy through meeting universal needs for variety and interest.

Prosthetic supports: Everything in our environment that helps us and supports us to do what we need to do better is prosthetic. Is the treatment garden maximally prosthetic, without appearing to be prosthetic? Are there enough places to sit? To lean on? Is the garden oriented in such a way that the sun will shine in during the winter, but there will be shade during the hot summer? Have steps been avoided? And what about ramps and inclines that might be slippery when wet? Every element–from the height and width of informal sitting places like stone walls and planter box edges, to the height and shape of planned sitting places, must be considered in terms if their prosthetic qualities. Even the lowly bird feeder might be leaned on for support and has to be stable enough to take someone's occasional weight.

Residential and normal: A treatment garden is first a garden and only then a treatment for an illness. Garden users include family members, visitors, young people and students, staff members, and people in different stages of life with Alzheimer's. Each person using the garden will be influenced by his or her perception of the garden's beauty and comfort, and how welcoming it feels. The more institutional it seems, and planned-for-sick-people, the less the garden will have these effects. The more like a residential front yard or back yard, the garden looks and feels like, and the more like a normal public park the garden seems, the more those using it will themselves feel normal; and the more they will treat each other–both ill and not ill–as normal.

IMPLICATION FOR DESIGN TEAM ORGANIZATION

Design teams organized to plan environments for people living with Alzheimer's must include architects, interior designers, and landscape or garden designers from the very beginning of the process to the very end. For someone living with Alzheimer's, the relationship in their mind and brain of exterior to interior, garden to living areas, and daytime to evening becomes more and more complex. Environments that actually complicate these relationships in the built world exacerbate the problem of living with Alzheimer's. The only way to be as certain as possible this is not the result of a disjointed design process is to join at the hip interior design, building design, and garden design from the start of the design process to the end.

THE POWER OF DESIGN TO TREAT

Nature and planned gardens that provide healthy opportunities to be in nature–even if just a grassy patch of lawn with a place to sit and enjoy the sun in winter and shade in summer–can immeasurably improve the quality of life of people living with Alzheimer's. As neuroscience knowledge become increasingly linked to environmental design, the impacts of nature on people becomes increasingly evident. With this knowledge, designers have a new responsibility, namely to do their best to make sure this happens. Just as those in the medical profession can treat and heal; so do designers. With this power comes the responsibility among designers to make the commitment to learn everything they can about how people living with Alzheimer's experience the world, and use all their design skills to make sure this knowledge is translated into exceptional treatment gardens.

REFERENCES

Grant, Charlotte (2003). "Chapter III: Hearthstone at New Horizons" in *Factors Influencing the Use of Outdoor Space by Residents with Dementia in Long term Care Facilities*. PhD Thesis, Georgia Institute of Technology, UMI Dissertation Publishing (disspub@umi.com: www.umi.com)

Lynch, K. (1960). *The Image of the City*. Cambridge, MA: MIT Press.

Norman D.A. (1988). *The Design of Everyday Things*. New York: Doubleday/Currency.

Zeisel, J. (2006) *Inquiry by Design: Environment / Behavior / Neuroscience in Architecture, Interiors, Landscape, and Planning*. New York and London: W. W. Norton

ADDITIONAL READINGS

Tyson, M.M. (1998).*The Healing Landscape: Therapeutic Outdoor Environments*. New York: McGraw Hill.

Zeisel, J., Hyde, J., & Levkoff, S. (1994) Best practices: an environmental-behavior (E-B) model for Alzheimer special care units. *Am J Alzheimer's Care and Related Disorders & Research, 9(2)*, 4-21.

Zeisel, J. & Tyson, M. (1999) Alzheimer's Treatment Gardens, in Clare Cooper Marcus and Marni Barnes (Eds), *Healing Gardens: Therapeutic Benefits and Design Recommendations*, New York: John Wiley & Sons.

Zeisel, J. & Raia, P. (2000) Non-pharmacological Treatment for Alzheimer's disease: A mind-brain approach *American Journal of Alzheimer's Disease and Other Dementias* November-December 2000, 15(6), Abstract published in *The Journal of Neuropsychiatry and Clinical Neurosciences, 12(1)*.

Zeisel, J. Silverstein, N., Hyde, J., Levkoff, S., Lawton, M. P., & Holmes, W. (2003) Environmental Correlates to Behavioral Outcomes in Alzheimer's Special Care Units, *The Gerontologist*, November, 43(5), pp. 697-711.

Zeisel, J & Welch, P. (1981) *Housing Designed for Families: A Summary of Research*. Cambridge, MA: Joint Center for Urban Studies for MIT and Harvard.

doi:10.1300/J081v21n01_02

Outdoor Wandering Parks
for Persons with Dementia

Jiska Cohen-Mansfield

SUMMARY. *Purpose:* This study aimed to characterize the features of outdoor areas for persons suffering from dementia, and to clarify the relationship between design features, utilization and satisfaction with these areas.

Methods: A national survey of long-term care facilities with outdoor areas investigated the characteristics and features of these areas, and how those relate to their perceived impact on their users.

Results: The majority of the respondents rated outdoor spaces as very useful, and as having a great benefit for users. The perceived benefit was related to the presence of more design features, such as the presence of gazebos and to the number of activities offered in the area. Despite these positive findings, respondents stated the areas were not used as much as possible and indicated several problems, mostly related to the safety of

Jiska Cohen-Mansfield, PhD, is affiliated with the Research Institute on Aging Hebrew Home of Greater Washington, and also George Washington University Medical Center.

Address correspondence to: Dr. Jiska Cohen-Mansfield, Research Institute on Aging, Hebrew Home of Greater Washington, 6121 Montrose Road, Rockville, MD 20852.

This article is taken from Cohen-Mansfield, J. & Werner, P. (1999). Outdoor wandering parks for persons suffering from dementia: A survey of characterization and utilization. *Alzheimer's Disease and Associated Disorders–An International Journal*, *13*(2), 109-117. Sections are printed here with permission from Lippincott Williams & Wilkins.

Available online at http://jhe.haworthpress.com
doi:10.1300/J081v21n01_03

the residents.

Conclusion: The results of this survey can assist facilities in better designing or improving their outdoor areas to increase utilization and satisfaction. doi:10.1300/J081v21n01_03 *[Article copies available for a fee from The Haworth Document Delivery Service: 1-800-HAWORTH. E-mail address: <docdelivery@haworthpress.com> Website: <http://www.HaworthPress.com>*

KEYWORDS. Sheltered areas, environmental design, nursing home, cognitive functioning, dementia, wandering park

INTRODUCTION

In the past, nursing homes landscaped whatever land they had with sufficient shrubs, trees, and grass to fit comfortably into the surrounding neighborhood. The land was not intended for recreational use by residents, staff, or neighbors, but served as a backdrop for the building. Only ambulatory, independent residents regularly ventured outside, and they were often forced to sit in the front of the building, if benches were available. If benches were not available, residents rarely left the building.

In the last two decades, nursing homes have been allotting space for the construction of courtyards, parks, patios, and gardens. Lawton's thesis of "environmental docility" (Lawton & Nahemow, 1973; Lawton, 1981) contributed greatly to this change. Briefly stated, Lawton posited an inverse correlation between the competency of a person and the impact of the environment. While the environment may have a minimal impact on the functioning of a competent person, it has a major impact on a person with limited competency. Consequently, if chaotic space can disorient confused patients, then well-ordered space, with cues, can be "prosthetic," improving residents' lives. And outdoor space, with its opportunities for pleasant visual, tactile, olfactory, and auditory stimuli, can be especially prosthetic. Such spaces are often used as gardens for persons with dementia who wander and with the goal of improving sleep and independent function in nursing home residents (Zeisel, 2005).

Believing that being outdoors will help residents, nursing homes have responded by building outdoor areas. "Special care units" geared toward dementia patients have been developed featuring these outdoor spaces in their therapeutic regimens (Calkins, 1987; Coons, 1987; Zeisel, Hyde, & Levkoff, 1994).

Several studies have shown some positive effects among those with dementia using an outdoor walking area (Mather, Nemecek & Oliver, 1997; Carillon, 2000; Cohen-Mansfield & Werner, 1998). Mather et al.'s small sample (n = 10) measured disruptive behaviors with the Dementia Behavior Disturbance Scale across seasons and compared indoor and outdoor use of a walled garden. While there was no significant change in disruptive behaviors with garden use, the study showed a trend toward less sleep disruption and less overall disruptive behaviors among the resident who used the garden most often. The study at Carillon Nursing and Rehabilitation Center found that a daily 30 minutes outdoor nature walked with nursing home staff resulted in a decrease in wandering (especially during meal times) and a decrease in sleep disturbances among participating residents based on nurse reports. In a study that aimed to investigate the utility of visits to outdoor garden area for nursing home residents suffering from dementia who tend to pace or wander, Cohen-Mansfield & Werner (1998) found that escorting nursing home residents who pace frequently to an outdoor area proved to have positive effects on mood and pacing behaviors. Trespassing and exit-seeking behaviors, the most difficult types of pacing related behaviors, decreased during the intervention compared to baseline. Several barriers to the intervention were encountered: the weather; residents' requiring one-to-one supervision; residents' fear of going outside; and accessibility of the outdoor areas.

The literature on what constitutes the ideal prosthetic outdoor space is both intuitive and prescriptive, offering checklists for administrators as they plan what these spaces should look like, and what should happen inside them. Unfortunately, the advice is often confusing. On one hand, residents need an array of therapeutic stimuli; on the other hand, residents suffering from dementia need a "peaceful, calm quiet environment" (Hiatt, 1979; Skolalski-Pelliteri, 1983; Peppard, 1986, Rauma, 2003). The open spaces should encourage movement–indeed, wanderers benefit from the opportunity to walk unimpeded. Yet space should be enclosed to prevent residents from getting lost, with definite circular pathways to permit continuous walking. Similarly, although ophthalmological research shows that the aging eye loses the ability to distinguish pastels (hence, people can better appreciate primary colors), a survey of residents of a retirement facility found that elderly residents preferred pastel, not primary, colored flowers (Gignoux, 1987).

The gerontological literature offers no thorough overview of the kinds of spaces constructed, their purposes, their uses, and finally, their usefulness. Cohen and Day (1994) surveyed 20 facilities, pointing out successful features of environments for people with dementia; and Zeisel et al. (1994) interviewed 50 special care units to construct a heuristic Environment-Benefits model, but no large-scale surveys have documented the kinds of outdoor spaces that facilities have been constructing. Architects (Calkins, 1987; Cohen & Day, 1994, Rauma, 2003), landscape architects (Lovering, 1990; Randall, Burkhardt, & Kutcher, 1990), interior designers (Brawley, 1992), and environmental and gerontological consultants (Hiatt, 1980, Zeisel et al., 1994) have drawn model blueprints, with advice on trees, plantings, pathways, fences, sitting, and activities. Most advice, however, has been based largely on intuition.

This study aims to complement their work through a survey of facilities which have constructed outdoor areas for their residents. The purpose of this survey is to describe the experience of long-term facilities with outdoor areas. This experience may guide other institutions willing to develop such areas.

METHODS

A nationwide list of 672 facilities with outdoor areas was obtained from the National Evaluation of Special Care Units (Leon & Siegenthaler, 1994). Three mailings of the questionnaire were sent, with the last two being directed to those facilities who did not respond to previous mailings. For about 15% of the facilities we attempted phone interviews. At each mailing, one questionnaire was sent per institution. Information was obtained for 320 facilities, yielding a response rate of 48% of surveyed nursing homes. Sixty-six percent of the respondents (n = 211) were directors of nursing, 13% were administrators, 16% occupied other positions, such as social worker, and 6% did not specify their position. Respondents worked at their facility for an average of 5.4 years (SE = .33).

The survey questionnaire included close-ended questions, i.e., questions with specific response options, as well as the option "other," as well as queries for objective numerical data, such as number of beds. For options "other," a request was included to specify the details of that choice. An open ended question queried about features which the respondents would like to add to their outdoor area. The questionnaire was developed on the basis of survey of the literature, discussions with architects of outdoor areas, and users of such areas. The questions pertained to the following: their operating characteristics (number of beds, occupancy, ownership, location); the design of the outdoor area, including size, site, landscaping, safety features, etc.; the activities that occur there; its usage (for whom it was created, who actually uses it, when is it available, how often it is used, accessibility); its limitations and its benefits to the facility. Perceived impact was rated on a 4-point Likert-type scale: positive, slightly positive, no effect, and negative effect. Ratings of perceived impact were obtained concerning impact on the following: cognitively intact residents, cognitively impaired residents, wanderers, families and visitors, staff members and volunteers, children from the neighborhood, public relations, and marketability of the facility. Areas of limitations queried included costs and safety.

RESULTS

Facility Characteristics

The facilities varied by ownership, size, and location. They included 61% for-profit facilities (compared to 67% nationwide; Cowles, 1995), 17% non-profit facilities, as well as 7% religious and governmental facilities (Veterans' Homes, other federal, state, city, and county). A majority of the facilities (60%) were part of a chain ownership. Facilities were split between suburban (42%), rural (35%), and urban (23%).

The mean number of skilled beds was 104.5 (with a range from 0 to 559), compared to 106.9 nationwide (Cowles, 1995). The mean number of intermediate beds was 92.6 (with a range from 0 to 333), and the mean number of residential beds was 37.7 (ranging from 0 to 206). Facilities ranged from campus-style arrangements of up to 9 buildings to one-building sites. The mean number of buildings was 1.3. Similarly, some facilities had buildings with as many as 7 floors, although the mean was 1.6. The mean number of units per facility was 4.9. The mean number of residents in the 216 facilities who provided the appropriate information was 124.1 (SE = 4.30; range 12–412).

Establishment of the Outdoor Area

The majority of the facilities (74%) reported that the outdoor areas were built with the facility's funding. Other funding sources included: private donations (6% of the facilities), private foundations (3%), and the government (1%).

Almost thirty percent of the facilities were built by the facility's maintenance crew, other facilities used local landscapers (27%), private contractors (20%), or a combination of the two (15%). The age of the outdoor areas ranged from a few months to 44 years, with a mean of 6.1 years.

Availability of the Outdoor Area

Facilities reported that their outdoor areas were open from 8:00 a.m. (modal time) until 8:00 p.m. (modal time). The majority of the facilities (88%) had flexible hours, with 60% reporting that the outdoor areas were open all day and night.

A quarter of the respondents (25%) reported that the residents are free to enter the outdoor area from their rooms. An additional 23% reported that residents have to be escorted to the outdoor area, and 38% reported a combination of both methods. Fourteen percent mentioned other ways of going outside such as being free to exit from any other area of the facility, and having to notify nursing staff members before going outside.

Design

The outdoor spaces varied widely in their designs. The majority of the facilities characterized their outdoor area as a "courtyard" (76%) or a "patio" (52%). Other definitions used included "garden" (16%) and "park" (11%).

Size

The mean size of the outdoor area was 38.2 yards long (range = 3-330) by 29.1 yards wide (range = 1-168; SE = 2.71 and 1.91 respectively), for a mean area of 1111.6 square yards. The facilities estimated that their outdoor areas could hold a range of from 6 to 400 people; the mean capacity was 42.8 (SE = 2.62).

Exterior Design

A majority of the facilities (68%) had separate outdoor areas for cognitively intact and cognitively impaired residents. All the facilities described their outdoor areas as enclosed. The most common enclosures were a wooden fence (46% of the facilities), buildings (37%), a chain link fence (31%), and bushes or hedges (12%). The least commonly used alternatives were a brick wall or a plexiglass fence. The mean height of the enclosure was 7.2 feet (SE = 0.22), with a range of 3 to 30 feet. Facilities used different elements to discourage residents from exiting the enclosures: 49% used a fence; 20% used plants; 13% used a combination of different elements, and another 13% used other types of camouflage such as an iron fence, and an additional fence on top of the regular one. Four percent of the facilities did not use any method to prevent exit.

Almost half of the facilities (49%) reported having their outdoor spaces exposed to the sun all day; 47% reported their outdoor area being exposed to the sun for half the day. Only six facilities reported their courtyards as being rarely or never exposed to the sun.

The main view from the outdoor area was a fence for 41% of the facilities; in the others, residents could view a residential neighborhood (30%); buildings (23%); woods (21%); a street or highway (14%) or an interior courtyard (11%). Fewer than ten percent reported a view of lawns, playground, school, parking lot, or farm. Obviously, in many of the facilities, the view included more than one of the possible views.

Interior Design

Available features. The distribution of interior design features in the surveyed facilities are summarized in Table 1. All the facilities reported walkways (usually made of concrete–78.1%) as part of their *landscaping*, as well as trees (83.5% of the facilities), flowers (79.4%), and bird feeders (59.4%). The most common *seating features* were: lawn furniture (84.8% of the facilities), picnic tables (68.9%), and benches (24.4%). A few facilities (15%) integrated water into their outdoor area designs, with fountains/waterfalls (12.4%), fish ponds (4.1%), and brooks (1.6%).

Few facilities provided *convenience features* that could facilitate their use by elderly persons, such as handrails (present in 13.3% of the facilities), easy access to a bathroom (11.1% of the facilities), a drinking fountain (available in 4.8% of the facilities), or a coffee bar/snack cart (1.3%). As many as 41.6% of the facilities had lights for evening use.

The main type of *protection against sunlight* was umbrella tables (present in 48.9% of the facilities). While 83.5% of the courtyards had trees, only 18% saw them as protection against the sun. Gazebos were used by 28.6% of the facilities. Only 15.6% of facilities provided awnings and 7.3% provided trellises. Only a minority of the facilities had playground equipment (5%).

Over a third (35%) of the facilities had pets in the outdoor area; 21.6% of the facilities mentioned having birds. Other common pets mentioned were cats and dogs. Three facilities (1%) reported including wall murals (see Table 1).

Essential and desired features. In addition to the features available, participants were asked what design features they considered essential in an outdoor area. The five features considered most essential by the respondents were: lawn furniture (14% of the facilities); a gazebo (14%); trees (12%); picnic tables (12%); and flowers (12%). Fifty-five percent of the facilities wanted to add features to the outdoor areas. The most common features desired were: raised gardens for wheel-chair access (19% of the 176 facilities which stated that they wanted to add some feature), lawn furniture (11%), bird feeders (10%), trees (9%) and easy access to a fountain (9%).

Problematic features. Few facilities stated that any of the features were problematic. The five features considered most problematic were: Concrete walkways (13% of the facilities); lawn furniture (3%); fences (2%); raised gardens (1%); and flowers (1%). Of those facilities reporting problems, almost

TABLE 1. Distribution of the Main Interior Design Features of the Outdoor Areas

		n	%
LANDSCAPING			
	Walkways	320	100.0
	of these:		
	concrete	250	78.1
	natural dirt	11	3.4
	brick	7	2.2
	wood	2	0.6
	other[a]	21	6.6
	combination	29	9.1
	Trees	263	83.5
	Flowers	250	79.4
	Ground level gardens	180	57.1
	Raised gardens	124	39.4
	Decorative objects	64	20.3
	Rock gardens	34	10.8
WATER -RELATED FEATURES			
	Bird feeders/baths	187	59.4
	Fountains/waterfalls	39	12.4
	Fish ponds	13	4.1
	Brooks	5	1.6
	Bridges	3	1.0
SEATING			
	Lawn furniture	267	84.8
	Picnic tables	217	68.9
	Curved benches	77	24.4
	Game tables	11	3.5
	Swings	4	1.3
CONVENIENCE FEATURES			
	Lights for evening use	131	41.6
	Handrails	42	13.3
	Easy access to bathroom	35	11.1
	Storage area	23	7.3
	Easy access to drinking fountain	15	4.8
	Coffee bar/Snack cart	4	1.3
PROTECTION FROM SUN			
	Umbrella tables	154	48.9
	Gazebos	90	28.6
	Awnings	49	15.6
	Trellis	23	7.3
PETS			
	Birds	68	21.6
	Cats	39	12.4
	Dogs	23	7.3
	Fish	7	2.2
	Other pets	24	7.6

n = 320 for walkway characteristics n = 315 for all other features
[a] Such as: grass and asphalt.

n = 320 for walkway characteristics; n = 315 for all other features
[a]Such as: grass and asphalt.

60% explained that the cause was that they threatened the safety of the residents.

Safety features. In most of the facilities, the key safeguards for residents were not alarm systems (used in 26% of the facilities), television monitors (used in 2%), or physical supports (17%), but the fact that staff accompanied residents outside (69%). Similar to accompanying the resident, some facilities assured safety by visual contact with the resident in the garden (15%). Safety features mentioned by fewer than 10% of facilities included use of a buzzer, a speaker system, a fence, and signs.

Although all outdoor areas were enclosed, only 5% of the facilities considered the enclosure to be a safety precaution. The mean ratio of staff to residents in courtyards was one staff member for 8.2 residents. It is interesting that although maintaining the safety of the residents should be of primary concern, 11% of the facilities did not report any safety devices. However, only 10% of the facilities said that they did not secure the gates, while 67% of the facilities secured gates with locks. Many options were used in the continuum between locked and open gates, including code buttons, camouflage of gates, alarms, latches, and clasps. Each of these options were used by a small minority of the facilities (5% or fewer).

Activities

The participating facilities reported a wide variety of activities held in the outdoor areas. An average of 5.1 activities (SE = .13) were reported. 86% of the respondents reported using the outdoor areas for eating and barbecues, 62% for exercise, 55% for private parties, 46.5% for communal gardening, and 44% for individual gardening. Other activities conducted in the outdoor area included: sports (42%), concerts (33%), reality orientation (29%), crafts (21%), and physical or occupational therapy (18%). Low frequency activities included use of pets, reading, and story telling.

Utilization of Outdoor Areas

Intended Users

Most of the outdoor areas were originally created especially for cognitively impaired residents (84.6% of the facilities) and wanderers (76.8%). Fewer facilities (36.6%) designed their outdoor areas to serve non-ambulatory residents, the hearing-impaired (21.9%), or the visually impaired (20.3%). Only 12.4% of the facilities said that they designed their areas for "all types of residents" (see Table 2).

TABLE 2. Type of Intended and Actual Users of Outdoor Areas

| | Number of Facilities | | | |
| | Intended (n=306) | | Actual (n=319) | |
	n	%	n	%
Cognitively impaired	259	84.6	273	85.6
Wanderers	235	76.8	262	82.1
Cognitively intact	148	48.4	162	50.8
Family/Visitors	141	46.1	197	61.8
Non-ambulatory	112	36.6	167	52.4
Staff/Volunteers	86	28.1	142	44.5
Hearing impaired	67	21.9	122	38.2
Visually impaired	62	20.3	119	37.3
Children	14	4.6	18	5.6
Other	21	6.9	16	5.2
All types of residents	38	12.4	-	-
No response	14	4.4	1	.3

Actual Users

In the majority of the facilities, the intended beneficiaries were indeed those using the outdoor areas. In over 80% of the facilities, residents with dementia and wanderers were those using the space, although they were not the only users. Half the facilities reported that cognitively intact, as well as non-ambulatory residents were using the space.

Although only 46.1% of the facilities created outdoor spaces with family/visitor recreation as a key goal, in 61.8% of the facilities, families and visitors were using the space, as were staff and volunteers (44.5% of the facilities), even though they, too, were not the intended beneficiaries (see Table 2).

The average number of users per day ranged between 12.9 (SE = .60) for cognitively impaired residents to 6.9 (SE = .86) for visually impaired residents.

Rate of Outdoor Area Utilization and Reasons For Nonuse

As expected, the outdoor areas were used most frequently during the summer (77% were used everyday, and 98% at least several times a week). Conversely, rates of utilization were lowest in the winter, in which 46% of the facilities reported to use the outdoor area rarely, and only 23% reported using it every day. Rates reported for the spring and fall indicate an everyday use by about half the facilities, and use by the vast majority (over 90%) at a rate of at least several times a week.

In response to the question, "Is the outdoor area used as much as it could be?" as many as 62% of the facilities responded "no." The main reasons provided for this included: weather-related problems (e.g., too hot, too windy, or too sunny)–31.3% of the facilities; accessibility problems (e.g., area not accessible, heavy doors leading out, and residence buildings too far from outdoor area)–25% of the facilities; design problems (e.g., no walkways, no benches, or too small)–22.8% of the facilities; and supervision problems–8.5% of the facilities. Almost a quarter of the facilities (24.1%) stated that their outdoor area was not used as much as possible because the residents were not accustomed to going outside. However, the majority of the respondents reported that the existence of the outdoor area encouraged staff members (81%) and families (72%) to take residents outside at least more often than prior to having the enclosed area (see Table 3).

Benefits of Outdoor Areas

Outdoor areas demand staff time and attention; consequently, facilities must evaluate their overall usefulness and impact. When asked to rate their overall usefulness, all facilities rated the outdoor areas as useful, with 69% rating them "extremely useful," 26% "very useful," and 5% "somewhat useful."

In addition, facilities were asked to rate the impact of the outdoor spaces on 8 domains: on cognitively intact residents, on cognitively impaired residents, on nursing home residents who wander, on family and visitors, on staff members and volunteers, on neighborhood children, on the facility's public rela-

TABLE 3. Reasons for Non-Use of Outdoor Areas (n = 307)

WEATHER (31.3%)	
Too hot	18.6%
Too windy	7.2
Too sunny	5.5
ACCESSIBILITY (25.0%)	
Heavy doors leading out	7.8
Not accessible	6.8
Area not convenient	5.2
Residence far from outdoor area	2.9
Need to use stairs, elevators	2.3
OUTDOOR AREA'S DESIGN (22.8%)	
Nothing to see	8.8
No benches	6.2
No walkways	3.9
Too small	3.9
SUPERVISION PROBLEM (8.5%)	
Not enough staff	8.5
OTHER REASONS	
Resident not used to going outside	24.1
Not specified	28.3

TABLE 4. Ratings of Perceived Impact of Outdoor Areas

	Positive	Slight Positive	No Effect	Negative Effect	No Response	
		(% of those responding)			n	%
Cognitively intact	84.6	8.4	6.3	0.7	34	10.6
Cognitively impaired	72.1	23.7	3.9	0.3	12	3.8
Wanderers	77.0	15.4	5.6	2.0	15	4.7
Families/Visitors	84.4	11.4	3.9	0.3	13	4.1
Staff/Volunteers	76.2	15.2	8.3	0.3	17	5.3
Neighborhood children	17.0	5.7	73.6	3.8	108	33.8
Public relations	76.0	15.3	8.3	0.3	32	10.0
Marketing	82.7	12.5	4.4	0.3	25	7.8

Percentages do not add up to 100 due to rounding.

tions and on their marketability. Almost all facilities (range 84.6%–72.1%) perceived a positive impact on the residents who use the outdoor area (see Table 4).

Attributes of Outdoor Area Which Affect Perceived Impact

In order to clarify which attributes of the outdoor areas were related to the perceived impact, *t*-tests comparing impact between facilities which do and do not have specific attributes were conducted. The *t* values and significance levels describing the relationships between areas' activities and design features for impact on the cognitively impaired resident, the cognitively intact resident, and for wanderers are presented in Table 5. Because of the use of multiple tests, only those which were significant at the .01 level are presented. Similar to the *t*-tests, correlations of perceived impact with the number of activities offered, number of design features utilized, and number of design problems (e.g., nothing to see, accessibility problems, no benches, too small) were all significant at the .01 level, though their magnitude was moderate (ranging from .15 to .29, with *n*'s ranging from 286 to 308).

Similar *t*-tests were calculated comparing the areas' perceived impact on the facilities' public relations and marketability for areas with and without specific features. As can be seen in Table 6, similar features are related to the facilities' public relations and marketability. Impact on public relations and marketability were also significantly (p < .001) related to number of activities, number of design features, and number of design problems (with correlations ranging from .23 to .36).

Problems with Outdoor Areas

Fifty-five percent (n = 160) of the facilities reported having encountered problems with the areas. The most common problems were: problems related

TABLE 5. Comparisons of Facilities With and Without Attributes Concerning Activities in the Outdoor Area and Design Features of the Outdoor Areas: Significance Level of t-Test Comparisons.

	Cognitively Intact	Cognitively Impaired	Wanderers
ACTIVITIES			
Sports		.005	.000
Physical therapy			.001
Exercise		.000	.001
Crafts		.001	.000
Gardening (Individual)	.002	.005	
Gardening (Communal)		.000	.007
Private Parties	.001		
Reality orientation			.007
DESIGN FEATURES			
Gazebo		.001	.002
Lights		.006	
Fountains	.002		
Trellis		.000	.000
Storage Features	.001		.001
Raised Gardens	.000		
Rock Gardens	.001		
Playground equipment		.001	.001
Lawn furniture		.009	
Pets	.001		
Easy access to bathroom		.000	
Easy access to fountain			.001

TABLE 6. Comparison of Facilities With and Without Different Attributes on Public Relations, and Marketability: Significance Level of T-test Comparisons

	Public relations	Marketability
ACTIVITIES		
Sports	.002	
Physical therapy	.001	.000
Exercise		.001
Eating	.003	
Concerts	.008	
Reality orientation		.006
DESIGN FEATURES		
Gazebo	.004	.002
Lights		.004
Bird feeders or bird baths	.004	.008
Rock Gardens		.001
Curved Benches	.009	.007
Trees	.009	
Pets	.000	.001
Easy access to bathroom	.000	

to the safety of the residents (58% of those who encountered any problem), and insect pests (34%). A quarter of the facilities (26%) with specific difficulties mentioned problems with residents, another 10% mentioned problems with staff, and 6% said the area was too costly.

DISCUSSION

Nursing homes, particularly those with dementia units, have acknowledged the utility of outdoor spaces for residents and have incorporated "courtyards" and "patios" into their facilities. Although the gerontological literature stresses the prosthetic benefits of outdoor spaces (Cornbleth, 1977; Hiatt, 1980; Randall et al., 1990; Brawley, 1992), no information is available concerning the characteristics of these areas, and how they are related to the relative perceived impact the areas have on their users. Results of this national survey of long-term care facilities with outdoor areas show that although some of the guidelines and advice provided by architects, designers, and researchers have been incorporated, several problems remain. It is hoped that these results, especially the descriptions of the specific features and problems, will aid facilities in planning and designing new outdoor areas.

The majority of the facilities included walkways, trees, and flowers as part of their landscaping. However, only 40% included elevated gardens, and a mere 20% included decorative objects, which have been cited as features encouraging participation in activities and evoking positive behaviors (Hiatt, 1980; Calkins, 1987). Similarly, although almost half of the respondents reported using umbrella tables to protect from the sun, only 30% had gazebos, which are considered a better protection from the vagaries of the weather (Calkins, 1987). Indeed, as many as a third of the respondents linked non-use to weather related reasons (such as: "too hot" or "too sunny"). While facilities cannot change the setting of their outdoor areas, they can use more features to provide protection from the weather, such as extended roofs, trellises, and awnings.

Although the items listed by facilities can provide ideas for other facilities regarding possible features and their *desirability*, caution should be taken in utilizing them. For example, lawn furniture was considered one of the most essential features, and one of those most desired by facilities. On the other hand, lawn furniture was also mentioned, albeit by a small number, as a problem in outdoor areas. Lawn furniture per se is not sufficient; it needs to be tailored for the needs of the residents, as it relates to convenience (e.g., height of seats), safety, location, aesthetic quality, and other design features.

The view from the outdoor area has been mentioned as very important because it provides stimulation (Lovering, 1990; Brawley, 1992). Despite this, 41% of the respondents reported that the main view from their outdoor space is a fence. Only a minority reported having scenery, buildings, or other surroundings that may arouse the residents' curiosity and interest. A stimulating view with activity is probably most desirable, especially one in which residents can view daily life, as they might do sitting on the porch at home. Indeed, lack of appropriate view or activity ("nothing to see") was one of the problems cited with some of the outdoor areas.

Safety is well known to be of primary importance as problems may arise due to lack of available staff or fears on the part of staff or family members that residents may hurt themselves while in the gardens (Heath, 2004). In a study exploring the preferences of older persons in a retirement center for the landscape of outdoor spaces, Gignoux (1987) found that the main concern of these elderly people was safety. Given its importance, it is surprising that as many as 11% of the respondents reported having no safety measures in place. Furthermore, 69% rely on residents being accompanied by staff members. This type of safety feature poses an inordinate cost on the facility, because much staff time is required to optimize the use of the outdoor area. An alternative strategy is the use of safety measures. One such example is use of an enclosed area to which residents have free access and monitoring of residents by visual contact or TV monitors. This type of arrangement also enhances the residents' autonomy and sense of control. In a somewhat similar setting, Namazi and Johnson (1992) demonstrated that the number of agitated behaviors observed in 22 nursing home residents decreased during an unlocked door condition compared to a locked door condition. These results confirmed that with appropriate measures, it is possible to increase the residents' well-being without endangering their safety. Therefore it is disappointing that such a small proportion of the facilities relied on safety measures such as visual contact or alarm systems.

Most facilities have integrated at least some of their activities into the outdoor space. The most frequently cited activities include: barbecues, exercise, private parties, and gardening/horticultural therapy (Jarrott & Gigliotti, 2004). Although inter-generational programs that expose nursing home residents to children, and vice versa, are praised (Hiatt, 1980), few homes cited such activities, and few included playground equipment or game tables in their spaces. Indeed, only 18 of the facilities utilized the outdoor areas for children. Some of these facilities may have day care services for children on the premises and utilize the outdoor area for both purposes. Further study on this use is needed. Furthermore, the extent of utilization of the outdoor area by children who visit the elderly resident rather than by neighborhood children needs to be explored in future research.

Although one of the main difficulties cited in the literature concerns the accessibility of the outdoor space, results of this survey show that this remains a problem. As many as 25% of the respondents cited an accessibility reason for non-use of their spaces. Additionally, only a minority of the facilities mentioned convenience features such as easy access to a bathroom and easy access to a drinking fountain. Given the great difficulty that moving residents from their units imposes on staff members, solving the problem of accessibility is of utmost importance. Administrators designing new areas should consider accessibility in their list of priorities. Those who already have such areas should think about imaginative and creative ways of improving the access to the outdoor spaces. Possibilities include adding features, such as handrails, to ease the move of frail elderly, or to use the help of volunteers (adults and children) in transporting residents to the open space.

On the positive side, findings of this survey show that outdoor spaces are not only used by those for whom they were originally built (mainly cognitively impaired residents and wanderers), but also by intact residents, family members, visitors, staff members, and volunteers. Indeed in this study, respondents unanimously rated their outdoor spaces as "useful", with over half calling them "extremely useful". Outdoor areas were reported to have a positive impact on all the users, as well as on the public relations and marketability of the facilities. The extent of this perceived positive impact was related to the presence of design features, such as gazebo, or benches, and to the number of activities offered at the outdoor area. This finding is supported by Bengtsson (2005) whose focus groups found that staff members appreciated the outdoor parks and gardens surrounding their workplace and found them important to everyday life. Heath (2001) also showed that 97% of participants surveyed liked or strongly liked a therapeutic garden in their nursing facility, although opinions on specific features of the garden varied.

The survey includes 47.6% of the facilities with outdoor areas at the time of the survey, comprising of 320 facilities. Although this number represents only a small portion of nursing homes, they are quite representative of nursing homes in general with 60.8% for-profit nursing homes, similar to the 66.6% national average, and with an average of 104.5 skilled beds where the national average is 106.9. The facilities also represent a wide variation in other characteristics, such as ownership, location, number of buildings or number of residents, and seem to be representative of nursing homes nationwide, in characteristics other than having an outdoor garden. Therefore lessons from these facilities are likely to be directly applicable to other nursing homes.

A number of related research questions follow the examination of outdoor areas in nursing homes. For example, what solutions have been used by multiple story, or inner city facilities, where an outdoor area is less feasible? Outdoor areas are intended to allow nursing home residents to get out of the unit environment and get a sense of the light, air, and other features of the outdoors. Have facilities used innovative balconies? How did they secure them, and how did they maximize the sense of outdoors. Similarly, an area for research is optimizing the accessibility and utility of gardens. What type of access between the unit and the outdoor garden will optimize utilization? For example, would a glass door, or large windows next to a door be more enticing to residents? What innovative solutions can be suggested for the problem of weather? Do facilities use glasshouses with vegetation in the winter? Furthermore, the impact of outdoor areas needs to be investigated directly, rather than only relying on the perceptions of caregivers. Although some such information exists (e.g., Namazi & Johnson, 1992; Cohen-Mansfield & Werner, 1998), additional questions need to be answered: Is simply getting off the unit as beneficial as actually using the garden? What is the impact of having control over using a door vs. the actual access to a garden? Answers to these issues will aid caregivers in finding the best practice of care which is also feasible for them.

Several limitations of the study should be considered. First, the survey included only nursing homes with special care units. Second, the response rate was close to, but less than half of the facilities contacted. This may decrease the generalizability of the results. Another concern is that the relationships between outdoor area impact and its characteristics was explored through multiple *t*-tests. Although we tried to control for the risk of finding significant relationships by chance because of the use of multiple tests by using a .01 significance level, the use of multiple tests does increase the risk of such errors. Although we considered using multivariate analyses, we felt that this was an exploratory study, and later studies with better designed outcome measures would be necessary to examine the complex relationships between the different characteristics of an outdoor area, the characteristics of the nursing home, its usage, and its impact. Finally, we believe that the use of outdoor areas for persons with dementia has increased in recent years, and the survey does not reflect the most recent trends.

In summary, the findings of this survey serve as guidelines for those facilities interested in developing new outdoor spaces or those willing to change their current ones. The variability in design features used in the different facilities can be used by other facilities to develop an outdoor area to fit their specific needs and resources. There is a need to attend to specific design principles which will allow better utilization of the area. Once these principles are taken into account, more people can become users and enjoy outdoor spaces.

The design of the spaces should be adapted to the specific needs of the expected users, because the users are less likely to adapt to the demands of the environment. Although the location of the open space may have an important effect on its use (Randall et al., 1990), this should not be the only consideration. Possibilities may be created by extending rooms into the exterior, constructing porches, or protected balconies. It is the combination of adherence to known principles and continuous creativity which would promote solutions to foster the well-being of the elderly person who suffers from dementia.

ACKNOWLEDGMENTS

The data was based on a study supported in part by grant AG11502 from the National Institute on Aging. Portions of this paper were taken with permission from Lippincott, Williams & Wilkins Publishing and previously published in: Cohen-Mansfield, J. & Werner, P. (1999). Outdoor wandering parks for persons suffering from dementia: A survey of characterization and utilization. Alz Dis & Assoc Dis; 13(2):109-117.

REFERENCES

Bengtsson A. Outdoor Environments at Three Nursing Homes Focus Group Interviews with Staff. Journal of Housing for the Elderly 2005;19(3/4):49-69.

Brawley E. Alzheimer's disease: Designing the physical environment. Am J Alzheimer's Care Rel Disord & Res 1992;7:3-8.

Calkins MP. Outdoor Spaces. In: Calkins MP, ed. *Design for Dementia: Planning Environments for the Elderly and the Confused*. National Health Publishing, 1987: 109-112.

Carillon Nursing and Rehabilitation Center. Nature walk: from aimless pacing to purposeful walking. Nursing Homes Long term Care Management, 2000;49(11):50-4.

Cohen U, Day K. Emerging trends in environments for people with dementia. Am J Alzheimer's Care Rel Disord & Res 1994;9:3-11.

Cohen-Mansfield J, Werner P. Visits to an outdoor garden: Impact on behavior and mood of nursing home residents who pace. In Vellas, B. J., Fitten, G., & Frisconi (Eds): *Research and practice in Alzheimer's disease intervention in gerontology*. Serdi Publishing: Paris, France, 1998, pp. 419-436.

Coons D. Designing a residential care unit for persons with dementia. Congressional Office of Technology Assessment, Washington D.C., 1987.

Cornbleth T. Effects of a protected hospital ward area on wandering and nonwandering geriatric patients. J Gerontol 1977;32:573-7.

Cowles CM. Nursing Home Statistical Yearbook. The Cowles Research Group, Takoma, WA, 1995.

Gignoux LC. Executive Summary: The landscape design preferences of older people. Study conducted at Wheatland Hills Retirement Center, Radford, VA, 1987.

Heath Y. Evaluating the effect of therapeutic gardens. Amer J Alz Dis Other Dement 2004;19(4):239-57.

Heath Y, Gifford R. Post-occupancy evaluation of therapeutic garden. Activities, Adaptation & Aging 2001; 25(2):21-42.

Hiatt LG. Environmental considerations in understanding and designing for mentally impaired people. In: McBride H ed. *Mentally Impaired Aging: Bridging the Gap.* Washington D.C., American Association of Homes for the Aging 1979:33.

Hiatt LG. Moving outside and making it a meaningful experience. Nurs Homes 1980, (May/June):34-9.

Jarrott SE, Gigliotti C. From the garden to the table: Evaluation of a dementia-specific HT program. Acta Horticulturae 639, ISHS 2004: XXVI International Horticultural Congress: 139-44.

Lawton MP. Sensory deprivation and the effect of the environment on the management of the patient with senile dementia. In: Miller N, Cohen G Eds. *Clinical aspects of Alzheimer's disease and senile dementia.* New York: Raven Press, 1981, pp 227-251.

Lawton MP, Nahemow L. Ecology and the aging process. In: Eisdorfer C, Lawton MP Eds. *The psychology of adult development and aging.* Washington D.C.: American Psychological Association, 1973, pp. 619-674.

Leon J, Siegenthaler LA. Perspectives on the major special care units surveys. Alzheimer Dis Assoc Disord 1994;8(Suppl. 1):S58-S71.

Lovering MJ. Alzheimer's disease and outdoor space: Issues in environmental design. Am J Alzheimer's Care Rel Disord & Res 1990;5:33-40.

Mather JA, Nemecek D, Oliver K. The effect of a walled garden on behavior of individuals with Alzheimer's. Amer J Alz Dis 1997;Nov/Dec:252-7.

Namazi KH, Johnson BD. Pertinent autonomy of residents with dementias: Modification of the physical environment to enhance independence. Am J Alzheimer's Care Rel Disord & Res 1992;7:16-21.

Peppard NR. Special nursing home units for residents with primary degenerative dementia: Alzheimer's disease. J Gerontol Soc Work 1986;9(2):5-18.

Randall P, Burkhardt S, Kutcher J. Exterior space for patients with Alzheimer's disease and related disorders. Am J Alzheimer's Care Rel Disord & Res 1990;5:31-7.

Rauma P. What makes a healing garden? Nursing Home Long Term Care Management 2003;52(10):50-4.

Skolaski-Pellitteri T. Environmental adaptations which compensate for dementia. Phys Occup Ther Geriatr 1983;3(1):31-44.

Zeisel J. Treatment effects of healing garden for Alzheimer's: A difficult thing to prove. Edinburgh Garden Paper 2005; retrieved on June 20, 2006 from; http://www.openspace.eca.ac.uk/conference/proceedings/PDF/Zeisel.pdf.

Zeisel J, Hyde J, Levkoff S. Best practices: An Environment-Behavior model for Alzheimer special care units. Am J Alzheimer's Care Rel Disord & Res 1994;9:4-21.

doi:10.1300/J081v21n01_03

Housing and Connection to Nature for People with Dementia: Findings from the INDEPENDENT Project

Grant Gibson
Garuth Eliot Chalfont
Pamela D. Clarke
Judith M. Torrington
Andrew J. Sixsmith

SUMMARY. This paper reports on the qualitative findings of the first phase of the INDEPENDENT Project, an EPSRC funded EQUAL 4 consortium project in the UK that aims to investigate enabling environments for people with dementia. The overall project focus is on wellbeing and quality of life for people in different types of housing, with particular focus on the possible roles technology can play in maintaining the person's independence as long as possible. Connection to nature, access to the outdoors, and participation in nature-based activities were among a wide range of enjoyable activities reported by study participants living in their

Grant Gibson, MA, Pamela D. Clarke, MA, MSc, and Andrew J. Sixsmith, PhD, are affiliated with the Division of Primary Care, University of Liverpool, Whelan Building, Brownlow Hill, Liverpool, L69 3GB, United Kingdom, (E-mail: g.gibson@liv.ac.uk).

Garuth Eliot Chalfont, PhD, and Judith M. Torrington, BArch, RIBA, are affiliated with the Department of Architecture, University of Sheffield, Arts Tower, Western Bank, Sheffield, S10 2TN United Kingdom (E-mail: g.chalfont@sheffield.ac.uk).

[Haworth co-indexing entry note]: "Housing and Connection to Nature for People with Dementia: Findings from the INDEPENDENT Project." Gibson, Grant et al. Co-published simultaneously in *Journal of Housing for the Elderly* (The Haworth Press, Inc.) Vol. 21. No. 1/2, 2007, pp. 55-72; and: *Outdoor Environments for People with Dementia* (ed: Susan Rodiek and Benyamin Schwarz) The Haworth Press, Inc., 2007, pp. 55-72. Single or multiple copies of this article are available for a fee from The Haworth Document Delivery Service [1-800-HAWORTH, 9:00 a.m. - 5:00 p.m. (EST). E-mail address: docdelivery@haworthpress.com].

Available online at http://jhe.haworthpress.com
doi:10.1300/J081v21n01_04

55

own homes or in residential care. First, an overview of connection to nature for people with dementia and the importance of this connection within their home environments are given. Secondly, the research study is described and data from interviews with people with dementia and from focus groups with family and professional carers including access to, and preferences for nature are summarized. Multiple factors enabling or challenging a person's participation in nature-related activities included personal factors, formal support, social networks, as well as cultural and spiritual aspects. These factors are briefly described and compared. Lastly, factors of the built environment and differences between building types are presented and conclusions drawn. doi:10.1300/J081v21n01_04 *[Article copies available for a fee from The Haworth Document Delivery Service: 1-800-HAWORTH. E-mail address: <docdelivery@haworthpress.com> Website: <http://www.HaworthPress.com> © 2007 by The Haworth Press, Inc. All rights reserved.]*

KEYWORDS. Dementia, nature, home, residential care, gardens

INTRODUCTION

The INDEPENDENT Project is a three year consortium research project funded in the United Kingdom by a project grant from the Engineering and Physical Sciences Research Council (EPSRC) as part of the EQUAL 4 programme, focused on improving quality of life for older and disabled people. The multidisciplinary team includes the Division of Primary Care at the University of Liverpool, the School of Architecture at the University of Sheffield and the Bath Institute for Medical Engineering (BIME) at the University of Bath, in partnership with Northamptonshire Social Services, SheffCare (care housing provider), Huntleigh Healthcare and Dementia Voice. INDEPENDENT investigates the enabling role that technology can play for people with dementia from three specific perspectives–person, place and pleasure. Person: the research is user-led by consulting people with dementia directly and through their carers. Place: the housing and the built environment are considered in all aspects of the research and design. Pleasure: the project intends to increase opportunities for older people with dementia to experience enjoyment, pleasurable activities and social interaction, the focus of the technology being on design for well-being and quality of life rather than on safety, security and monitoring. The project intends to design, develop, install and evaluate technological responses to the needs and desires expressed by persons with dementia. This paper reports on this first phase of work, the needs analysis.

BACKGROUND AND CONTEXT

Dementia; the Person the Disease Has

Dementia means a loss of intellectual abilities or impairment of mental powers (literally meaning 'away' and 'mind'). It is a word describing a group of symptoms including memory loss, confusion, and disorientation, which are caused by brain diseases–the two most common being Alzheimer's and vascular dementia. While the cause and the cure for dementia remain unknown, it is clear that one's environment can offer support for cognitive impairment, hence the ongoing interest in the design of living environments. Research into dementia, drawing upon the social model of disability, increasingly recognizes that people with dementia, rather than being defined by the presence of the disease, are individuals themselves, each with their own opinions, feelings and desires (Kitwood, 1997). For many individuals, having some form of connection to nature can have important beneficial effects upon cognitive function, a sense of well-being and on quality of life. Connection to nature can be understood in many forms, from passive stimulation by natural sensations, made possible by simply stepping outside or opening a window (e.g., the wind, sunshine or birdsong), to more active and interactive participation with the natural environment, such as going for a walk through a bluebell wood. Beyond physical sensation, nature can provide a person with stimulation that is mental, emotional and spiritual, with potential for positively impacting upon wellbeing.

Connection to Nature & Dementia

Nature is an abundant source of multi-sensory stimulation (MSS). Providing access to nature as a form of MSS has been shown to be particularly beneficial within controlled settings in dementia care (Cohen Mansfield & Werner 1998, Baker et al., 2001; Burns et al., 2002, Lovering et al., 2002). Multi-sensory Environments (MSEs) (formerly known as Snoezelen) have been used in dementia care for relaxation, recreation, enjoyment, and stimulation of the senses (Pinkney, 1994; Hope, 1997). However, while MSEs continue to offer 'unrealized potential for improving the quality of care of older people with dementia' (Hope, 2004), the benefits of the stimulating natural world for people with dementia are largely un-researched. Nature-related activities are often an essential aspect of a person's cultural heritage, which is known to be currently underused as a therapeutic resource in environments for people with dementia (Day & Cohen, 2000). Such activities may involve physical exercise which has been shown to 'significantly and substantially improve cognitive ability'

(Lindenmuth & Moose, 1990). The authors attributed this to an improvement in cardiovascular factors and 'emotional stimulation' (increased sensory input).

Connection to nature also extends to people's interactions with animals. Companion animals and pets have been shown to have a beneficial effect upon people with dementia, particularly in terms of promoting stimuli for meaningful social interaction between individuals, professional and informal carers and relatives (Richeson, 2003; Baun & McCabe, 2003). Pet-assisted therapy with people with dementia facilitates interaction between the person with dementia and others, assists in the recall of memories, and facilitates temporal sequencing of events (Roth, 1999).

Natural environments such as gardens can have a positive therapeutic impact upon older people, their general health and their quality of life (Kaplan, 1973; Kaplan & Kaplan, 1990; Milligan et al., 2004). Gardening as an activity affords both passive and interactive stimulation; this may explain its current popularity as a therapeutic tool. There is a growing literature on the design of gardens for people with dementia (Pollock, 2001; Lovering, 1990; Lovering et al., 2002), on examining gardens within the context of outdoor activities (Cobley, 2002; Archibald, 1999), and on adapting activities in the garden for people with dementia (Kwack et al, 2005). Most difficulties encountered during gardening activities are related to sensory (visual, olfactory, tactile, auditory) impairment, mobility, access to the activity areas in the garden and ability to use tools or techniques. However, if such difficulties can be overcome, providing opportunities to be active in the garden can contribute towards improved self-confidence and social interaction, feelings of self worth, hopefulness, and enjoyment (Kwack et al., 2005).

Nature, Dementia and Home Environments

Design literature increasingly recognises and promotes the physical living environment as essentially therapeutic (Day et al., 2000; Teresi et al., 2000). Connection to nature is an aspect of an overall therapeutic approach which includes retaining links with the healthy and familiar, supporting functional ability through meaningful activity, providing natural light and plants indoors, and accessible outdoor spaces for planting, walking and sitting (Cohen & Weisman, 1991). Domestic, small scale, non-institutional or 'homely' environments 'in which therapeutic care can be delivered easily, efficiently and economically' (Phippen, 1998; p. 19) are therefore desirable in dementia care facilities. However such environments are often difficult to achieve. Residential care settings may be limited by health and safety regulations in areas such as furnishings and materials, eating food grown on site, water features and on keeping pets. By eliminating natural elements from daily life it is argued that care environments 'exclude people with dementia from the pleasurable sensory experiences most of us enjoy every day' (MacDonald, 2002).

Within the United Kingdom, approximately 80% of people with dementia continue to live within their own homes. Of these, a third is estimated to have severe dementia (Blackman et al., 2003). Home has been shown to have an increased importance to people as they age, with most people desiring to be supported in their own homes in the event of illness or infirmity (Sixsmith 1986; 1990; Blackman et al., 2003). Living at home has been shown to provide individuals with a sense of familiarity, privacy and control, a link to events in the past and continued membership within a local community (Sixsmith, 1990; Fogel, 1992). The concept of 'home' is a central concern of health and social care for older adults, as seen in current UK Department of Health policy, which encourages people to remain in their own homes for as long as possible (Department of Health, 2001). However, while providing opportunities for people to remain within their own homes can promote independence, such a policy may not support inclusion in society, as individuals may be unable to go outdoors to enjoy local amenities without assistance. The hesitancy of some participants to go outside is examined in recent research into use of outdoor environments conducted by Oxford Brookes University (Mitchell et al., 2004). The study found that people with dementia tend to have problems recognising and understanding where they are and remembering where they are going, compounded by normal aging factors such as frailty, sensory impairment, poor mobility and reduced strength and stamina. The research produced guidelines for dementia-friendly neighbourhoods. Likewise, dementia-friendly buildings can contribute to participation by allowing the person to operate at their best possible level cognitively while not adding to their impairments (Marshall et al., 2000).

QUALITATIVE STUDY OF USER NEEDS ANALYSIS

Settings

This stage of the project involved conducting qualitative interviews with people with dementia living either within their own homes or within residential care homes, as well as with family and professional carers. For the purposes of this study, living in a person's own home was defined as living either in privately owned or rented accommodation, or within sheltered housing.

Study participants were recruited through project partners involved in housing provision. Participants living in their own homes were located in a large town in the Midlands and a major city in the North West of England. Those either living in residential care homes or attending day centre in the care homes were recruited from a major city in the North of England. Those in the Midlands were currently receiving assistive technology devices as part of a project linked to the local county council providing these technologies (Frisby & Woolham, 2002). Individuals living within the North-West were recruited with the assistance of the local branch of the Alzheimer's Society.

Residential care homes in the UK are communal living environments for older people who are unable to remain living at home, but who are not in need of nursing care. They differ in size and configuration, depending on the building regulations and care standards in effect at the time, and can usefully be compared to assisted living in the USA. Within a care home a number of beds, often a 'wing' or 'corridor', may be designated EMI (elderly mentally infirm) for people with dementia or other mental health needs, for whom a higher level of care and security is provided. The two homes participating in the research were situated in urban working class neighbourhoods of a city in the North of England. They were built originally in the 1970s as local authority sheltered housing. Today they are 40 bedded care homes for people who are older and frailer than the building was original designed for, some with severe mobility limitations. Adaptations and upgrades to meet fire regulations resulted in compartmentalization of the corridors and stairwells. Facilitated in part by these changes plus a growing need for EMI beds, both homes now have at least one dementia care corridor for ten residents. A purposive sample was recruited from these corridors in each home.

Participants

The perspective of the person with dementia is often ignored in the research process when indeed, 'much can be gained from a systematic study' of their views regarding their illness and care(Cotrell and Schulz, 1993). Involving people in this way is a main priority of the research and the ethical protocols have been informed both by a growing body of literature (ASTRID, 2000; Cantley, 2001; Hughes, et al., 2002) and by ongoing consultation with project partner Dementia Voice.

To be included in this study, individuals must have received a diagnosis of dementia of any type. *Twenty six* people with dementia, *twenty three* informal carers, and *eighteen* service professionals were involved across the three study sites, forming a total sample size of sixty seven people. The sample was divided into two basic cohorts, those living in their own homes and those in residential care homes. Sixteen people with mild to severe dementia living at home were interviewed (N = 8 in the North-West, N = 8 in the Midlands); nine females and seven males. Four were living alone and twelve with an informal carer, usually a spouse. Informal carers also took part in the interview if people with dementia could not participate due to the severity of dementia, or where their presence was requested. This occurred in most cases (N = 15). In one case the husband and daughter of a person with severe dementia were interviewed in order to gain a proxy account. Interviews lasted from 15 minutes to two hours; written informed consent was sought from all individuals and was continually reaffirmed throughout the interview (Bartlett & Martin, 2002). Ten family carers and eight service providers also took part in four focus groups.

Within the two residential care homes a total of ten individuals with dementia were interviewed, three of whom were day centre clients living at home. Classification of the degree of dementia of the residents was taken from personal records, care plans, case worker knowledge and/or written reports of diagnoses from their general practitioner. Residents were experiencing mild to severe dementia and day centre clients were experiencing memory loss and confusion. Thirteen family carers and ten professional carers participated in focus groups, bringing the total study participants in residential care (or day care) to thirty-three.

Methods

Connection to nature is one aspect of a quality life. The INDEPENDENT Project investigated many aspects of life for the person with dementia in order to inform the design process in which the project team is now involved. The data presented in this paper represent a small part of the data collected during this first phase of the work. To determine if and how nature was important to people with dementia, semi-structured interviews and focus groups invited discussion on a range of activities people with dementia took part in and enjoyed, either currently or in the past, both from their own perspective and that of their carers. Further probes also investigated any difficulties individuals may have in participating in such activities, and the individualised meanings that may be derived from participation. Questions were broad and open-ended such as 'What do you (the resident) enjoy doing?' or 'What makes your mum (or the person you care for) happy?' All interviews were audio taped and subsequently transcribed. The transcript data were then analysed using a thematic analysis technique drawing upon the principles of grounded theory (Charmaz, 1995). This involved coding the transcript data for references to nature and the outdoors and then clustering the data relevant to the building and from the person's perspective. From the data, 'nature' was identified from dictionary definitions as elements of the earth that are living and animate (such as plants and animals), geographic (land, sea and sky) or solar and climatic such as rain, sun, stars, wind and snow. Connection to nature therefore can be achieved while indoors or outdoors since it involves sensory stimulation from, or interactive participation with, natural elements. Results are presented briefly in Tables 1A & 1B.

One important methodological difference between data gathered from people living in their own homes and those in residential care, was the use of extended observation. Such observation was not possible within private homes due to issues of privacy and intrusiveness. The use of written notes and photographs illuminated the many factors impacting a resident's ability and success in a range of activities. Such factors, once identified, informed the team's decision criteria for technological design possibilities and led to an understanding of the rich complexity of 'environment'. Clearly, an activity can be denied a person if any of a number of factors challenge rather than enable its success. Therefore, the data analysis process involved a template approach in which these various environmental factors were mapped against the set of activities identified as important by the participants.

FINDINGS

A wide range of activities contributing to wellbeing were enjoyed by people living either in dementia care environments or in their own homes. Of these activities, many involved nature and the outdoor environment. Tables 1A & 1B categorizes the activities; geographically by where they actually occurred (indoors, outdoors near the home, or outdoors while going somewhere); temporally by whether they occurred in the past and are being recollected or whether they are believed by the person to occur now (imaginary ongoing participation); and by whether they were done alone or socially. Tables 2A & 2B summarize factors enabling and/or challenging participation in nature related activities within both environments. Finally, Table 3 compares factors relating to the built environment, which may impact upon participation across the two settings.

DISCUSSION

Homes are complex environments. Both domestic environments and residential care settings may have distinct advantages depending upon the individual, the level of cognitive decline they are experiencing, and their particular care needs. Individuals living in their own home appeared to be more likely to enjoy nature and the outdoors, having more opportunities to go outside. These opportunities were contingent on the availability and willingness of informal carers to assist the person with accessing gardens and other outdoor spaces. Gardens and indoor spaces were also more likely to be arranged according to the particular preferences of an individual (e.g., decoration) or as a result of their particular care needs (e.g., adapting furniture or rooms). Gardens played an important part in their experience of nature, being the primary site in which they could experience and interact with natural stimuli.

TABLE 1A. Nature-related activities participated in by people with dementia LIVING IN THEIR OWN HOME

	Done alone	Done socially
Indoors	Counting cars Having a view out of window) observing nature, flowers, trees, birds being nosey, keep an eye out seeing/feeling the sunshine	Owning a pet Enjoying plants & animals
Going Outdoors	Gardening (digging, planting, potting plants, weeding) Enjoying the garden (looking at or sitting in the garden) 'Pottering' Feeling weather, sunshine, breeze Going for a walk	Garden: enjoying wildlife; watching the birds Physical: playing sport with grandchildren Visiting friends walking the dog Going for a walk having a party in the garden talking to neighbors
Going Somewhere	Going shopping Walking (for transport; recreation; or to & around the shops) Going to the pub	Attending day centre, community centre or church Being outdoors, going for walks Going on holiday/vacation Going to the shops, cinema, hairdressers Going to football matches Playing golf Going on day trips with carers Going to the pub Visiting local park, boating lake
Reminiscing	countryside, the outdoors, fishing	Working life holidays and travel Past places lived
Imagining	Playing golf Pottering in the garden	Going to golf clubs Going out with carer Travelling to other countries Playing football with grandchildren Going to church

TABLE 1B. Nature-related activities participated in by people with dementia LIVING IN RESIDENTIAL CARE

	Done alone	Done socially
Indoors	looking, watching out of the window having a view feeling weather, sunshine or a breeze bird / squirrel watching or listening keeping, touching or caring for pets	Handicrafts with leaves, flowers, pine cones, etc. Gardening, planting Reminiscing about going places, gardening, walks, or driving through the countryside
Outdoors	observing nature, flowers or trees sitting in the sunshine (done 'alone' meaning seated by themselves, not outside by themselves)	using an edge space (porch, balcony, doorway...) walking the dog going into town, shopping or the post office going for a walk going outside, going into the garden
Going Out	(none)	day trips, outings, local place of interest or farm meeting someone for a drink, coffee or meal going to the countryside going to the day centre; church
Reminiscing	keeping, touching or caring for pets walking the dog going to work Tidying or pottering in the garden gardening, potting plants or weeding	community gardening travelling abroad; flying; barge trip going dancing, tea dances, cinema, show, concert going for fish & chips, ice cream cone going on honeymoon talking to the neighbours, locals, shop keepers going to the countryside; going to a football game going out with friends; riding the bus or tram visiting a family member's house or grave going on holiday, to the seaside
Imagining	Tidying or pottering in the garden gardening, potting plants or weeding observing nature, flowers or trees walking	Swimming going to the park, common, or bowling green going for a walk fishing

TABLE 2A. Factors enabling or challenging participation in nature-related activities
LIVING IN THEIR OWN HOME

	ENABLING	CHALLENGING
Personal	Being in good physical health Being mobile, Being able to use tools or equipment, being dextrous. PwD retaining their own interests and desires e.g. seeking out gardens: Desire to get out and about on own, go to particular places, see particular people Desire to take part in exercise Preventing social isolation & loneliness	Being in poor physical health Having difficulty with walking; being unable to walk Having difficulty with accessing transport Having no interest in going outside. Needing to be motivated or coerced into going outside Wanting to stay at home all the time Losing any tools/equipment needed to do things outside (e.g. gardening) Lessened ability/desire to be active Having difficulty with using tools/equipment e.g. in garden. Forgetting about having gone outside recently. Forgetting about going out. Becoming lost outside, having difficulty with way finding. Depression & sadness Fear of falling

Formal Care	Assistance in home from professional carers.
	Assistance in home from family - informal carers
	Support from day centre as a place for PwD to go to.
	Providing motivation & encouragement
	Respite services as providing a break;
	   providing a change of scenery/holiday for PwD.
	   providing a break from care duties for informal carers.
	Professional carers acting as friends of PwD –involving person in activities in house, garden, outside.
	Providing choice & control
	Accepting levels of participation
		Demands on professional and informal carers time
		Limited availability of formal support from care providers
		Negative perceptions of formal support & formal care agencies.
		Unwillingness amongst some carers to use respite services
		Worry about PwD becoming lost or separated from carers when outside

Social network	Having a strong network of friends & family
	Providing accompaniment for PwD:
	   make PwD feel more secure and safer
	Car ownership amongst relatives:
	   able to take people on longer distances
	Ability to use public transport e.g. buses, either accompanied or unaccompanied
	Contacts within local community:
	   providing assistance and support in local area.
	   maintain position and standing within local area
	Stimulation from contact with friends/family.
		Unwillingness amongst some cares to go on trips:
		   difficulties in organising going out,
		   forgetting about trips shortly after they ended.
		Poor access to public/private transport
		Declining social network and relationships
		Difficulties with walking and mobility
		PwD may be unwilling, unable of fearful of going outside
		Forgetting about friends or relatives
		   forgetting about taking part in events with friends

Cultural & Spiritual	Stimulation from contact with friends/family
	   Setting of events e.g. in garden
	Enjoyment from contact with animals and pets
	   Passive – watching birds through window
	   Active – playing with a pet.
	Stimulation of conversation from contact with animals
	Contact with plants, flowers and appreciation of beauty
		Persons reactions to presence of animals or pets
		   May be negative due to severity of dementia
		Inability to cope with events or surroundings

Amongst those living in residential care, access to nature was restricted by frequency of family visits and by the time and resource demands placed upon care workers. Health and safety regulations and risks of physical harm, falling or walking away from the home were cited and perceived by carers to impose the greatest constraint on connection to nature for residents. Building configuration also influenced access to nature in both environments. The orientation of rooms within a building and their subsequent use may influence interaction (e.g., whether a window faces onto a garden or the street). Similarly, configuration of furniture may restrict viewing possibilities or may have an aspect conducive to feeling a breeze or the sunshine. Access through doorways to the

TABLE 2B. Factors enabling or challenging participation in nature-related activities
LIVING IN RESIDENTIAL CARE

	ENABLING	CHALLENGING
Personal	Memory – remembering they used to enjoy doing something long ago, remembering the answer to a question boosts self confidence and reinforces desire to participate; Physical – strength & agility, dexterity in hands; Sensory abilities – hearing, seeing; Automatic responses are still possible Use of walking frame, wheelchair; may still read but may not comprehend written words; Think they are younger than they are; Enjoy doing fun things, laughing; May enjoy walking about often; If they enjoy socializing, nature activities involving other people will encourage them to participate; Giving opportunities for people to pay their way; May respond positively later to a rejected suggestion due to changes in mood.	Forgetting they enjoy something; getting bored and/or losing concentration with an activity and stopping it. Forgetting to need or how to do something; Inability to initiate; perceived 'lack of initiative' Boredom – not remembering what they do and so thinking they do nothing may lessen desire or undermine self confidence that they are able Thinking they won't like doing something and resist doing it; Don't like to go too far away Physical disability, frailty, sensing the cold, pain, fatigue, Sensory disability – deafness or blindness Depression and sadness, teariness Unsettled, wants to 'get back' Fear of falling; Feeling distances are too far for them to walk wayfinding - may not know left from right, understand directions, recall the way back home;
Formal Care	Carers recognized from daily contact & providing encouragement; Allowing the person to keep a pet, have a bird feeder outside their window; Carer interests in person; what the person was like and what their passions used to be; Allow outdoor tasks such as sweeping, serving and tidying up; provide time & space for 'pottering'	Not enough activities scheduled or happening
Social network	Choice & feeling of care home – building feels full of light & fresh air Connection to local neighbourhood Visits from friends/family Bringing flowers and plants Taking PwD to visit their own garden Having somebody to go out with Visitors providing contact to residents other than own family/friends;	Memory – if they don't remember doing things (trip, activity), did they (will they) benefit? Family disappointment if they put on a special event and the person forgets it, doesn't even recognize themselves in photos afterwards; Not wanting to go outside: 'They just want to be inside, warm and safe'
Both formal and social care	Insisting they participate if known PwD enjoys activity Going along with 'their rules' if playing a game Providing transport Taking them for a walk outside Offering choices to the person Providing encouragement Providing prompting and reminders Accepting participation 'at a certain level' Encouraging discussion about past enjoyed activities Having correct information about dementia informs actions and efforts; Giving person choice and control;	Professional carers lacking time & resources needed to take people outside
Cultural & Spiritual	Activities that are gender and age appropriate; Familiar and recognizable activities Peer support for traditions & values 'Time frame identity' (how old they think they are) affects participation in activities	Through stigma of dementia or on advice from psychiatrist, the person is not allowed to 'live in the past' - if they talk about activities they can no longer do as if they are still doing them, they are 'pulled back into the present';

outside may also be restricted (e.g., by a perceived step or decline in gradient caused by different coloured surfacing).

As noted, most people with dementia also have other health complaints. This was true for people living in both settings. Problems with walking and mobility had the most serious impact upon access to the natural environment and were often viewed as being more detrimental to well-being than the dementia itself. Initiative and concentration also affected ability to access nature. Although many were willing to engage with nature of their own volition, several required encouragement and cajoling before engaging with an activity

TABLE 3. Built environment factors impacting participation in nature-related activities by people with dementia: A cross-setting comparison

	LIVING IN THEIR OWN HOME	LIVING IN RESIDENTIAL CARE
Indoors	View of outside from the window – garden environment or roadside view, rural or urban settings. Types and layout of furniture in room Layout & use of room in home (e.g. as living room, bedroom) Adaptations made to home – equipment (lounge chair, handles) Adaptations made to home through spatial changes in rooms (e.g. downstairs bedroom, inclusion of 'treatment' room) may change how house is used and subsequent access. Decorations in room, potted plants, pictures & paintings etc.	Seating & standing space near windows Moveable seating - can pull near to a door Views out - people, cars, community, action Doors the person can open to the outside An outside area meant for residents to use Windows that are opened routinely with multiple adjustable panes; Automatic door openers Rooms and spaces specific to activities help reinforce meaning and prompt participation; Presence of natural materials, living things
Outdoors	Access to the garden via edge spaces in home Layout & design of garden e.g. steps in garden, pathways through/around garden. Height of flower beds. Furniture/tools in garden Access to tools in garden. Boundaries to garden Protection from elements. View of garden from home – via windows. Proximity to neighbours Access to common spaces in local area Wheelchair access to home	Access to the toilet Microclimates create sunny places, protect from cold, wind Proximity to neighbours - talking over the fence develops relationship, communication Locked, blocked doors Something nearby outside to walk to Wheelchair access to garden areas Visibility from indoors of outdoor areas Secure perimeters of outdoor spaces Ground floor, level access to outdoors Seating of different sizes, materials & types Tables, umbrellas, small tables to put things on Planters & pots, trellis, arbor, greenhouse
Going Out	Existence of and proximity to local places nearby Environment enables wayfinding, provides ways to return safely if person becomes separated from carer Local area – rural or urban. Implications for PwD and carers/relatives if PwD goes outside alone	Existence of local places nearby, fabric of the neighbourhood - farm, river, park, field? Problems with continence, transferring & travel sickness; Transportation is difficult for family to manage (telling Dad to stand still while I go and park the car) Person becomes agitated, needs to get back to the home

from which subsequent enjoyment was gained. Thus, ensuring access to nature in terms of improving well-being may require more flexible approaches in which the first answer a person gives may not truly reflect their needs and desires (Wells, 2004).

For most individuals living in residential care, daily physical access to nature was limited to the amount of time spent in various rooms in the home, programmed use of accessible and comfortable outdoor spaces, building location and occasional trips away from the home. Interestingly, some people perceived their access to nature differently, as well as reminiscing about outdoor activities some believed they still participated, despite declining ability and limited opportunity. When asked, 'Do you go outside?,' the response was often 'yes,' although the reality was 'no'. When asked, 'Do you want to go outside?,' they normally declined, expecting they would be cold.

One advantage of the residential home buildings themselves over private homes relates to the size, configuration and placement of the building on the site. Both of the residential homes in this study are set back from the property lines and are surrounded by open space. Daylight comes into the EMI corridors from all directions, illuminating different rooms at different times of day.

A person moving through the rooms can orient themselves according to time of day and season of the year based on sun angle in the sky and quality of the light visible from views out of the building (Torrington, 2004).

An inter-relationship between formal and social support was identified that may enable or hinder access to nature. Within residential care both social and professional carers could and did enable activities, often liaising with each other to ensure participation. Amongst people living in their own homes, relatives acted to meet care needs both in providing for instrumental activities of daily living (IADL's) and through providing social support by enabling activities that may promote enjoyment. Professional carers also provided important social support such as communication and friendship for the person with dementia.

The study found that imagined participation in an activity both amongst care home residents and amongst people living in their own homes can play a role in their well-being. This raises ethical concerns. Clearly, imagined participation in something such as golf lacks the benefits of actual participation (i.e., fresh air, physical exercise and contact with real nature) and is no substitute. Neither do the authors support the position that people with dementia should be lied to by reinforcing misconceptions about actual participation in activities. Perhaps we can simply recognize the creative ability of the participants to enjoy themselves in the face of impairment by imagining they still do the things they love. Maintaining one's self identity and body image is a powerful antidote to depression in the face of serious illness from the natural abandonment of self (Shaver, 2002)

Some limitations of this study have been identified. Individuals within different types of housing provision were identified and approached. However, due to the design of the project and problems with access we were unable to reach individuals living either in extra-care or sheltered housing, or people with more severe levels of dementia living in nursing homes. Therefore the experiences of two large cohorts of people with dementia, who may have very different experiences of nature, were omitted from this study. Secondly, as a result of differences in the levels of dementia amongst participants, their ability to take part in the research varied. Some individuals were unable to take part in an interview due to the severity of their dementia. In order to include their views, either observational methods were used, or proxy accounts were gained from professional or family carers. However this may not provide a true account of their 'voice'. Similarly, the sample size of people with dementia living within residential environments is smaller than that of people living within their own homes. This is offset to some degree by extended observation in the care homes of a total of twenty persons with dementia of varying degrees of severity.

CONCLUSIONS

People with dementia are people first, with their own interests, experiences and opinions. While such experiences may be transformed as a result of dementia, this does not preclude their existence, nor the benefit they can gain from being given the opportunity to participate in them. The natural environment was particularly powerful as an arena for these experiences, giving people with dementia the opportunity to be stimulated through increased sensory input, and to continue with pastimes they enjoyed.

Several key factors were identified in both settings which enable or challenge interaction and connection with nature. Those relating to the building included connections between the indoor and outdoor environment, architectural features such as windows and doors, building and room configuration, proximity to outdoor resources, proximity to natural scenery and habitat, climate, weather and views. Relating to social support, involvement from carers was in most cases the primary force for ensuring access and connection with nature. For people living at home, this included gaining access to nature and the outdoors through accompanied leisure activities and providing assistance with activities while outdoors. In the care homes, going outside was only accomplished if level access to a secure area was available and its use was programmed into the weekly routine. Personal factors concerned memory loss, personal preference, physical ability, bodily comfort, initiative, concentration and focus. Some carers were less willing to take part in activities due to the person forgetting the activity after it had happened. Thus, although the activity was enjoyed in the moment, carers questioned the benefit of something so easily forgotten, which impacted on their willingness to plan further trips or activities.

Providing opportunities to experience and actively engage with nature and the outdoor environment can be an important and possibly overlooked element of providing housing choices. The natural environment has been shown to have important therapeutic outcomes, it can provide a context for meaningful interactions between people with dementia and their carers, offering opportunities for individuals to engage with nature, and it can improve self-perceived well-being and quality of life (Pulsford, 1997; Lovering et al., 2002). However, many people with dementia, like many older people, have chronic, long-term and multiple conditions, including high levels of mental confusion and impaired sight and hearing, all of which place increasing restrictions on their activities (Froggatt, 2004) and increasing challenges on environmental design (Keen, 1989; Marshall, 1998; Valla & Harrington, 1998; Cohen-Mansfield & Werner, 1998). Access to nature in itself is not always positive as older people experience discomfort from glare, draughts and cold. People with dementia are especially vulnerable as they are less able to modify their environment. Therefore, access to the natural world and participation in nature-related activities benefit a person with dementia to the extent that their real needs are understood and addressed.

This research provides further support to the growing work which includes people with dementia within research, and of the valuable role they can actively play within research into their illness (Gibson, 2004). Further research is required to examine the potential of nature and the natural environment to enhance their well-being. Through listening to people with dementia, and through understanding the ways they desire to interact with nature, we can continue to develop strategies to integrate within housing this fundamental part of our life.

REFERENCES

ASTRID (2000). *ASTRID: A guide to using technology within dementia care.*

Archibald, C., Murphy, C., Stevenson, L. & Allan, K. (1999). *Activities and people with dementia: Involving family carers.* Stirling, Dementia Services Development Centre, University of Stirling.

Bartlett, H. & Martin, W. (2002) Ethical Issues in Dementia Care Research. In Wilkinson H. (ed) (2002) *The Perspectives of People with Dementia: Research methods and Motivations.* London: Jessica Kingsley.

Baun, M.M & McCabe, B.W. (2003) Companion Animals and Persons with Dementia of the Alzheimer's Type. *American Behavioural Scientist.* 47. (1) 42-51. DOI: 10.1177/0002764203255211.

Blackman, T., Mitchell, L, Burton, E., Jenks, M, Parsons, M., Raman, S., Williams, K. (2003) The accessibility of Public Spaces for People with Dementia: new priority for the 'open city'. *Disability and Society* 18 (3) 357-371. DOI: 10.1080/0968759032000052914.

Burns, A., Byrne, J. Ballard, C., Holmes, C. (2002). "Sensory Stimulation in Dementia." *British Medical Journal* 325: 1312-3. DOI: 10.1136/bmj.325.7376.1312.

Cantley, C. (2001). *A handbook of dementia care.* Buckingham, Open University Press.

Charmaz, K. (1995). Grounded theory. Smith, J.A., Harre, R., Langenhove, L.V. (Eds.) *Rethinking Methods in Psychology* (pp. 27-49). London: Sage.

Cobley, M. (2002). "Using outdoor spaces for people with dementia–a carer's perspective." *Working with older people* 6 (2): 23-30.

Cohen, U., Weisman, G. D. (1991). *Holding on to home: Designing environments for people with dementia.* Baltimore, Johns Hopkins University Press.

Cohen-Mansfield, J., Werner, P (1998) The effects of an enhanced environment on nursing home residents who pace. *The Gerontologist.* 38. 199-208.

Cotrell, V. Schulz, R. (1993). "The perspective of the patient with Alzheimer's disease: A neglected dimension of dementia research." *The Gerontologist* 33(2): 205-211.

Day, K., Cohen, U. (2000). "The role of culture in designing environments for people with dementia: A study of Russian Jewish immigrants." *Environment & Behavior* 32(3): 361-399. DOI: 10.1177/00139160021972577.

Day, K., Carreon, D., Stump, C. (2000). "The therapeutic design of environments for people with dementia: A review of the empirical research." *The Gerontologist* 40 (4): 397-416.

Department of Health (2001) *National Service Framework for Older People*. London: Department of Health.

Fogel (1992) Psychological aspects of staying at home. *Generations: Journal of the American Society on aging*. 16, 15-20.

Frisby, B., Woolham, J. (2002) *Safe at Home–Using Technology to Support People with Dementia in their own homes in Northamptonshire*. Northampton: Northamptonshire County Council Social Services.

Gibson, G., Timlin, A., Curran, S., Wattis, J. (2004) The scope for qualitative methods in research and clinical trials in dementia. *Age and Ageing*. 33 (4) 422-426. DOI: 10.1093/ageing/afh136

Hope, K. (1997). "Using multi-sensory environments with older people with dementia." *Journal of Advanced Nursing* 25: 780-785. DOI: 10.1046/j.1365-2648.1997. 1997025780.x

Hope, K., Waterman., H. (2004). "Using Multi-Sensory Environments (MSEs) with people with dementia: Factors impeding their use as perceived by clinical staff." *Dementia* 3(1): 45-68. DOI: 10.1177/1471301204039324

Hughes, J. C., Hope, T. Savulescu, J., Ziebland, S. (2002). "Carers, ethics and dementia: A survey and review of the literature." *International Journal of Geriatric Psychiatry* 17(1): 35-40. DOI: 10.1002/gps.515

Kaplan, R. (1973) Some psychological benefits of gardening. *Environment and Behaviour*. 5. (2) 145-162.

Kaplan R., Kaplan. S., (1990) Restorative experience: the healing power of nearby nature. In Francis M, Hester, R.T. (1990) *The meaning of gardens*. Cambridge: MIT Press.

Keen, J. (1989) Interiors: Architecture in the lives of people with dementia In *International Journal of Geriatric Psychiatry* 4. 255-272. DOI: 10.1002/gps.930040504.

Kitwood, T. (1997) *Dementia Reconsidered: The person comes first*. Buckingham: Open University Press.

Kwack, H., Relf. P. D., Rudolph, J. (2005). "Adapting Garden Activities for Overcoming Difficulties of Individuals with Dementia and Physical Limitations." *Activities, Adaptation & Aging* 29(1): 1-13.

Lindenmuth, G. F., Moose, B. (1990). "Improving cognitive abilities of elderly Alzheimer's patients with intense exercise therapy." *The American Journal of Alzheimer's Care and Related Disorders and Research* 5(1): 31-33.

Lovering, M. J. (1990). "Alzheimer's disease and outdoor space: Issues in environmental design." *The American Journal of Alzheimer's Care and Related Disorders and Research* 5(3): 33-40.

Lovering, M.J., Cott, C.A. Wells, D.L. Schleifer-Taylor, J., Wells, L.M. (2002) A study of a secure garden in the care of people with Alzheimer's Disease. *Canadian Journal on Aging/ La revue canadienne du viellissement*. 21(3) 417-427.

MacDonald, C. (2002). "Back to the real sensory world our 'care' has taken away." *Journal of Dementia Care:* 10 (1) 33-36.

Marshall, M. (1998) Therapeutic buildings for people with dementia. In Judd, S., Marshall, M., & Phippen, P. (1998) *Design for Dementia.* London: Journal of Dementia Care.

Marshall, M., Stewart, S., Page, A., Laurie, C. (eds.) (2000). *Just another disability, making design dementia friendly: A strategic brief and audit tool for houses and flats for people with dementia.* Glasgow.

Milligan, C., Gatrell, T., Bingley, A. (2004) 'Cultivating Health': Therapeutic landscapes and older people in Northern England, *Social Science and Medicine,* 58, 1781-1793. DOI:10.1016/S0277-9536(03)00397-6

Mitchell, L., Burton, E., Raman, S. (2004). *Neighbourhoods for Life.* Oxford, Oxford Centre for Sustainable Development, Department of Architecture, School of the Built Environment, Oxford Brookes University.

Phippen, P. (1998). Interpreting 'home', the architect's dilemna. Design for Dementia. In Judd, S., Marshall, M., Phippen, P. (eds) (1998) *Design for Dementia* London, Journal of Dementia Care.

Pinkney, L. (1994). Snoezelen–an evaluation of an environment used by people who are elderly and confused. In Hutchinson, R. & Kewin, J.. *Sensations and Disability: Sensory Environments for Leisure, Snoezelen, Education and Therapy.* Chesterfield, Rompa: pp 172-183.

Pollock, A. (2001). *Designing gardens for people with dementia.* Stirling, Dementia Services Development Centre.

Pulsford, D. (1997) Therapeutic Activities for people with dementia–what, why . . . and why not? *Journal of Advanced Nursing* 26, 704-709.

Richeson, N. E. (2003). "Effects of animal-assisted therapy on agitated behaviors and social interactions of older adults with dementia." *Am J Alzheimers Dis Other Demen.* 18(6): 353-8.

Roth, J. (2000), Pet therapy Uses with Geriatric Adults, *International Journal of Psychosocial Rehabilitation,* 4, 27-39.

Shaver, W.A. (2002). "Suffering and the Role of Abandonment of Self at End of Life". A poster presented at the 14th International Congress on Care of the Terminally Ill, Montreal, Canada, October 5-10, 2002.

Sixsmith A.J. (1986) Independence and home in later life. In Phillipson, C., Bernard, M., Strang, P. (1986) *Dependency and interdependency in old age–theoretical perspectives and policy alternatives* Croom Helm: British Society of Gerontology.

Sixsmith A.J. (1990) The meaning and experience of 'home' in later life. In Bytheway, W.R., Johnson, J. (1990) *Welfare and the ageing experience.* Aldershot: Avebury.

Teresi, J.A., Holmes, D., Ory. M.G. (2000). "The therapeutic design of environments for people with dementia: Further reflections and recent findings from the National Institute on Aging collaborative studies of Dementia Special Care Units." *The Gerontologist* 40(4): 417-421.

Torrington, J. (2004). *Upgrading buildings for older people.* London, RIBA Enterprises.

Valla, P., Harrington, T. (1998) Designing for older people with cognitive and affective disorders *Archives of Gerontology and Geriatrics* Suppl. 6 515-518. DOI 0167-4943/98.

Wareing, L-A., Baker, R., Bell, S., Baker, E., Gibson, S., Holloway, J., Pearce, R., Dowling, Z., Thomas, P., Assey, J. (2001). "A randomized controlled trial of the effects of multi-sensory stimulation (MSS) for people with dementia." *British Journal of Clinical Psychology* 40 (1) 81-96.

Wells, S. (2004) Edith's weekend away: Issues for advocates in dementia care. In *Journal of Dementia Care.* 12 (4) 18-20.

doi:10.1300/J081v21n01_04

Restorative Dementia Gardens:
Exploring How Design
May Ameliorate Attention Fatigue

Keith Diaz Moore

SUMMARY. Recent neuropsychological research suggests that attention function has significant predictive value in diagnosing dementia in the preclinical phase. Given this ongoing, and presumably progressively declining function in people with dementia, it makes sense to more fully understand the ways in which natural settings may restore attentional capacity. This article explores the design implications of Kaplan's Attention Restoration Theory (ART) for restorative gardens aimed to serve those with dementia. It does so by engaging in an interpretive exploration of a qualitative data set regarding expert commentary on a set of gardens nominated for their design quality and responsiveness. The interpretation attempts to connect the design concepts identified by the expert panel with the four properties of restorative environments cited in the Attention Restoration Theory, thereby making theoretical connections for consideration in the design and subsequent evaluation of such places. doi:10.1300/J081v21n01_05 *[Article copies available for a fee from The Haworth Document Delivery Service: 1-800-HAWORTH. E-mail address: <docdelivery@haworthpress.com> Website: <http://www.HaworthPress.com> © 2007 by The Haworth Press, Inc. All rights reserved.]*

Keith Diaz Moore, PhD, AIA is Associate Professor of Architecture, School of Architecture and Urban Planning, University of Kansas.

[Haworth co-indexing entry note]: "Restorative Dementia Gardens: Exploring How Design May Ameliorate Attention Fatigue." Diaz Moore, Keith. Co-published simultaneously in *Journal of Housing for the Elderly* (The Haworth Press, Inc.) Vol. 21, No. 1/2, 2007, pp. 73-88; and: *Outdoor Environments for People with Dementia* (ed: Susan Rodiek and Benyamin Schwarz) The Haworth Press, Inc., 2007, pp. 73-88. Single or multiple copies of this article are available for a fee from The Haworth Document Delivery Service [1-800-HAWORTH, 9:00 a.m. - 5:00 p.m. (EST). E-mail address: docdelivery@haworthpress.com].

KEYWORDS. Healing gardens, dementia, Alzheimer's, design, directed attention, fatigue

The connection between nature and healing is not a new idea. Certainly one can look back at least as far as the monastic cloister gardens of the twelfth through fourteenth centuries where herbs, daylight, fresh air and reflection were the prescribed regimen for healing. The Ancient Greek Asklepion was a place of healing organized along an east-west axis with full exposure to the southern sun and a courtyard that sat to the south. Again, themes of daylight, air, and direct connection with nature are found. While not a new found relationship, over time, the Western approach to healing became reliant on more technical approaches which proved highly successful in addressing acute conditions. However, chronic health issues have proven more difficult to address as often the issue is not cure but rather care.

In our aging society, a particularly vexing chronic condition is that of dementia. Dementia is a syndrome characterized by progressive decline in mental functioning that may have numerous causes including degenerative diseases such as Alzheimer Disease and Parkinson's, vascular constriction, head trauma and infectious diseases such as AIDS and Creutzfeldt-Jakob disease. The syndrome is characterized by compromised functioning in domains such as language, memory, visual or spatial abilities, or judgment severe enough to interfere with daily life. However, the disease is highly idiosyncratic with manifestations and trajectories varying from person to person. The most common form of dementia is Dementia of the Alzheimer's type (DAT), with the Alzheimer's Association (2006) estimating that approximately 4.5 million Americans currently have DAT, with a projection for as many as 16 million people by 2050. While recent research indicates a link between particular genes and Alzheimer Disease, currently, in about 90% of cases, no genetic link is found (Alzheimer's Association, 2006). Diagnosis remains based upon observable manifestations with typical warning signs being memory loss, difficulty with routine tasks, disorientation to time and place and misplacing items.

Often design responses stem from a desire to respond to these manifestations. Gardens that utilize familiar backyard plants are thought to be more recognizable, potentially cuing memory. Continuous looping paths are thought to allow wandering or exploring behavior in a safe and secure manner. Zeisel and Tyson (1999) discuss numerous such design suggestions for gardens serving those with dementia.

Yet recent neurological research reflects growing interest in attempting to identify those cognitive functions that seem most likely to precipitate the development of Dementia of the Alzheimer's Type. Two functions of particular interest are that of executive function and attention. Executive function is what controls the execution of complex, goal-directed activities. If a task requires numerous acts be taken in particular sequence in order for success, executive function orchestrates that sequencing. When executive function is compromised one may witness manifestations of forgetfulness, disorientation and agitation. Attention, on the other hand, is the cognitive ability to focus; to suppress extraneous stimuli and attend to that stimuli which is directly related to the task at hand. Classic dementia manifestations such as short attention spans, distractibility and impulsivity suggest on-going attentional impairment.

In an important finding from the Berlin Aging Study, Rapp and Reischies (2005) found that both attention and executive function tests have significant predictive value in diagnosing DAT in the preclinical phase of Alzheimer Disease. There is growing suspicion that these cognitive abilities may be the first to be compromised on the progressively declining glide path that characterizes the dementia experience. However, these two functions are not distinct nor hierarchically equivalent. Directed attention theoretically supports executive functioning (Lezak, 1982; Perry & Hodges, 1999), and therefore if directed attention is compromised, so too will executive function. Chiu, Algase, Whall and colleagues (2004) have conducted the only environment-related study that has explored the relationship between directed attention and behavioral outcomes, reporting that among people with dementia, "getting lost behavior" (GLB) in both familiar and unfamiliar environments was significantly predicted by the attentional impairments described above.

ATTENTION RESTORATION THEORY

While cursory, the growing interest in the role of directed attention in the manifestations that characterize the dementia experience provide an interesting theoretical connection for those interested in therapeutic gardens that serve this population. The reason for this is that directed attention is a key concept within the Attention Restoration Theory of Stephen Kaplan (1995). While stress reduction is an oft-cited goal of therapeutic or restorative gardens (c.f. Ulrich, 1999), Kaplan (1995:178) makes the important observation that "insufficient attentional resources will often be an antecedent of stress." Thus if one were able to support or restore such resources, the resulting stress would be ameliorated or, perhaps if such resources were replenished in time, may not even occur.

Chiu and colleagues (2004: 175) describe directed attention as a "global inhibitory mechanism which is under voluntary control and functions to suppress distraction." Directed attention is essential to selection and inhibition in perception, thought and action. However, directed attention requires effort and therefore is susceptible to fatigue. As is known from studies on sleep and performance, fatigue of directed attention explains much human error and ineffectiveness (Parasuraman, 1990). Momentary lapses, such as when behind the wheel of an automobile, may have dire consequences.

If we accept that directed attention is as critical to executive functioning and human performance, in general, as described above, maintenance of this cognitive mechanism is essential. Yet the increasing interest in attention and executive functioning in people with DAT is due to the fact that both functions are compromised early in this degenerative process. This is particularly true for the selection and command, or inhibition, dimensions of directed attention (Sieroff & Piquard, 2004). Discovering interventions that restore fatigued directed attention has particular salience within this context.

A significant body of research provides evidence that natural settings appear to provide a means for restoring attentional capacity; hence, the use of the phrase "restorative environments" (Hartig, Mang & Evans, 1991; Herzog, Maguire & Nebel, 2003; Tennessen & Cimprich, 1995). Kaplan's Attention Restoration Theory, for which the above studies provide empirical support, suggests that there are four conceptual properties associated with the experience of these environments that make them restorative: being away, fascination, extent, and compatibility. These four properties are defined by Kaplan (2001: 482) as follows:

> Being Away: being distinct, either physically or conceptually, from the everyday environment; Fascination: containing patterns that hold one's attention effortlessly; Extent: having scope and coherence that allow one to remain engaged; and Compatibility: fitting with and supporting what one wants or is inclined to do.

This chapter engages in an interpretive exploration for the presence of these four properties in a set of therapeutic gardens designed for people with dementia that an expert panel has nominated for consideration as exemplary. This research is an outgrowth of an effort spearheaded by the Acer Institute to identify a set of exemplary gardens designed for people experiencing dementia so as to inform better design and therapy practice. While it is too early in the process to identify the discussed gardens as exemplary, the case studies do provide a rich data set with which to engage in a meaningful content analysis as is done here. It is the hope of this chapter to raise the awareness of Attention Restoration Theory and its potential implications for designing garden environments and horticultural therapies for people experiencing dementia.

THE EXEMPLARY DEMENTIA GARDEN PROJECT

In 2005, the Acer Institute, in conjunction with Legacy Good Samaritan Hospital in Portland, Oregon, convened a one day symposium that aimed to build a knowledge community and knowledge base that would inform the development of "standards of practice for therapeutic gardens" (Acer Symposium, 2005). Participants ranged from designers to horticultural therapists to medical doctors to social workers. One of the concepts discussed was the need for moving the knowledge base beyond the anecdotal and subjective toward the objective. In between these two conditions is the consensual realm, which as described by Lawton and colleagues (1997: 195), may be considered "a characteristic of the environment, based on the reasoning that the judgments of multiple individuals will converge on the actual properties of the environment." While the implementation of rigorous, multi-site objective studies utilizing psychometrically validated instruments has proven onerous (e.g., time consuming, lack of funding and resources) within the therapeutic garden domain, it was felt that a project that called upon recognized experts in the field to identify exemplary gardens through consensus would move the knowledge base of the field in a positive direction. Hence was born the Exemplary Dementia Garden Project.

Beginning with some attendees of the Acer Symposium who volunteered to participate, the expert panel enlarged through snowballing, where experts identified additional experts to be included. The panel is constituted of twelve recognized experts in the field.[1] Assuming that the experts collectively possessed the best repository of knowledge regarding these gardens, they were asked to nominate gardens they felt might be considered exemplary in how they serve people with dementia. Over two dozen gardens in the United States were nominated and at minimum seconded. Through a Delphi process, the expert panel then developed a survey protocol that asked not only for design information but information regarding use as well. This protocol was sent out to the appropriate individuals associated with the nominated designs, and a rich dataset was developed. It is this dataset that the following analysis engaged.

FIVE THERAPEUTIC DEMENTIA GARDENS

There are five nominated therapeutic gardens designed for people experiencing dementia that are the focus of this inquiry. They are: The Alzheimer's Association Memory Garden at Monroe County Hospital (Rochester, NY), Cathedral Village (Philadelphia, PA), Converse Home (Burlington, VT), Portland Memory Garden (Portland, OR), and Sedgewood Commons (Falmouth, ME).

Alzheimer's Association Memory Garden at Monroe County Hospital

This garden is 1.5 acres and serves a county hospital with 500 long-term beds and a 34-resident special care unit for people with dementia. This large site was divided into four areas, sequentially linked by a walking path. The design provides for a covered pavilion for outdoor activities and three gardens of differing character. The Garden of Valor has a brick paver compass bordered by rhododendron and shade gardens, the rose garden and benches and abuts the pavilion. The Garden of Peace is a large serpentine perennial garden and the Circle of Hope has a circular brick walkway circumscribing shade provided by a mature deciduous tree, bordered by familiar plantings and sitting areas.

Cathedral Village

This Garden serves both an assisted living as skilled nursing residence housing about 150 residents. It is designed with both a pergola and gazebo offering sheltered social space linked by a meandering looping path that takes the user past several planting areas, including an herb garden that triggers reminiscence, and variously configured sitting areas. The garden is a retrofit of an existing site that opened accessibility to the outdoors for residents and provided outdoor program space for an ambitious horticultural therapy program.

Converse Home

The garden at Converse Home serves the 50 assisted living residents by providing three distinct garden settings in a rather narrow area, left over after the architectural design (as is common in many such projects). This design maximizes the potential by creating a clear sense of oasis with a tall enclosing fence buffered by plantings of various sizes and foliage. The design is informed by an ambitious effort to actively program the space by Converse Home staff, providing a setting for social events (the Public Garden with tables and chairs), horticultural therapy (the Working Garden with a lawn, raised planters and workshed) and for contemplation (the Native Garden with rich foliage, shade trees, trellises and benches).

Portland Memory Garden

This garden is a public garden situated within a city park in Portland, Oregon. This garden provides a rich array of plants providing visual and olfactory stimulation and do so in a mix of ground level and raised planters. The raised planters are at a height appropriate for sitting, providing access as well as choice in seating locations. It maximizes the impact of the existing mature trees by using them as a sense of enclosure from the larger parker and the busy streets. The path has a clear sense of entry with a looping path that returns visitors back to the point of origination.

Sedgewood Commons

Sedgewood Commons is a 108-bed assisted living residence serving solely people with varying levels of dementia. This design is actually three gardens, each serving a different level of cognitive impairment. The Hawthorne garden is designed for those with mild impairment which provides a rich array of choice for engagement, ranging from a lawn court and basketball net to a clothesline and raised planting beds. The Longfellow garden serves those with mid-stage dementia and is based upon a cloister garden, providing a pergola that secures as well as orients attention to a central focal point. Plantings that provide rich sensory stimulation include rhododendrons, azaleas, lilacs, honeysuckle and roses. Finally, the Millay garden serves those with advanced dementia and is the most reflective and passive garden with a strong sense of enclosure, a gently, winding strolling loop and plantings that attract wildlife.[2]

RESTORATIVE PROPERTIES IN THERAPEUTIC DEMENTIA GARDENS

Having briefly introduced the five case studies that are the focus of this inquiry, this section analyzes the data gathered to date on these gardens in relation to the four restorative properties identified by Kaplan. The qualitative data reflect the concepts shared by the expert panel, although the specific comments may originate from not only expert panel members but the designers of the gardens as well as the administrator's of the gardens. The comments selected are those that best capture the spirit of the discussion that has taken place among the expert panel members to-date as reflected by an analysis conducted according to standard thematic analysis techniques (Denzin & Lincoln, 1998).[3]

Being Away

The comments that capture this concept of being distinct from the everyday environment are largely related to the notions of contrast and shelter or enclosure. Contrast is referenced in almost every case study with the garden recognized as contrasting with the assumed institutional character of indoor life within these various care facilities. The simple change in type and amount of stimulation that an outdoor environment provides in settings of congregate care help to create this sense of being distinct from the quotidian. The designer at the Monroe County Hospital discusses a desire for the garden to "provide a calming effect for those experiencing dementia," implicitly suggesting a distressing indoor environment. The Executive Director at Converse Home eloquently stated that "one comment we hear repeatedly is that the garden really feels like another world. It provides visual and spatial relief from the inside." This "other-worldliness" character of therapeutic gardens assists in creating a sense of being away.

So, too, does provision of enclosure. One expert wrote, "I am not sure people are attracted to gardens that are too open. Attention may be brought to elopement potential and/or a sense of security may be compromised." Another expert said that there were two essential criteria for any dementia garden, one being a closed boundary. Comments about most of these gardens spoke positively about those elements that created a sense of enclosure. One exception to this was Sedgewood Commons which was critiqued by one expert as providing too much visual access to the surrounding environment (in one garden using only a low fence for a boundary), losing its sense of oasis. At the Portland Memory Garden, two elements working together were assessed at creating a positive sense of enclosure and hence, of being away. Here, both a low enclosing wall as well as the presence of mature trees around the perimeter create a sense of the garden being bounded (see Figure 1). The designer for the Converse Home garden had a specific goal to "create an oasis within the given framework." This is created by crafting an elegantly-designed eight-foot high enclosing fence which is then buffered by dense vegetation which softens the effects of the fence. The way in which each distinct garden at Converse is surrounded by plantings creates a sense of threshold where the walking path pierces the plant growth. Threshold is an important concept related to the experience of differentiation, or being distinct.

Fascination

In many ways, natural environments are inherently fascinating by Kaplan's definition as natural settings are riddled with patterns, whether they be created by natural forces (wind, water, sun), seasonal change, or other dynamics intrinsic to the natural world. Within this discussion, at both the Portland Memory Garden and the Monroe Community Hospital, the use of *existing mature trees* was seen as a real benefit in this regard. The designer at the Monroe Community Hospital clearly identifies the desire to provide variation in shade, shadow and sun conditions and these are promoted by the presence of a mature canopy. An expert states that shade areas are an essential ingredient to any ex-

FIGURE 1. Enclosure is created by both a low wall as well as the inclusion of existing mature trees.

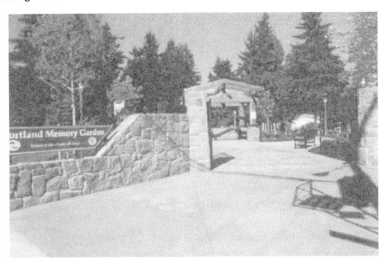

emplary dementia garden. The dynamic patterns created by sun and shadow create visual intrigue that hold an observer's attention rather effortlessly. Seasonal or climatic change is addressed in several designs in different ways. Again, at the Monroe Community Hospital, there is an intention to select and locate plants based upon their look and time of bloom, recognizing that this adds to fascinating variety. Sedgewood Commons carefully considered the serene beauty of a New England winter landscape by providing framed views from the interior that can be quite lovely whatever time of year (see Figure 2).

The expert discussion of Converse Home however, raises another characteristic of fascination and that is detail. One expert identifies the understanding this designer has for how a garden can absorb one's attention effortlessly by being constantly intrigued. In this garden, the detailing of a small bubble fountain, an ornamental grate for a necessary maintenance drain and other artfully executed details enrich the patterns of engagement to the finest grain. Other gardens may have executed this sense of detail as well, but it was Converse Home that highlighted this captivating concept related to fascination.

Extent

The property of extent may easily be confused with variety in stimulation, but the core of the concept goes beyond the richness in stimuli to demand also coherence in stimuli to the degree that the experience engages a substantial portion of one's mind. The expert comments focus on both sensory as well as

FIGURE 2. A restorative scene of an archetypal New England winter afforded by the garden design at Sedgewood Commons.

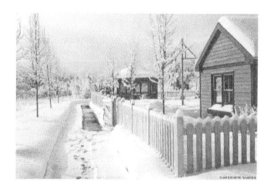

activity stimulation that these gardens foster, but the true focus seems to be on the haptic system which "involves the integration of many senses, such as touch, positional awareness, balance, sound, movement, and the memory of previous experiences" (O'Neill, 2001: 3). Comments in regard to both Monroe Community Hospital and Cathedral Village highlight the range of senses engaged by the garden design. The responding care professional from Monroe Community Hospital discusses the visual stimulation provided by the rich array of the flora palette, the olfactory stimulation of plants such as lilacs, and the auditory and tactile stimulation of rustling grasses. Aromatherapy is specifically referenced by the administrator of the Converse Home, but is implicit in comments regarding Cathedral Village as well. One expert stated that no other nominated garden provided the rich array of stimulation present at the Portland Memory Garden.

Sensory stimulation is perhaps the most immediately perceived attribute of therapeutic gardens, but research indicates that active engagement is very important to enhance the degree of therapeutic benefit of most psycho-social interventions. As such, the activity stimulation referenced in the expert comments is also a critical aspect for extent. At the Converse Home, the creation of distinct gardens, each with their own "personalities," with the provided resources matching that personality, was viewed as critical to several experts. One identified how such clear and coherent articulation of the purpose of each place assisted in those places serving as therapeutic mnemonics, cueing what is expected. Another identified how such differentiation no doubt in and of itself assists in orientation. Providing for a range of activity levels was also mentioned as important, so each individual might find an appropriate fit. This was mentioned in regard to Cathedral Village that provides both large and intimate social settings within the garden, but is perhaps exemplified at Sedgewood Commons with its provision of diverse activity options within each garden designed for a different level of impairment.

One final dimension that emerges from the expert commentary in regard to extent, is the importance of stimulation from other people. Without fail designers, care professionals and the experts all refer to the importance of the presence and engagement of other people. Several discuss the engagement of staff, family members (especially on weekends) and other residents as important drivers to facilitating sustained engagement with the natural setting. One must consider that self-initiation for people with dementia is often compromised and that dementia residents often follow, not lead. If there are a couple of residents able and interested to engage the garden on their own, others are likely to follow. In the larger picture however, this highlights the need for care organizations to recognize such gardens as alternative program spaces that demand programming in order to affect the restorative potential theorized by ART.

Extent demands both richness and coherence that here, it might be suggested, engages the holistic, experiential aspect of stimulation sensed by the haptic system (c.f. Bloomer & Moore, 1977). One horticultural therapist captures the essence of this restorative property when she responded, "The garden is a place that is stimulating to the senses with numerous planters containing colorful flowers which attract butterflies and hummingbirds . . . . It is a place to enjoy the dance of sunlight, the sound of birds singing and the movement of ornamental grasses in the breeze . . . .The garden gives the residents a destination, a pleasant experience".

Compatibility

This last property of restorative environments addresses both the issue of fit–of providing the necessary resources for what one wants to do–as well as with support–provision of what one needs. Beginning with what this user group needs, the data from these five cases provides a rich set of recommendations that are enumerated repeatedly. To organize these suggestions, it is useful to use the taxonomy of Diaz Moore and colleagues (2006) which discusses environmental interventions as involving physical components and sensory and spatial properties.

Physical Components. Several components are mentioned as essential in therapeutic gardens for people with dementia. Wide, level, non-glare paving was ubiquitously cited in the cases as was the provision of a range of sitting options, including movable chairs, chairs with tables, benches and sitting-height planter walls (e.g., Cathedral Village, Portland Memory Garden). Seating should be selected on the basis of the ergonomic needs of the aging body. Plants were discussed quite often with a seeming desire for gardens to have a high ratio of softscape to hardscape, with a great diversity of plants that are introduced to the garden in a variety of ways–planting beds on grade, raised beds, trees, hedges, trellises with vine and so forth. Paving, planters, benches and whatever else may be specified in the design should be easy to maintain with irrigation of planting beds a recurrent concern (e.g., Cathedral Village, Converse Home). The toilet provided in the Portland Memory Garden was hailed as very responsive to the issue of incontinence which is not uncommon to those with dementia.

Sensory Properties. In regard to the visual, both glare and contrast were significant issues to the experts. Regulating both is essential in the design of these gardens, although it appears there may be differences of opinion on how optimally to accomplish this. There was clearly appreciation for those designs (e.g., Monroe Community Hospital, Portland Memory Garden) that took advantage of existing mature trees to provide shade from the sun, thereby creating a diurnal drama of change in the garden. A great variety of visual attributes in the selected plantings is advocated, particularly when seasonal variations are clearly considered (e.g., Monroe Community Hospital).

The other senses are a bit more difficult to assess solely through documentary evidence, but the comments make clear that olfactory, tactile and auditory stimulation are considered as much as visual stimulation. Smells are discussed as particularly powerful for reminiscence (e.g., Cathedral Village, Converse Home) where highly scented flowers such as rhododendrons and herbs such as basil are utilized. Tactile engagement is thought to occur through therapeutic interaction with dirt and plants, but also brushing ornamental grasses, but is also considered in relation to the thermal delight offered by the sun, or for others, the shade.

Spatial Properties. While there is general consensus that dementia gardens should be simple in configuration and circulation, there is debate as to what simple is. Clearly there seems to be a preference for designs where one enters at a particular point and a main pathway leads one throughout the garden but returns to the point of origin without any dead ends or confusing choices (e.g., Converse Home). Choices in spatial qualities was also reinforced, although those choices should be clear, simple to make, and limited in number so as not to overwhelm. These choices should include places for social interaction as well as places for solitude; places for active participation, and places to be passive. These spatial properties should be executed with an understanding of the cultural heritage of the users and a responsiveness to climate. These conditions are well-exhibited in the Hawthorne Garden of Sedgewood Commons. There is also a desire for outdoor spaces to be at an intimate, human scale. Monroe Community Hospital goes to great lengths to discuss how the design is broken down from an overwhelming 1.5 acres into a series of distinct gardens linked by a path system (see Figure 3).

CONCLUSION

There is increasing interest in the role natural settings play in human health, to the point where some believe "that in the twenty-first century, the healing garden will be seen as an essential, intrinsic component of every healthcare setting" (Cooper Marcus & Barnes, 1999: 24). In order for this to become a reality however in our outcome-oriented world, increasing research needs to be conducted on how interaction with nature results in a set of positive outcomes. If this is peeled back, it is evident that greater theoretical understanding of the mediation between environment and observable outcomes is essential. Stress is the most common intermediating construct used in this area of research but remains a rather global construction demanding further refinement. Kaplan

FIGURE 3. Using plants to create a sense of enclosure and threshold help to create a meaningful series of transitions at the Monroe Community Hospital

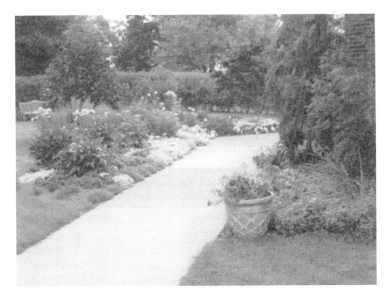

suggests that an important antecedent of stress is directed attentional fatigue. Literature reflects that attention and its relation executive function, are both compromised early in the dementia process and therefore it stands to reason that the resources these individuals have for attention are exhausted much more readily than for those without such cognitive impairment. Thus attention restoration and maintenance may play an important role in reducing some of the negative outcomes associated with stress in people experiencing dementia.

If this hypothesis is true, the salience of Kaplan's Attention Restoration Theory to the design of environments for people with dementia is self-evident. This paper explored the design implications that stem from the four properties of restorative environments identified by Kaplan: being away, fascination, extent and compatibility by engaging in content analysis of comments from experts, designers and administrators about garden designs nominated as potentially exemplary by a panel of experts in the field of therapeutic garden design for the cognitively-impaired. Being away is associated with the design concepts of design and enclosure with threshold being an important mediator. Fascination was found to be linked with the diurnal and seasonal changes found in natural environments as well as with the concept of detail. Extent was associated with sensorial, activity and interaction-related types of stimulation. When this stimulation arouses and engages the haptic system, suggesting an all-encompassing involvement of the senses, the property of extent is likely to be manifested. Compatibility is linked with a whole range of design components and properties including plants, paving, elements that engage the whole range of senses and spatial properties such as accessibility, simplicity and the provision of options.

Those design concepts identified with compatibility are those most typically used to inform the design of gardens for people with dementia as the issue of fit that underlies compatibility also is foundational to the typical user needs approach. What is interesting about examining ART, is the enriched sense one has of what such a garden should be like if indeed the intent is to restore attentional abilities. The importance of sustaining engagement with the garden becomes much more evident and may assist in hypothesizing why some gardens are thought to be more restorative than others.

This study should be viewed as a very early exploration of the implications ART has on the design of gardens for people with dementia. However, from it follow intriguing research questions. Can attention be restored in people with dementia as with the general population, and if so, to what degree? Is it possible to enhance their cognitive performance due to enhanced directed attention faculties due to engagement with such a garden? How does one conceptualize, operationalize and measure being away, fascination, extent and compatibility properties of the environment? Are all four properties equally as salient or is there a hierarchy of salience for restoring directed attention? If a garden measures well in regard to all four properties, does it perform better than the garden that measures best in compatibility?

If the intention is to design and advocate for gardens that enhance the well-being of people with dementia, it is necessary to articulate the hypothesized relationship as to how that is done. In applying Attention Restoration Theory, it is suggested that gardens designed to create the four properties of being away, fascination, extent and compatibility will assist those experiencing the garden to restore their attentional, and subsequently their executive functioning, capacities, thereby easing one antecedent of stress, namely attention fatigue. With stress thereby reduced, the various negative physical, psychological and behavioral manifestations of stress will be reduced and that many of these manifestations (e.g., agitation, anxiety) are commonly associated with the etiology of dementia. If this hypothesis were to hold, it would provide increased evidence for Gubrium's (1978: 28) observation that dementia is not solely etiological, but rather "who or what behavior is spoken of or recorded as senile depends on place.

NOTES

1. The author wishes to thank all 12 members of the expert panel who selflessly have shared their wisdom in therapeutic garden design for people with dementia: Elizabeth Brawley, Design Concepts; Margaret Calkins, IDEAS; Jack Carman, Design for Generations; Nancy Chambers, New York University; Nancy Chapman, Portland State University; Teresia Hazen, Legacy Health System; Rob Hoover, HBLA; David Kamp, Dirtworks; Annie Kirk, Acer Institute; Patrick Mooney, University of British Columbia; Martha Tyson, Design Consulting; and Joanne Westphal, Michigan State University.

2. Additional information on the design of this garden is available in Hoover, 1995.

3. Quotes utilized are from either the completed facility surveys or from the email dialogue between experts. This raw data is available from the author.

REFERENCES

Acer Symposium (2005). *Proceedings of the 2005 Acer Symposium.* June 17, 2005 in Portland, OR. Portland, OR: Acer Institute.

Alzheimer's Association (2006). Retrieved June 12, 2006 from www.alz.org

Bloomer, K. & Moore, C. (1977). *Body, memory and architecture.* New Haven, CT: Yale University Press.

Chiu, Y., Algase, D., Whall, A., Liang, J., Liu, H., Lin, K. & Wang, P. (2004). Getting lost: Directed attention and executive functions in early Alzheimer's Disease patients. *Dementia and Geriatric Cognitive Disorders, 17*(3): 174-180.

Cooper Marcus, C. & Barnes, M. (1999). *Healing gardens: Therapeutic benefits and design recommendations.* New York: Wiley.

Denzin, N. & Lincon, Y. (1998). *Collecting and interpreting qualitative materials.* Thousand Oaks, CA: Sage.

Diaz Moore, K., Geboy, L.D. & Weisman, G.D. (2006). *Designing a Better Day: Guidelines for adult and dementia day service centers.* Baltimore, MD: Johns Hopkins University Press.

Gubrium, J. (1978). Notes on the social organization of senility. *Urban Life, 7*(1), 23-44.

Hartig, T., Mang, M. & Evans, G. (1991). Restorative effects of natural environment experience. *Environment and Behavior, 23*(1), 3-26.

Herzog, T., Maguire, C. & Nebel, M. (2003). Assessing the restorative components of environments. *Journal of Environmental Psychology, 23*(2): 159-170.

Hoover, R. (1995). Healing gardens and Alzheimer's disease. *American Journal of Alzheimer's Care and Related Disorders and Research,* March/April, 1-9.

Kaplan, S. (1995). The restorative benefits of nature: Towards an integrative framework. *Journal of Environmental Psychology, 15:* 169-182.

Kaplan, S. (2001). Meditation, restoration, and the management of mental fatigue. *Environment and Behavior, 33*(4): 480-506.

Lawton, M. P., Weisman, G., Sloane, P. & Calkins, M. (1997). Assessing environments for older people with chronic illness. In J. Teresi et al. (Eds.), *Measurement in elderly chronic care populations.* New York: Springer.

Lezak, M. (1982). The problem of assessing executive functions. *International Journal of Psychology, 17:* 281-297.

O'Neill, M. (2001). Corporeal Experience: A Haptic Way of Knowing. *Journal of Architectural Education, 55*(1): 1-8.

Parasuraman, R. (1990). Event-related brain potentials and human factors research. In J.W. Rohrbaugh, R. Parasuraman & R. Johnson, Jr. (Eds.). Event-Related Brain Potentials (pp. 279-300). New York: Oxford University Press.

Perry, R. & Hodges, J. (1999). Attention and executive deficits in Alzheimer's disease: A critical review. *Brain: A Journal of Neurology, 122*(3): 383-404.

Rapp, M. & Reischies, F. (2005). Attention and Executive Control Predict Alzheimer Disease in Late Life: Results From the Berlin Aging Study (BASE). *American Journal of Geriatric Psychiatry, 13*(2): 134-141.

Sieroff, E. & Piquard, A. (2004). Attention and aging. *Psychologie & Neuropsychiatrie Du Viellisement (Psychology and Neuropsychiatry of Aging), 2*(4): 257-269.

Tennessen, C. & Cimprich, G. (1995). Views to nature: Effects on attention. *Journal of Environmental Psychology, 15:* 77-85.

Ulrich, R. (1999). Effects of gardens on health outcomes: Theory and Research. In C.C. Marcus, C.C. & M. Barnes (Eds.), *Healing gardens: Therapeutic benefits and design recommendations.* New York: Wiley.

Zeisel, J. & Tyson, M. (1999). Alzheimer's treatment gardens. In C.C. Marcus, C.C. & M. Barnes (Eds.), *Healing gardens: Therapeutic benefits and design recommendations.* New York: Wiley.

doi:10.1300/J081v21n01_05

The Garden-Use Model–
An Environmental Tool for Increasing
the Use of Outdoor Space by Residents
with Dementia in Long-Term Care Facilities

Charlotte F. Grant
Jean D. Wineman

SUMMARY. The Garden-Use Model is the result of a multi-case study involving five sites that was designed to develop a better understanding and holistic description of the interrelationship among organizational/ programming policies and spatial/physical attributes of the outdoor space in influencing how much this space was used by residents with dementia in long-term care facilities. The protocol replicated at each site involved an initial site analysis, distribution of staff questionnaires, and behavior observations for six days, including five weekdays and Saturday at every site but one. The results of the study discussed the alignment and findings based on descriptive analysis and collected data at each site regarding the following factors: organizational policy, staff attitudes, visual access, physical access and garden design.

This paper summarizes the results of the study related to the above

Charlotte F. Grant, PhD, is affiilated with MAKING PLANS–custom landscape design, Greensboro, GA.

Jean Wineman, DArch, is Professor, Taubman College of Architecture and Urban Planning, University of Michigan, Ann Arbor, MI.

[Haworth co-indexing entry note]: "The Garden-Use Model–An Environmental Tool for Increasing the Use of Outdoor Space By Residents with Dementia in Long-Term Care Facilities." Grant, Charlotte F. and Jean D. Wineman. Co-published simultaneously in *Journal of Housing for the Elderly* (The Haworth Press, Inc.) Vol. 21, No. 1/2, 2007, pp. 89-115; and: *Outdoor Environments for People with Dementia* (ed: Susan Rodiek and Benyamin Schwarz) The Haworth Press, Inc., 2007, pp. 89-115. Single or multiple copies of this article are available for a fee from The Haworth Document Delivery Service [1-800-HAWORTH. 9:00 a.m. - 5:00 p.m. (EST). E-mail address: docdelivery@haworthpress.com].

factors and use of available outdoor space. The ultimate focus and conclusion of the paper addresses findings and recommendations for designers, healthcare administrators and others interested in achieving optimal use of the outdoor space among residents with dementia in long-term care facilities. The theoretical framework diagrammed in the "Garden-Use Model" is based on data collected and rich description at each of the five sites that made up the study. This model is presented and serves as the structural basis from which discussion of the factors influencing use of outdoor space ensues. The Garden-use Model also serves in the paper as a tool for facilities that seek to increase garden use among residents and to offer a means for evaluation such facilities. *doi:10.1300/ J081v21n01_06 [Article copies available for a fee from The Haworth Document Delivery Service: 1-800-HAWORTH. E-mail address: <docdelivery@ haworthpress.com> Website: <http://www.HaworthPress.com> © 2007 by The Haworth Press, Inc. All rights reserved.]*

KEYWORDS. Dementia, environment, garden, long-term care, outdoor space

INTRODUCTION

In response to the increasing number of individuals diagnosed with Alzheimer's disease and related dementias in this country, designers, planners and caregivers are searching for effective environmental models designed to meet the needs of these individuals, improve their quality of life, and to create settings that foster dignity, a sense of independence and well-being (Day, Carreon & Stump, 2000; Zeisel et al., 2003). This response has been realized in part through the proliferation of special care units created to specifically address the needs of residents with dementia primarily through unique facility design and activity programming. Another aspect of this response has been the increased interest and incorporation of specially designed outdoor space associated with these long-term care facilities. This study addresses the latter setting–the garden–and offers a means to increase use of available outdoor space by residents in long-term care facilities.

This paper is based on a case study analysis of outdoor space use by residents with dementia in five long-term care facilities (Grant, 2003) and is founded on the assumption that it is beneficial for demented elderly individuals to spend time outside (Calkins, 1989; Cooper Marcus, 2005; Cooper Marcus & Barnes, 1999; Hiatt, 1988; Lovering, 1990; Zeisel & Tyson, 1999). In association with the Atlanta VA Rehab Research & Development Center

(Connell et al., 1998, 1999), we conducted several studies exploring the relationship between spending time outdoors and benefits to the long-term care residents with dementia. In fact, we found that in each facility few residents frequented available outdoor space. In every instance, we attributed our lack of significant findings to the residents' under-utilization of outdoor space–either independently or with staff. In response to the VA findings and to other studies that addressed the importance of "motivators" in promoting the use of outdoor space by Alzheimer's residents (Lovering, 1990), this study was designed to fill a need in the body of literature addressing use of outdoor space by this population. Our holistic approach has attempted to better understand and describe factors that interrelate to influence the amount of outdoor space use by individuals with dementia in long-term care facilities.

METHODS

A multi-case study design involving five different facilities was developed to gain a better understanding of the interrelationships among the factors influencing use of outdoor space by elderly residents with dementia in long-term care facilities. A research protocol was developed focusing on the following factors: organizational policy, staff attitudes, visual access, physical access and garden design. Our methodology involved an initial site analysis, distribution of staff questionnaires, and behavior observations for six days, including five weekdays and Saturday at four sites. At one site our observations were done on weekdays.

Three types of observations were developed to measure use of the outdoor space among the residents and were conducted by one of the authors from 9:00 am until 5:00 pm, with a break from 12:00–1:00 pm, during each study day. For the first type of observation (called "inside narrative"), the observer was positioned inside the facility near the door to outside space for one 20-minute segment each hour. These observations focused on the number of times a resident entered the outdoor space or exited (came indoors from the outdoor space; whether those who entered or exited the outdoor space were alone or with others; and whether this action was part of a programmed activity, related to staff involvement or independently (assumed to be self-motivated). The second type of observation (called "outside narrative") was also conducted for one 20-minute segment each hour and was identical to the first with the exception of the location of the observer being in the outdoor space with a clear view to the garden entry from within the facility. The final type of observation was behavior mapping, which entailed the observer doing a walk-through of the outdoor space, following a pre-determined route, at 20-minute intervals. The behavior mapping focused on the features and spaces in the garden being utilized by residents, whether residents were alone or with others, and whether residents were deemed to be located in a specific area as part of a programmed activity, due to staff initiative or independently.

Residents' use of outdoor space was regarded as being under independent, staff-initiated, programmed or enabled conditions. "Independent conditions" involved residents' apparent self-motivated with no evident influence by others; "staff-initiated conditions" were defined as situations when residents' behavior related to the outdoor space were physically, verbally or in some observable way influenced by staff; "programmed conditions" included scheduled group activities or group events under staff leadership planned for the residents as a component of the programming policy; and the "enabled" category included instances when a resident initiated the move to enter or exit the outdoor space and was aided by any other person, who might help with a door, for instance.

Results of the study form the basis of a theoretical framework diagrammed in the Garden-Use Model. This model serves as a summary of the findings as well as a tool for facilities that seek to increase garden use among residents.

Factors Influencing the Use of Outdoor Space

The factors influencing the use of outdoor space were selected and defined by the authors prior to the study.

Organizational policy was defined in this study as the stated goal of the facility regarding use of the outdoor space by residents with dementia. This stated goal was founded on the following: a mission statement or similar document presented by the facility, available literature and brochures, the education and training of staff, interviews with facility directors or administrators, and programming philosophy.

Staff Attitudes involved the overall staff mindset regarding the importance of the available outdoor space and the benefits that spending time outside offered residents. Staff attitudes were evaluated in this study by analyzing their responses to the Garden Use Questionnaire developed by Martha Tyson (Tyson, 1998). This instrument included a range of questions designed to evaluate such aspects of garden use as residents' access to available outdoor space, the effect of the garden on residents' moods, and residents' abilities to utilize the garden and its features. Staff at each facility who consistently spent time with the residents were asked to complete the questionnaire.

Visual Access was defined as encompassing views to the garden entry and to the garden from the interior of the facility.

Physical Access was the entry from the unit to the outdoor space including the immediate area surrounding the threshold both inside and outside.

Garden Design included the spatial layout of the garden, circulation routes, and the features or amenities within the space, including pertinent distances between them, and the garden access.

Site Selection

The selection of cases at five sites in the United States was based on the opinions of fifteen experts in research and design fields related to the outdoor environment for the cognitively impaired elderly. These experts were each sent a cover letter explaining the purpose of the study and were asked to name the "best-designed outdoor space" for demented residents in a long-term care facility in this country. The resulting list was narrowed to five sites based on the frequency of selection by the experts and availability of the facility for the study. By narrowing the selected sites to the "best-designed" outdoor spaces, the assumption was that these sites would provide a rich database to study design features that might affect space use. The names of the sites have been changed for the purposes of this paper. Of the five sites, four of the cases involved assisted care facilities with residents in early to mid stages of dementia–most of whom were ambulatory and required little or no assistance to move about the unit and outdoor space. The exception was Cedar Lawn, a day-care facility in Michigan, which was included due to its exceptional outdoor space.

CASE STUDIES

Oak Park

Description of Facility and Resident Population

Oak Park was a continuum of care community founded in 1994 to house residents in all stages of dementia. Located in a former convent facility in a Massachusetts town, Oak Park also incorporated a day care program, which was typical of all five of the sites in this study. Generally, Oak Park utilized the three-story structure by placing those residents in early stages of dementia or with mild cognitive impairment on floor two, those in middle to late stages of dementia on floor one, and encouraged all of the residents who were able and the day care participants to spend most of the day on the ground floor where activities and dining occurred.

Analysis

In our view, Oak Park felt non-threatening both indoors and in the enclosed outdoor park-like space. This was likely due to several factors, including the legibility of the spaces and the consistent presence of activities and movement, which appeared to create a friendly atmosphere and an appropriate amount of stimulation.

Oak Park actively encouraged residents' use of the outdoor space through its activity programming. This was reflected in the high percentage of programmed and staff-initiated outdoor activities. In fact, the mission statement, staff attitudes, physical access to the garden, the layout of the garden, and the observation data addressing residents' use of the outdoor space at Oak Park all appeared to align positively toward a goal of residents' spending time outdoors. Perhaps the only questionable area was visual access. Though there were ample windows facing the garden from the well-used portions of the Oak Park facility, the views were somewhat impeded in the dining room by furnishings, which also inhibited one drawing physically near the windows, and in the living room by sheer window coverings.

The layout of the garden (see Fig. 1) offered a variety of opportunities for residents; however, it did lack covered areas near the entry, which might have allowed more independent and programmed use. On the whole, staff responses to the "Garden Use Questionnaire" indicated a positive perception of the garden and its benefits to the residents. When asked on the questionnaire to rate potential reasons "if residents do not use the outdoor space," the highest mean response (1.78 of a possible 4.00) was for the response "the area is exposed to sun, wind, etc." Though this response is not significant in itself, it seemed to indicate that when pressed to name a potential negative influence on

FIGURE 1. Oak Park garden plan

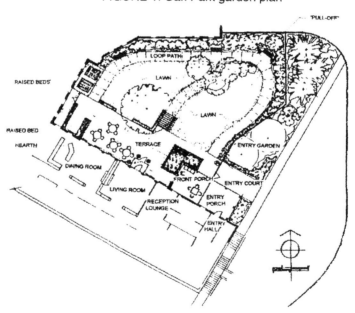

outdoor use by residents, staff selected a lack of shelter from harsher weather conditions.

Though residents at Oak Park went outside under all conditions (independent, staff-initiated, programmed or enabled by others), the numbers indicated a strong staff involvement with encouraging residents to use the outdoor space (see Table 1). Similarly, behavior mapping observations illustrated significant staff involvement (including the presence of residents outside due to programmed activities or staff initiative) with residents being outside 59% of the time due to staff during these observations.

Residents used the terrace the most (75%) including all conditions (see Table 6). Interestingly, the seating area away from the building was second in frequency of use during the programmed and independent conditions. This would indicate that residents were willing to venture to a distant portion of the garden to a seating area that was appealing to them. At Oak Park, the seating in the "pull-off" offered some shade, privacy, and a sense of "being away." However, the "pull-off" was also a place where small programmed activities took place on occasion, which could have influenced residents in the group to later feel comfortable returning independently to this area.

Maple Ridge

Description of Facility and Resident Population

Maple Ridge, located in a small Ohio community, was also a continuum of care facility dedicated solely to the care of individuals with dementia. It was founded in 1987 and occupies a one-level building, which was formerly an el-

TABLE 1. Summary of observations–Oak Park

	TYPES OF USE				TOTAL
	Independent	Staff-initiated	Programmed	Enabled	
RESIDENTS EXITS TO OUTSIDE					
Residents	54	36	71	3	164
Residents w/ Staff	1				1
Residents w/ Others	6				6
Sub-Total	**61**	**36**	**71**	**3**	**171**
RESIDENTS ENTRIES TO INSIDE					
Residents	85	44	15	8	152
Residents w/ Staff	8				8
Residents w/ Others	4				4
Sub-Total	**97**	**44**	**15**	**8**	**164**

ementary school. The study took place on the assisted living unit of the facility for those individuals in early stages of dementia. The residents on the assisted living unit were also joined several days a week by the participants in the day program.

Analysis

In our opinion, the assisted living unit of Maple Ridge felt very quiet for the most part and, possibly due to this absence of activities and motion, also had an institutional atmosphere. It was legible, or simple to read and discern recognizable options and main routes within the facility, and included two residential halls and one administrative hall radiating from the central public hub. While there was no fear of getting lost, there was also no "place" to go. The friendliest and warmest area of the unit was the sunroom, which had comfortable porch-like furnishings, an entertaining pet bird, and a wonderful view to the garden.

Maple Ridge presented a very unusual situation regarding the relation of the operating philosophy, staff attitudes, physical and visual access to the garden, the design of the garden, and use of the garden among the residents of the assisted living unit (including the day program participants). The mission statement and its stated goals along with the brochures prepared by Maple Ridge and statements by the director were all compiled to define the operating philosophy of the facility. Interestingly, these sources all aligned in presenting objectives and other descriptions related to maximizing the functioning of the residents, providing a daily and varied activity program, encouraging independence, promoting self esteem, and promoting "freedom of movement through the large, friendly open areas and outdoor gardens." However, in direct conflict with these stated goals was the number of programmed activities for the residents and physical access to the garden from the assisted living unit.

The door to the garden (as well the door to the rest of the facility) from the assisted living unit remained locked at all times during the study and was accessible only to those who could work the code pad near the door. The residents who went out to the garden most often were those who either kept the written code with them or the few who could remember the numbers of the code required to unlock the door to the garden. Although the facility offered residents a clear and expansive view of an appealing outdoor environment (see Fig. 2), such as the view of the garden from the sunroom on the assisted living unit, physical access was denied for many because of a locked door.

During the study period, there were also no instances of programmed activities in the outdoor space for the assisted living residents at Maple Ridge. The majority (79%) of the assisted living residents who went outside did so under

FIGURE 2. Maple Ridge garden plan

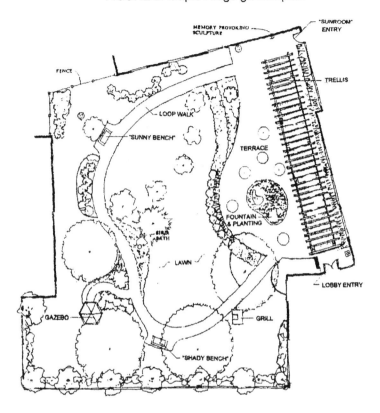

independent conditions (see Table 2); while 9% of these residents went out-side due to staff initiative.

During the behavior mapping observations, there were no instances of these residents being outside due to programmed activities, and most (94%) seen outside were under independent conditions (see Table 6). The majority of residents were seen on the terrace, and the next most utilized area by the as-sisted-living residents was loop walkway. The only covered area was the ga-zebo, which was used very little. Similar to the Oak Park staff responses to the "Garden Use Questionnaire," Maple Ridge staff were generally positive in their answers related to the use of the garden. When asked about possible rea-sons why residents might not utilize the outdoor space, the Maple Ridge staff also responded that "the area is exposed to sun, wind, etc." (highest mean rat-ing (1.79 out of 4.00) of the possible answers). However, it was interesting that

TABLE 6. Summary of observations–Maple Ridge

	TYPES OF USE					TOTAL
	Independent	Staff-initiated	Programmed	Enabled		
RESIDENTS EXITS TO OUTSIDE						
Residents	70	8		11		**89**
Residents w/ Staff						
Residents w/ Others	3					**3**
Sub-Total	**73**	**8**		**11**		**92**
RESIDENTS ENTRIES TO INSIDE						
Residents	65	4		12		**81**
Residents w/ Staff	4					**4**
Residents w/ Others	5					**5**
Sub-Total	**74**	**4**		**12**		**90**

only one staff member rated "entrances locked" as a "very likely" potential reason for residents not using the outdoor space.

Willow Run

Description of Facility and Resident Population

Willow Run was also a free-standing, one-story continuum of care community devoted entirely to the care of people with Alzheimer's and related dementia. It was opened in 1994 in a small town in Maine near the coast and had three different "houses" or wings each with its own enclosed garden to serve residents in varying stages of dementia. The houses were identical in layout, but each of the respective gardens was created to meet the unique needs and cognitive levels of the residents (see Fig. 3). This study took place in the residential care unit for individuals in early to mid stages of the disease. Similarly to the other sites, Willow Run also offered an adult day program. During the study there were two day-program participants who joined the residential care unit when they came in for the program.

Analysis

The atmosphere at the residential care unit of Willow Run appeared to have an appropriate balance between stimulation and quiet. There were ongoing activities in the central area; small groups of residents gathered independently in

FIGURE 3. Willow Run garden plan

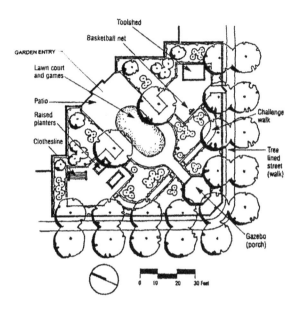

seating areas; residents gathered informally in the television room or in the small sunny hall adjacent to the garden entry; movement throughout the variety of public spaces and circulation routes within the unit; and areas for privacy. The unit had a warm feeling and, in our opinion, did not feel institutional. It was easy to imagine that one could feel comfortable and that he or she belonged in this setting.

The operating philosophy at Willow Run was defined by the mission statement, the statement of philosophy, and through our interview with the program director. The emphasis of these sources was upholding the dignity and self-respect of the residents, the rights of the residents, creating a home and atmosphere where individuals could achieve their highest well being in all aspects of their lives. Though the program director believed in the value of keeping residents busy with activities, she did not necessarily view the outdoor space as the venue for these activities. In fact, she expressed her philosophy that scheduled outside activities would take away from the garden as being a place of respite for the residents. Use of the garden by residents as well as staff responses to the "Garden Use Questionnaire" reflected this philosophy. Staff rated the garden as most successful in offering "easy access to the outdoors" and a place for residents' "visiting with family/friends" and in en-couraging the feeling among residents of "freedom to go outdoors."

Visual and physical access aligned positively with the operating philoso-phy and actual use of the garden by residents. Visual access to the garden was good from the central public area of the unit; and the door remained unlocked 100% of the observation periods and propped open 51% of the time during the observations. The behavior observations of residents' use of the garden also verified the operating philosophy. All of the residents who went outside were under independent conditions, and residents went outside over twice as much when the door was propped open as when it was closed. Residents went inside under independent conditions 96% the time and due to staff initiative 4% of the instances (see Table 3).

Similarly, during the behavior mapping observations, residents were seen outside under independent conditions 100% of the time during the study. The patio was the most used feature with 36% of residents observed in this loca-tion. The residents were located on the "clothesline terrace" (14%) and the loop path (14%) next most frequently (see Table 6).

Coinciding with staff responses to the "Garden Use Questionnaire" at Oak Park and Maple Ridge, Willow Run staff took a positive view of the garden and its benefits to residents; and when asked about potential reasons why resi-dents might not use the garden, staff at Willow Run also rated the most likely explanation as "exposure to sun, wind, etc." (with a mean rating of 2.00 out of a possible 4.00). As did Maple Ridge, Willow Run offered a unique look at how residents utilized the outdoor space under independent conditions–partic-

TABLE 3. Summary of observations–Willow Run

	TYPES OF USE					TOTAL
	Independent	Staff-initiated	Programmed	Enabled		
RESIDENTS EXITS TO OUTSIDE						
Residents	91					91
Residents w/ Staff						
Residents w/ Others	5					5
Sub-Total	**96**					**96**
RESIDENTS ENTRIES TO INSIDE						
Residents	82	4				**86**
Residents w/ Staff	1					**1**
Residents w/ Others	6					**6**
Sub-Total	**89**	**4**				**93**

ularly given that they had no prior experience of becoming acquainted with certain outdoor features during programmed activities.

Given the intentions of the landscape architect, we believe that the assisted living garden at Willow Run was successful in creating a "typical" New England residential setting. Some of the features were likely selected for visual effect rather than intended use. Based on the study observations, features such as the basketball goal, the game lawn, and the clothesline were not used frequently by the residents.

Pine View

Description of Facility and Resident Population

Pine View opened in 1988 as a residential care facility for individuals primarily in the early to mid stages of Alzheimer's disease and other forms of dementia and was located in a residential neighborhood in a small Maine town. There was a day care program at Pine View, and the fourteen day participants at the time of the study came in on varying days during the week. The clapboard one-level structure appeared more residential than institutional in style and blended easily with its surroundings. The interior of the facility was laid out with a large central activity and dining area, which was flanked on one side by a hall connecting administrative offices and the kitchen and on the other side by residents' bedrooms.

Analysis

When examining the interior plan of Pine View, it initially appears legible and conducive to wayfinding; however, in reality, the interior of the facility was not conducive to exploring. We felt that this was largely due to the doors from the front hall and the rear garden entry hall to the residential area of the unit remaining closed. Though our mission differed from that of the residents, the environment did not seem to draw one to move about the inside area. While the positive aspects of the large central activity/dining area were its centrality, openness and adaptability for a variety of functions; the negative aspect, in our opinion, was its impersonal nature.

The operating philosophy of Pine View, including the mission statement, philosophy of care statement and interview responses from the facility administrator, emphasized planned activity for the residents, individuality and independence of residents, encouraging residents to live to their fullest potential, and creating a homelike environment. The administrator believed the outdoor space to be a very important component of these goals. Staff attitudes, visual access and the garden design all aligned positively with these objectives as well. Physical access was easily managed by residents except during the 7% of the observation periods when the door to the garden was locked by staff. Actual use of the garden did not reflect the anticipated influence of programmed activities; however, many scheduled activities had been curtailed due to the unusually hot weather. The residents who went outside at Pine View did so most frequently (62%) under independent conditions (see Table 4). During the behavior mapping observations, however, residents were seen outside under independent conditions only slight more than due to programmed activities (see Table 6).

The patio was the most often used outdoor space during each category of conditions, and, interestingly, residents used the "shady chairs" the next most frequently under independent conditions. These chairs were not visible from

FIGURE 4. Pine View garden plan

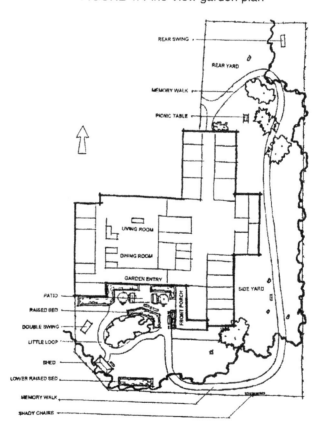

the garden entry or from most of the patio and were not used under pro-grammed or staff-initiated conditions; so, relative to the independent use of garden features, residents were willing to venture down the "memory" walk to this seating area although it was removed visually and physically from the pa-tio and garden entry. The Pine View garden was unique in its large size as well as its unusual configuration wrapping around much of the building (see Fig. 4). One had visual access only to the area immediately around the patio when entering the outdoor space, and it was necessary to walk nearly the length of the memory walk in order to view the entire outdoor space. As with previous staff responses to the "Garden Use Questionnaires," Pine View's staff re-sponded favorably regarding their garden and rated "the area is exposed to sun, wind, etc." as the most likely reason why residents might not use the outdoor space.

Cedar Lawn

Description of Facility and Day Client Population

Cedar Lawn was founded in 1991 as a non-profit organization dedicated to provide services and support for individuals and families affected by Alzhei-mer's disease and other dementias. It is located in a converted convent in a moderate-size Michigan city and, unlike the other facilities included in the study, was strictly a day care program for adults with dementia who came in to Cedar Lawn on varying days during the week.

TABLE 4. Summary of observations–Pine View

	TYPES OF USE					TOTAL
	Independent	Staff-initiated	Programmed	Enabled		
RESIDENTS EXITS TO OUTSIDE						
Residents	58	12	28	2		100
Residents w/ Staff	1					1
Residents w/ Others	10					10
Sub-Total	**69**	**12**	**28**	**2**		**111**
RESIDENTS ENTRIES TO INSIDE						
Residents	55	14	28	4		101
Residents w/ Staff	5					5
Residents w/ Others	9					9
Sub-Total	**69**	**14**	**28**	**4**		**115**

The portion of the first floor of the building used by the Cedar Lawn daycare program included a large activity space, that formerly served as the chapel for the convent, a kitchen, and administrative offices–all of which were on the side of the structure with no views to the garden. The atrium allowed natural lighting through its glass roof and had a running fountain, tile floors, a high ceiling and many live plants. During the study, staff and day clients ate lunch in the atrium most days. The conservatory, where the day clients enjoyed indoor horticulturally-oriented activities, overlooked most of the main area of the garden.

Analysis

This was an unusually large and beautiful garden, which was extremely well maintained and offered a wide range of opportunities for different experiences and activities for individuals of all cognitive and physical abilities (see Fig. 5). Covered areas providing shade included the covered glider in the

FIGURE 5. Cedar Lawn garden plan

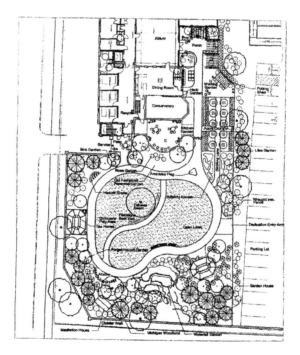

working garden, umbrella tables on the conservatory terrace, the tea house, and the summer house.

Cedar Lawn was a particularly unique site in this study as solely a day care program and with its magnificent and high budget garden. The objectives of Cedar Lawn centered on serving families and caregivers of those with Alzheimer's. Visual and physical accesses to the garden were removed from the primary activity area designated for the Cedar Lawn day program participants. Visual access to the main portion of the garden was only available from the conservatory, where horticultural activities took place, and physical access, likewise, was only offered from the areas near the atrium and conservatory.

The programming policy with regard to outdoor use was very controlled, and all outdoor use by day program participants was under programmed or staff-initiated conditions (see Table 5). During behavior mapping observations day clients were observed most frequently on the loop path followed in frequency of use by the garden house (see Table 6). There was a noticeable lack of correlation between the mission and objectives of Cedar Lawn and the behavior observations; there were no instances of family members or caregivers (other than Cedar Lawn staff or volunteers) seen in the garden.

DISCUSSION

The five sites studied during this research each offered a unique alignment of the factors influencing use of outdoor space among individuals with demen-

TABLE 5. Summary of observations–Cedar Lawn

	TYPES OF USE					TOTAL
	Independent	Staff-initiated	Programmed	Enabled		
DAY CLIENTS EXITS TO OUTSIDE						
Day Clients		3	61			**64**
Day Clients w/ Staff						
Day Clients w/ Others						
Sub-Total		**3**	**61**			**64**
DAY CLIENTS ENTRIES TO INSIDE						
Day Clients		3	29			**32**
Day Clients w/ Staff						
Day Clients w/ Others						
Sub-Total		**3**	**29**			**32**

TABLE 6. Comparative use of garden spaces

	Oak Park	Maple Ridge	Willow Run	Pine View	Cedar Lawn
Terrace/Patio					
Independent	60	29	25	13	
Staff-initiated	14	3		11	
Programmed	125			32	
Sub-Total	**199**	**32**	**25**	**56**	
Paths					
Independent	13	17	9	11	
Staff-initiated	1			3	
Programmed					36
Sub-Total	**14**	**17**	**9**	**14**	**36**
Garden Structures					
Independent	8	1	4		
Staff-initiated	5				3
Programmed					25
Sub-Total	**13**	**1**	**4**		**28**
Seating away from Bldg.					
Independent	21	3		23	
Staff-initiated	3				2
Programmed	10				8
Sub-Total	**34**	**3**		**23**	**10**
Raised/Garden Beds					
Independent	8		1	2	
Staff-initiated				1	
Programmed					
Sub-Total	**8**		**1**	**3**	
TOTAL	**268**	**53**	**39**	**96**	**74**

tia. The first study site, Oak Park, was the only one of the five that was strongly aligned in all factors positively influencing outdoor use and showed active use of the garden by residents. Maple Ridge was misaligned with regard to operating philosophy, physical access and actual use of its garden. The mission statement goals, which pointed to independence, the importance of activities, and the value of the garden, did not match the locked door to the garden and the absence of programmed outdoor activities. Willow Run was actually aligned in all factors related to outdoor use, like Oak Park, but simply did not take an aggressive approach to getting residents outside through programmed activities. Pine View had a particularly unique outdoor space in both its size and configuration.

Unlike the other long-term-care facilities in the study, only portions of the Pine View outdoor space could be seen from any given location within the garden, although this did not appear to affect its use. Programmed activities were apparently curtailed due to the unusually hot weather during the time of the study. Cedar Lawn was unique in every way–particularly its mission objectives being focused on the caregivers of individuals with dementia. The gardens of Cedar Lawn also have the most varied features and opportunities for a wide range of activities and movement patterns; however, all use of the garden by the day clients was staff-initiated or programmed.

Excluding Cedar Lawn, which had only staff-involved use of the outdoor space by day clients, Oak Park was the only site with a larger percentage of residents going outside under programmed situations than independent conditions. The other three sites, Maple Ridge, Willow Run, and Pine View, had considerably greater independent use of the garden among the residents than use due to programmed activities or staff initiative. The same results were seen during the behavior mapping observations. Though Pine View instances of programmed or staff-initiated (47%) outdoor use appeared to move closer to the independent use (53%), this was probably due to one instance of an activity group involving a large number of residents taking place on the patio. This study did not track specific residents or record objectively how the residents at each site utilized the available outdoor space, including how individual features were used, under independent conditions. However, in a subjective attempt to describe how the gardens were used by residents due to their own initiative, it was observed that in all cases (excluding Cedar Lawn, which had no independent use of the garden by day clients), under 50% of the residents typically utilized the available outdoor space under independent conditions.

At the first four sites, the terrace/patio near the garden entry was used by residents most often under all conditions (programmed, staff-initiated and independent). Maple Ridge and Willow Run had no instances of programmed activities. Cedar Lawn, on the other hand, which had no instance of independent use of the garden, had the greatest percentage of programmed use on the garden paths, followed by the garden house. There were several plausible reasons for the large percentage of residents seen on the terrace or patio during independent as well as programmed use of the outdoor space. In all instances where this occurred, the patio was nearest to the garden entry and also had the most seating. In all cases there was some sun protection offered by umbrella tables, and in all instances this area could be seen from within the unit. At Cedar Lawn, although there was a generous amount of seating and tables on the terrace for programmed activities such as bingo or group discussions, the largest percentage of day clients were observed in programmed activities on the loop paths. This lower level of terrace use may have been due to the separation of the terrace at this facility from the garden entry. Consequently, the terrace was not part of the inside/outside transition environment seen at other facilities.

Interestingly, when residents move outside independently, the location utilized most frequently after the terrace or patio was typically a location that was not necessarily closest to the terrace or the garden entry. At Oak Park, for example, residents were seen in the "pull-off" (a seating area in a shady niche off the loop path on the opposite side of the garden from the entry) for 19% of the instances of independent use. Similarly, in another of the large outdoor gardens Pine View residents were seen in the "shady chairs" (a significant distance down the memory walk from the garden entry) 21% of the time. At Maple Ridge, also considering only independent usage of the garden, 33% of the assisted living residents observed were seen on the loop path. At Oak Park and Pine View it would seem the nearness to the garden entry and visual access to a feature from within the unit were less important to the residents than was finding comfortable seating in a relatively private and shady part of the garden.

All of the facilities lacked a covered outdoor area near the garden entry. This could have inhibited outdoor use under any of the conditions during more extreme weather. Staff responses to the "Garden Use Questionnaires" support this view.

GARDEN-USE MODEL

On the basis of these results, a model has been developed to enhance the use of outdoor space in long-term care facilities. Recommendations focus on the five factors addressed in this study, organizational policy, staff attitudes, visual access, physical access and garden design, and are derived from the site analysis conducted at each facility, qualitative observations and discussion with facility staff, data compiled through systematic behavior observations, and the "Garden Use Questionnaires" completed by staff. Each of the factors was defined at the outset of the study for consistency and clarity; however, these factors were "re-defined" on the basis of data from each of the sites in terms of the qualities necessary for encouraging use of the outdoor space.

The Garden-Use Model illustrates the factors related to garden use among residents with dementia in long-term care facilities addressed in this study (see Fig. 6). These factors with their interpretations are represented in the column of boxes in the diagram. For increased garden use among the residents, the model proposes that each factor must be realized at a site in terms of the descriptives listed in each corresponding circle to the right of the arrow in the diagram. For a facility to produce optimal garden use among residents, the column of circles in the model must all be manifested and linked to one another.

The proposed model and underlying theoretical framework, which The Garden-Use Model depicts, are based on the data collected and rich description at each of the five cases making up the study. Though individual differences and abilities of residents have not been analyzed in this study, the model

FIGURE 6. The Garden-Use Model

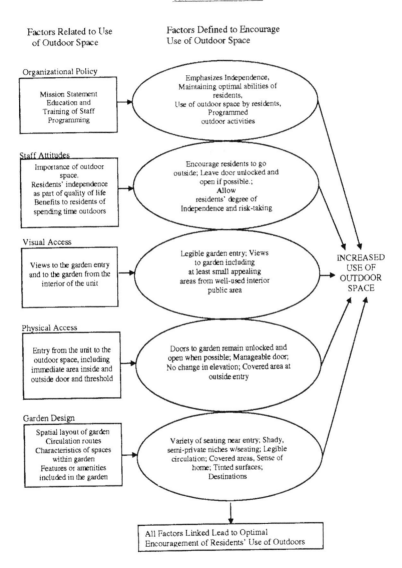

The Garden-Use Model

seeks to create optimal garden use for all residents within their range of capabilities. The purpose of the model is to serve as a guide for facilities that seek to increase garden use among residents and to offer a means of self-evaluation for such facilities.

Organizational Policy

Organizational policy was defined by such elements as facility mission statement, available literature and brochures, the education and training of staff, interviews with facility directors or administrators, and programming philosophy. To encourage use of the available outdoor space at a facility these elements should promote residents' independence and maintaining their optimal abilities; encompass a positive belief in the value of the outdoors for residents; and through programming reflect an active effort toward exposing residents to the outdoor space.

All of the sites incorporated an organizational policy very supportive of residents' using the outdoor space available to them and of the value of the outdoor area for the residents' well being. The Willow Run program director's philosophy that such programmed use of the garden would detract from the garden's being a place of respite was reflected in the absence of any programmed or staff-initiated use of the garden by residents. Based on this data, it seems probable that a change in this aspect of organizational policy to a more active influence on residents' use of the outdoor space through programmed group activities would increase the amount of overall use of the garden by residents. On the opposite end of the spectrum, Cedar Lawn had very controlled outdoor use by residents with no use of the outdoor space by day clients. Based on data gathered from behavior observations as well as the interview with the program director, it would seem that a modification of the organizational policy to encourage independent use of the garden by day clients would be advisable.

There were also instances during the course of the study when the organizational policy of the facility did not translate into the reality of the situation–particularly with regard to encouraging independence and including a variety of programmed outdoor activities. At Maple Ridge the absence of programmed outdoor activities (as well as the locked door to the garden during all observation periods) was in direct conflict with the stated goals of the facility. The programmed outdoor activities as evidenced by the behavior observation data at Pine View were also less than anticipated given the organizational policy; however, as discussed previously, this conflict was very likely due to the unusual heat wave at the time of the study. Based on observations, it seems likely that overall use of the gardens would be enhanced by increasing programmed outdoor activities at Maple Ridge and at Pine View. The other noticeable discrepancy between facility goals and reality involved use of the garden at Cedar Lawn by family members–a situation that could be resolved through the addition of activities involving the family of day clients or through other means of encouragement that did not alter the garden as a place of respite for the families.

Staff Attitudes

Staff attitudes involved the overall staff mindset regarding the importance of the available outdoor space and the benefits that spending time outside offered residents. In order to encourage use of the outdoor space, it became evident during the case studies that staff attitudes were an important ingredient in encouraging residents to go outside and allowing residents a degree of independence and risk taking. For instance, at Oak Park we observed an overall mindset among staff that going outside was beneficial for residents, and we felt that this attitude was reflected in resident's freely going outside; while at Pine View, we noted several instances where staff expressed concern about some residents' being outside without supervision and responded by locking the doors to the garden on occasion. Staff attitudes were evaluated in this study through responses to the Garden Use Questionnaires and generally took a positive view of the available outdoor space for residents; however, this research did not consistently demonstrate a strong link between staff attitudes as measured by responses to the questionnaires and use of the outdoor space by residents.

Visual Access

Visual access was defined as encompassing views to the garden entry and to the garden from the interior of the unit. After completing the studies at the five sites, it became possible to better define visual access in terms of encouraging use of the outdoor space. 'Visual Access' was expanded to include a legible garden entry, and characterization of views to the outside to include appealing areas, such as colorful flowers. At Oak Park, based on the descriptive site analysis as well as informal conversations with staff, it appears that independent use could be improved by increasing visual access (and possibly physical access) to the garden from the well used dining and living rooms of the ground floor of the unit. In the dining room, the furnishings could be removed from in front of the windows to the garden, and the sheer window coverings in the living room could also be removed to increase visual access to the garden from this area.

Because the relationship between visual access and garden use was not objectively measured in this study, the recommendations are founded on descriptive analysis and informal observation. Unfortunately, the site with the most encompassing visual access from the interior public area to the garden also had a locked door to the garden during 100% of the observation periods. From the sunroom of the assisted living unit at Maple Ridge, one had a nearly complete overview of the garden; however, only residents who could master the coded access pad were able to independently enter the garden. On the opposite end of the visual-access spectrum, Cedar Lawn, which had no visual access to the garden from the most used interior areas, also had only staff-controlled use of the outdoor space by day clients. Both of these situations, therefore, made it impossible to make judgments regarding visual access and garden use.

Physical Access

Physical access was the entry from the unit to the outdoor space including the immediate area surrounding the threshold. Not surprisingly, in order to encourage use, it became evident during the study that it was important to keep doors unlocked, have manageable doors and avoid changes in elevation. The recommendation for increasing outdoor use at Maple Ridge is obvious. It would undoubtedly increase independent use of the outdoor space to keep unlocked the door from the assisted living unit to the garden. This suggestion is based on descriptive analysis of the situation and systematic observations noting that this door remained locked during 100% of the observation periods. At Cedar Lawn, though there was an alarm connected to the doors which sounded if a door was opened without a key, the doors were not kept locked during the day. It is possible that the removal of the alarm as a deterrent to independent use would increase such usage by day clients. Also, though this would not be feasible in many climates, the observations at Willow Run pointed to a recommendation for all facilities. During the observation periods when the door to the garden was propped open on the unit, residents went outside independently over twice as much as when the door was closed. The observations also potentially link the relation of the spatial layout of the building and the location of the door to the garden to use of the garden by residents–particularly under independent conditions. It would seem that all facilities could increase outdoor use by eliminating as many physical barriers as possible between inside and outside.

Garden Design

Garden design was defined at the outset of the study to encompass the spatial layout of the garden, circulation routes, and the features or amenities within the space including pertinent distances between them and the garden access. Aspects of garden design to encourage use of the outdoor space were more specifically defined at the conclusion of the case studies to include a variety of seating near the entry, shady and semi-private niches with seating, legible circulation and covered areas.

A primary design recommendation for all the sites would be to include near the garden entry covered, protected areas with a variety of seating. This suggestion is supported in part at the first four sites by staff responses when asked on the Garden-Use Questionnaire, "if residents do not use the outdoor space" to rate potential explanations. Staff across these sites responded that "the area is exposed to sun, wind, etc." as the most likely explanation. The suggestion for covered seating areas near the entry is also derived from the descriptive analysis of each site. Such areas would not only encourage more independent use but also allow more programmed activities to take place on the terrace within easy access from the interior of the unit during harsher weather conditions.

This recommendation is also derived from observation data. Generally speaking, there appeared to be two main zones of independent use by residents–the terrace or area near the garden entry and a more private place removed from the garden entry. Primary examples of the private areas a distance from the patio/terrace were the "pull-off" at Oak Park and the "shady chairs" at Pine View. What was also exceedingly obvious was the absence of transition zones between the interior of the facilities and the outdoor space at all of the sites. All of the facilities would, therefore, benefit by adding such a zone that offered not only physical protection from inclement weather but would provide a necessary area for visual adjustment, particularly for the elderly individuals with sensitivity to glare.

Additionally, Willow Run could encourage more outdoor usage by residents and their guests by adding seating near the entry and could also offer the residents a more varied experience by adding seating to areas away from the building. The two main recommendations for Pine View would be to locate comfortable seating on the porch, unlock the door from the unit to the porch and add additional seating along the memory walk and throughout the entire outdoor space. Based on descriptive analysis and observation of garden use, Pine View would at least improve the quality, if not also increase garden use, of the outdoor experience with the addition of seating along the memory walk.

With regard to the garden design as well as the entire environment of each site, including the interior of the facilities, each of the long-term care facilities analyzed in this study stressed the importance of creating a "home-like" setting for the residents. This has been a trend in all such facilities in this country in recent years when the environment has taken on a new importance. There is no firm definition for this descriptive term, and, though there are likely common solutions at long-term care facilities, home-like qualities are uniquely realized at individual sites. This was certainly true in these case studies. The common element in an attempt to create a "home" for residents is to offer a sense of familiarity, belonging, freedom and warmth. Since all of the facilities and their gardens in this research were different from one another, each had a distinctive answer to creating a "home."

CONCLUSION

In sum, it would appear from these studies that independent use of the outdoor space among residents or day program participants in facilities for individuals with dementia is influenced primarily by physical access. Visual access is likely important at least to the degree that from inside the facility or through a door to the garden, there is enough of a view to illustrate an appealing outdoor area. Facilities with poor physical and visual access are necessarily more dependent on staff initiated and programmed group activities to realize significant use of the outdoor spaces. It appears that the mission statement affects use of the outdoor space only if an objective of encouraging residents to use the outdoor space is derived from it, clearly instilled among staff, and reflected in programming policy. The only facility that clearly exhibited this link from mission statement and objectives to outdoor use was Oak Park.

This research did not demonstrate a strong link between staff attitudes as measured by responses to the "Garden Use Questionnaires" and use of the outdoor space among residents. In several instances, the questionnaire responses did not correspond with the reality of the facility and its operating environment. Though we would not discount staff questionnaires as a viable means for measuring staff attitudes toward the garden and its use by residents, it appears that some future revisions and clarifications of this tool would be positive.

As illustrated in the Garden Use Model, it is proposed that the greatest amount of outdoor space use will occur in a facility in which the operating philosophy, including the mission statement, goals, and beliefs of administrators, are supportive of residents going outside; there exists adequate visual access to the garden entry and to at least a portion of the outdoor space that is pleasing; and has easy physical access–defined as being unlocked, having a manageable door, on one level. It is conceivable that the overall design is not as important as is the provision of legible spaces that are comfortable in terms of seating and shade. An additional hypothesis might be that the design of the space is more important for its effect on the length of time residents spend outside than for encouraging their going outside in the first place. There is little doubt, however, that a strong positive correlation between operating philosophy, outdoor activity programming, and visual and physical access to an outdoor space will encourage residents to utilize the outdoor space.

REFERENCES

Calkins, M. (1989). *Design for dementia: Planning environments for the elderly and confused.* Owing Mills, MD: National Health Publishing.

Connell, B.R., Sanford, J.A., Wineman, J., & Grant, C.F. (1999). *Benefits of going outdoors among ltc residents.* Unpublished study conducted by the Atlanta VA Rehabilitation Research & Development Center and the College of Architecture, Georgia Institute of Technology, Atlanta.

Connell, B.R., Sanford, J.A., Wineman, J., & Grant, C.F. (1998). Outdoor space in long term care settings. Unpublished study conducted by the Atlanta VA Rehabilitation Research & Development Center and the College of Architecture, Georgia Institute of Technology, Atlanta.

Cooper Marcus, C. (2005, March). No ordinary garden. *Landscape Architecture, 95,* 26-39.

Cooper Marcus, C., & Barnes, M. (Eds.). (1999). *Healing gardens: Therapeutic benefits and design recommendations.* New York: John Wiley & Sons.

Day, K., Carreon, D., & Stump, C. (2000). The therapeutic design of environments for people with dementia. *The Gerontologist, 40,* 397-416.

Grant, C.F. (2003). Factors influencing the use of outdoor space by residents with dementia in long-term care facilities. Unpublished doctoral dissertation, College of Architecture, Georgia Institute of Technology, Atlanta.

Hiatt, L.G. (1988). Environmental design and mentally impaired older people. In H. Altman (Ed.), *Alzheimer's Disease* (pp. 309-320). New York: Plenum.

Lovering, M.J. (1990, May/June). Alzheimer's disease and outdoor space: Issues in environmental design. *The American Journal of Alzheimer's Care and Related Disorders & Research,* 33-40.

Tyson, M.M. (1998). *The healing landscape.* New York: McGraw-Hill.

Zeisel, J., Silverstein, N.M., Hyde, J., Levkoff, S., Lawton, M.P., & Holmes, W. (2003). Environmental correlates to behavioral health outcomes in Alzheimer's special care units. *The Gerontologist, 43,* 697-711.

Zeisel, J., & Tyson, M.M. (1999). Alzheimer's treatment gardens. In C. Cooper Marcus & M. Barnes (Eds.), *Healing gardens: Therapeutic benefits and design recommendations* (pp. 437-504). New York: John Wiley & Sons.

doi:10.1300/J081v21n01_06

Effects of Therapeutic Gardens in Special Care Units for People with Dementia: Two Case Studies

Rebecca Ory Hernandez

SUMMARY. Researchers and designers have recently focused on design of Special Care Units and effects of the environment on people with dementia. However, empirical findings that question the effects of such units on people with dementia are limited. Smaller still are empirical studies with regard to the outdoor environment in facilities housing those in Special Care Units. This research explores the idea that "therapeutic garden" spaces may play an important role in therapeutic restoration of people with dementia, and questions how well such spaces are integrated into the designs of outdoor spaces for this population.

This research conducts post-occupancy evaluations of outdoor spaces of two special care units of assisted living facilities for people with dementia in a Midwest metropolitan area. Multi-method qualitative research techniques were employed including interviews, behavior-mapping, and observations using the AARS observation tool for dementia behavior interpretation. Residents, family members and staff from the two special care units were interviewed to explore the garden use. Additional interviews were conducted among administrators and design pro-

Rebecca Ory Hernandez, MS, is Development Director, Weber State University, 4018 University Circle, Ogden, UT 84408-4018 (E-mail: Rohernandez@weber.edu).

[Haworth co-indexing entry note]: "Effects of Therapeutic Gardens in Special Care Units for People with Dementia: Two Case Studies." Hernandez, Rebecca Ory. Co-published simultaneously in *Journal of Housing for the Elderly* (The Haworth Press, Inc.) Vol. 21, No. 1/2, 2007, pp. 117-152; and: *Outdoor Environments for People with Dementia* (ed: Susan Rodiek and Benyamin Schwarz) The Haworth Press, Inc., 2007, pp. 117-152. Single or multiple copies of this article are available for a fee from The Haworth Document Delivery Service [1-800-HAWORTH, 9:00 a.m. - 5:00 p.m. (EST). E-mail address: docdelivery@ haworthpress.com].

Available online at http://jhe.haworthpress.com

doi:10.1300/J081v21n01_07

117

fessionals.

This study is a first step in examining the effectiveness of gardens in special care units in order to advance present knowledge and to provide a more informed basis for design. The vast majority of people interviewed expressed positive responses when discussing the garden spaces in the facilities and recommended that gardens be a standard in all nursing home facilities. Themes were discovered that correlated with the level of physical and psychological activity.

This research concluded that there is a need for therapeutic gardens to be incorporated as a 'standard' complementary element in special care units for people with dementia. Such an inclusion directly impacts the quality of life for residents, staff and family members. doi:10.1300/J081v21n01_07 *[Article copies available for a fee from The Haworth Document Delivery Service: 1-800-HAWORTH. E-mail address: <docdelivery@haworthpress.com> Website: <http://www.HaworthPress.com> © 2007 by The Haworth Press, Inc. All rights reserved.]*

KEYWORDS. Outdoor environments, qualitative research, post-occupancy evaluation, gerontology, landscape architecture, health, dementia

INTRODUCTION

"Therapeutic garden" spaces may play an important role in therapeutic restoration of people with dementia. This research questions how well such spaces are integrated into the designs of outdoor spaces for this population. While there are documented design guidelines and recommendations on the design of outdoor spaces for people suffering with dementia, there is little information regarding post-occupancy evaluation and studies after installation of gardens within special care units for people with dementia (Cooper Marcus, 1999; Gerlach-Spriggs, 1999; Tyson, 1998).

Two case studies were performed to look at the effects of the "therapeutic garden" concept within the scope of the environmental design field. The studies analyzed the outdoor garden spaces of two special care units for people with dementia. The gardens are located within assisted living facilities identified as "Garden View" and "Sunshine Center" in the Midwest, USA. It was hypothesized that the gardens could serve as an example of applied research and demonstrate the therapeutic potential of outdoor environments in the care of people with Alzheimer's disease.

An estimated 4.5 million Americans live with dementia (Alzheimer's Association, 2006). Half of all nursing home residents have Alzheimer's disease

FIGURE 1. Garden in dementia care space at Garden View, June 2002 (Ory Hernandez).

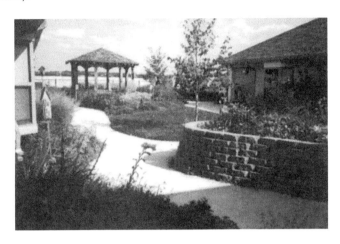

or a related disorder (National Center for Health Statistics, 1985). It is believed that many negative behaviors displayed by people with dementia can be attributed to the consequences of nursing homes and other institutional, non-therapeutic environments (Calkins, 1988; Cohen and Day, 1993; Lawton, 1991; Schwartz, 1996; Zcisel, 1999; Tyson, 2002). Though there are studies evaluating the success of housing and interior space-planning schemes for special care units for those with dementia, there are far fewer studies of post-occupancy evaluations of health care facilities and almost none of facility gardens (Cohen and Weisman, 1991; Cooper Marcus, 1995; Tyson, 1998).

RESEARCH DESIGN AND METHODS

Through qualitative research methods, this research investigated the impact, use (or lack of use) and possible benefits of gardens for residents with dementia, their families and staff of the facilities. Justification for using qualitative research methods corresponds to the research questions being based on searching for a *meaning* and an understanding of a process (Maxwell, 1996) which is inductive in approach. Qualitative research methods emphasize depth of understanding, attempt to tap the deeper meaning of human experience, and intend to generate theoretically rich observations embedded in context (Creswell, 1998; Maxwell, 1996; Rubin & Babbie, 1993; Patton,

2002). The effects of therapeutic gardens was explored by identifying the experiences and behavior of the residents in their setting, and interviewing staff members and families of residents.

Recent studies on the approach of changing nursing home culture have yielded promising results using medical and administrative indicators. However, these studies have limited outcomes on psychosocial issues that influence the quality of life for nursing home residents. This study addresses such limitations by conducting a more in-depth evaluation of the effectiveness of the garden spaces on nursing home residents' quality of life through observations and interviews.

Research Questions

The main research question was: What effect does the garden design have on the quality of life of residents living in special care units for people with dementia? More specific questions that supported the main objective are summarized in Table 1.

The study is grounded within the theoretical tradition of qualitative inquiry as it relates to ecological psychology and sociology. Ecological psychologists are concerned with the relationships between human behavior and the environment, and their research attempts to define and distinguish the elements of specific environments that makes them unique (Patton, 1990). The tradition of ecological psychology supports the framework for this qualitative study as it sees the relationship between humans and their environment as one that is interdependent (Barker, 1968; Barker et al., 1978; Lewin, 1936; Schoggen, 1978).

Interviews

Staff and families were interviewed (twenty to forty-five minute interviews) to find out whether they used the garden space and how the residents used the garden. Interviews with staff and family members provided the core of the data regarding the experience of working and living in the special care units. The interviews were tape recorded at the special care unit in a private area. Complete confidentiality was guaranteed, and participants were able to withdraw from the study at any time. Questions for family members included: What do you think about the garden in the facility? Do you support your loved one using the garden independently? What kind of affect do you think the garden has on the residents? Do the residents ever talk about the garden or outdoor areas? Are there favorite areas? Is there anything that you or the residents

TABLE 1. Research Questions and Methods Table

Research Questions	Methods
What effect does the garden design have on the quality of life of residents living in special care units for people with dementia?	
• What are the specific spaces within the garden that are being used? • How are they being used? • What are the emotional reactions of residents while in the garden?	• Behavioral mapping • Interview with staff • Interview with family • Apparent Affect Rating Scale (AARS)
• What value is placed on the garden space?	• Interview with staff • Interview with family
• What were the design criteria used to program the space? Does the criteria correspond to the special needs of the users?	• Interview with administrator • Interview with architect • Interview with landscape architect

do not like about the garden? Are there any areas that induce negative behaviors?

Questions for the staff included: Is the garden used as part of the residents' therapy? Can you explain how it is, or why it is not? How do the residents use the garden? Why do you use the garden? Do you ever go out into the garden to get away from the residents, or to have some quiet time? These questions were used as a starting point to initiate further conversation.

The architects and landscape architects were interviewed (thirty to forty-five minute interviews) to find out how they went about programming and designing the site. Examples of interview questions were: Can you take me through the steps of how you made decisions in designing the garden and outdoor areas? What criteria did you use to design the outdoor space? Have you done a post-occupancy evaluation to assess how the garden is being used?

Behavioral Mapping

Observations of daily life and resident/staff behavior in the garden were conducted through behavioral mapping. The outdoor area is considered shared or common space, (i.e., sitting areas under the awning off of the kitchen, benches, perennial garden spots, and the walking paths which wind around the perimeter of the property).

Sketches of the garden space site plan were systematically marked with a unique code to indicate who used the space, how the space was being used, how long that space was being used, etc. The behavioral mapping method was based on past studies by environmental designers that used a similar process (Cooper Marcus, 1998; Regnier, 1985; Schwarz, et al, 2001; Zeisel, 1981). The specific identity of residents was not indicated in the reports. Each resident, staff member or visitor was identified by a number or letter code. Frequency counts were then calculated for the number of residents, staff or visitors. The different types of activities (behavioral patterns) taking place in the garden were also identified on the map. Data was gathered over a nonconsecutive two-week summer and fall time period. Having time in the summer and later in the fall allowed for the different seasons to be taken into consideration. The weather in the Midwest is typically very hot in the summer (getting into the 100 degree Fahrenheit range in mid-afternoons) and very cold in the winter (below freezing temperatures in January and February). The timing of data collection was an important part of the behavior mapping segment. Naturally, field work in sites with a milder climate would optimize observing resident use of the outdoor space.

The behavior mapping was conducted during a minimum of five randomly assigned one-half hour periods from 7:00 AM–11:00 PM every day of the week, including weekends. Times and specific garden locations were also written on the behavior map. Selected behaviors (e.g., walking, sitting, standing, wandering, verbalizing) were recorded on the maps using symbols. The intention was to understand how residents, staff and families were using the garden space. After observing residents in the garden for a one-week period, it was believed that patterns would emerge. For example, if a person routinely visits the same areas day after day, or hour after hour, the pattern would reveal itself by the same "markings on the map," time after time.

Apparent Affect Rating Scale

The Apparent Affect Rating Scale (AARS) tool assists with interpreting emotional expression of people with dementia by looking at specific facial and body behavior (Lawton and Rubenstein, 2000, p. 102). The AARS entails rating three negative emotions (anger, anxiety/fear and depression/sadness) and two positive emotions (pleasure and interest) over a 5-minute period (unless another time frame is specified. Specific examples include pleasure (through smiling, laughing, singing) and anger (clenching teeth, grimacing, shouting, yelling, cursing). Patterns of relevance emerged based on places the residents returned to or avoided. Observing such behavior during common as well as uncommon hours from six to eight hour blocks of time were conducted until "saturation" was achieved.

Site Selection

The chosen sites were similar in value, but not identical in plan. Both were in urban areas and provided ample garden spaces intended for residents' use. Both were specifically designed as dementia-care facilities and showed evidence of Alzheimer's disease research considered as part of the design and construction of the facility. Both facilities advertise for dementia care and provide ambulatory residents the option of aging in place. Finally, both offer an option of a day stay program for people with dementia as part of their services. Garden View houses 24-34 residents, while Sunshine Center houses 35-45 residents in their special care units. All rooms are private rooms containing a private bathroom with a shower and a large window.

FIGURE 2. Garden View Site Plan

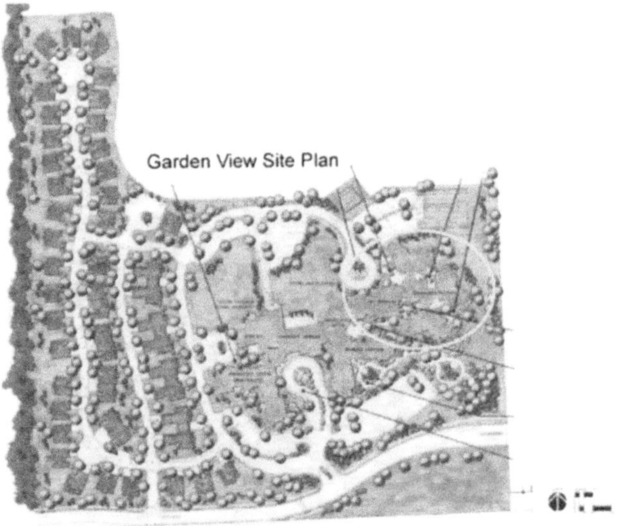

Garden View Site Plan

Note: circle indicates special care units

FIGURE 3. Entry to Garden View Dementia Suites

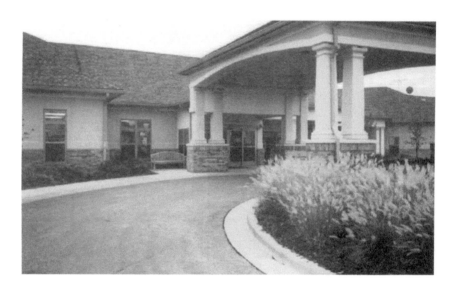

FIGURE 4. Floorplan of Dementia Suites at Garden View

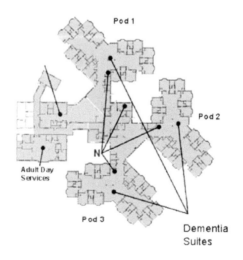

FIGURE 5. Location of garden site for Pods 2 and 3

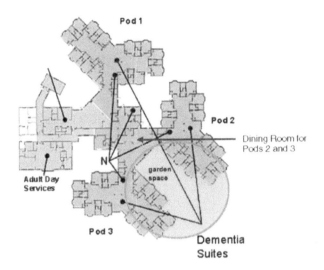

Garden View

The site of Garden View is located in an urban area within a major Midwestern city, but has the feel of a residential neighborhood. Garden View is a large retirement "campus" which contains detached retirement homes, enhanced living apartments, a full nursing home, adult day care services, and three wings of assisted living special care units specifically designed for housing people with dementia (see Figure 2). The dementia wings are arranged in clusters, which the facility terms "pods" which house twelve residents per pod, each with a private room and window (see Figure 5). Each "pod" or neighborhood suite is designed with the individual residents' stage of Alzheimer's or other cognitive illness in mind. The facility attempts to place residents from higher functioning to lower functioning in suites one through three. Residents who are highest in cognitive and physical functioning reside in "Pod 1" and tend to socialize with visitors who come for adult day services. Those people who have significantly limited cognitive abilities but can still function physically reside in "Pod 2." Finally, those people with late stage dementia and those in need of hospice care and more intensive private skilled nursing needs reside in "Pod 3."

The philosophy of care at Garden View is for residents to "age in place" instead of relocating to a nursing home. 'The Dementia Suites' are advertised in

FIGURE 6. Site plan of Sunshine Center illustrates houses and surrounding landscape (not to scale)

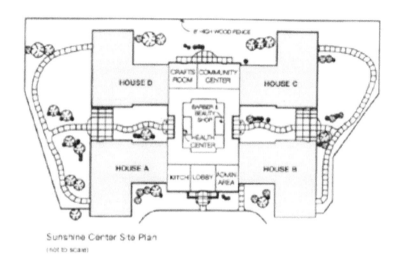

Sunshine Center Site Plan
(not to scale)

FIGURE 7. Entry to Sunshine Center

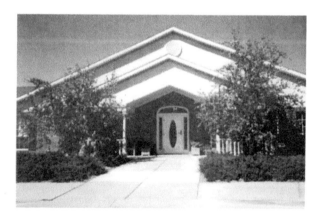

FIGURE 8. Floor plan of typical "house" in Sunshine Center

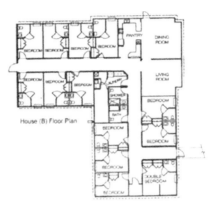

FIGURE 9. Typical space where residents and visitors sit outdoors to visit at Garden View. Area is shaded in the morning but fall sun in the late afternoon and early evening.

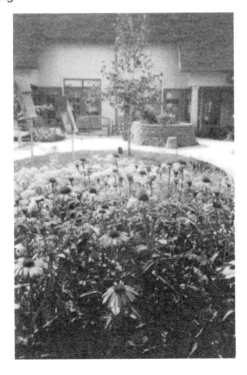

their marketing materials as being, "uniquely designed for seniors experiencing memory loss" and include a 'homelike' environment, including the feature of landscaped outdoor courtyards for strolling and sitting. Garden View is a private-pay non profit facility. However, they have been allocated several Medicaid beds to accommodate those in need.

Sunshine Center

Although the Sunshine Center is located in a busy urban area within a major Midwestern city, it is secluded by a surrounding wooden privacy fence. The facility is also located across the street from a small commuter hotel and is two buildings away from a preschool. Sunshine Center is stand-alone assisted living facility that features a "four-house" design model. The larger shell of the building is divided into four small neighborhoods that allow residents to move about safely (see Figure 6). Each of the four neighborhoods provides its own kitchen and dining area, along with a sitting/living room with comfortable furniture. The dining spaces have windows which look out onto the garden spaces. The residence features a floor plan that, according to their marketing material, "creates indoor wandering paths, safe outdoor areas and visual cues that keep residents from becoming overwhelmed or lost." Each resident has his or her own private room which includes a small bathroom and a window.

Nursing assistance and health services are provided as needed. Sunshine Center markets itself as a specialized living residence for the memory impaired. It does not provide nursing home care on site. Sunshine Center is a private pay facility without allocations for Medicaid beds.

Data Collection

Interviews were conducted with the following people: twenty-eight staff members, twelve family members, and five architects and/or designers. A total of forty-five people participated in forty-three interviews. Interviews with nursing staff members (CNA staff) comprised the core of data about what was happening in the special care units.

While spending time in each facility making observations, fieldnotes were taken in conjunction with the behavior mapping and AARS. When making observations, analytic memos and contact summaries were written (Miles & Huberman, 1984). Notes were made directly on the AARS form or on the behavior maps about what a person was doing while in the garden, albeit walking, sitting and talking to a friend, or gardening.

Many of the residents were high-functioning, inquisitive folks who had much to tell me about their thoughts about the garden and the facility in gen-

FIGURE 10. Bench along garden path for sitting and enjoying the garden. Lovely white floral interest that attracts butterflies.

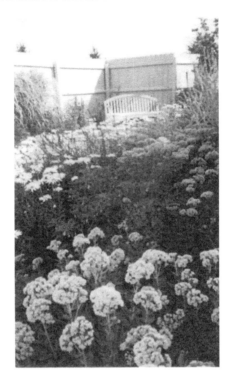

eral. Residents were opinionated and verbal about either liking or not liking certain areas of the garden spaces. At times they would point out things that didn't 'look right' to them. A common conversation was one that referred to what they liked and didn't like about their gardens in their previous homes. That information was documented by making memos.

Data Analysis

An abridged list of concepts was identified from an interview (Table 2). Three themes emerged through discussion as a result of analysis: (1) the garden as a therapeutic benefit both psychologically and physically, (2) facility operations and regulations and its impact on garden use, and (3) recommendations for improving the gardens in making it a more meaningful and/or useful space for residents, staff and families. Table 3 shows how concepts were organized according to the theme of *gardens as therapy*.

FIGURES 11 & 12. Gazebo as designated smoking space, Sunshine Center.

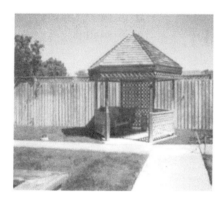 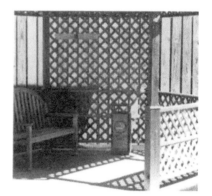

FIGURE 13. Resident out for a walk. Garden View, June 2002.

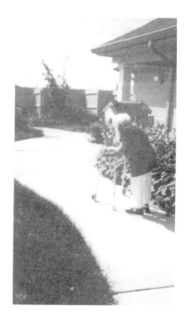

FIGURE 14. Residents came out to join gardeners. Sunshine Center.

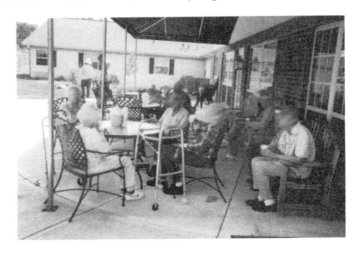

FIGURE 15. Residents outdoors in the gazebo talking. Garden View, Fall 2002.

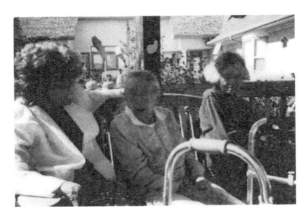

FINDINGS

Therapeutic Effects of the Gardens

Activity in the Garden

Positive comments were continually made about the garden spaces. Value was placed on the garden (or outdoor space) as a therapeutic tool for enhanc-

FIGURE 16. Resident at Garden View picking flowers. Note mailbox as a reminiscence tool.

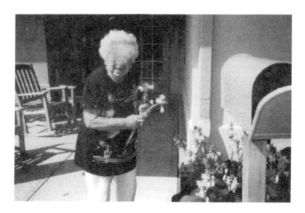

FIGURE 17. Mother (right) and Daughter (left) planting flowers in Memory Garden. Sunshine Center.

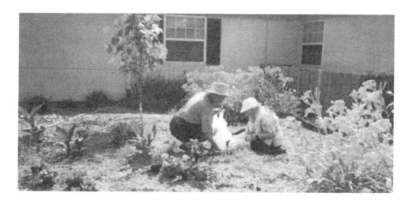

ing life quality. Staff and family members placed value on the garden space whether they could express that idea specifically or not. The responses were broken down into categories of low-level, mid-level and high-level activity.

Low-Level Activity (Passive)

Sitting Indoors Looking Out at the Garden

Francine, Family Member–Well, mother loves looking out her window at the new tulip tree we planted there for the 'memory garden.' She goes out-

FIGURE 18. Two Residents of Sunshine Center participating in planting and weeding.

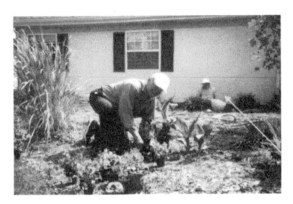

FIGURE 19. SE courtyard, Garden View. Landscape architect recommended an awning and tinted cement, but was not implemented due to budget constraints. Raised planter is not functional for residents (they can't reach inside to plant)–Photo also shows glare on sidewalk that becomes a problem in the afternoon and non-functional mailbox.

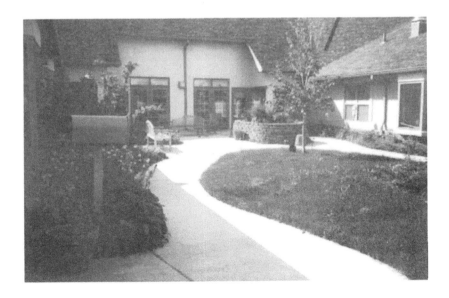

doors and walks around on a regular basis, but she also spends some time in her room . . . and she has a little bit of a view. I got her a little snowman birdfeeder which she asked me for last Christmas when we were at the store shopping. I think it's tacky, but she just loves it, and it brings her such joy to look out at it in the garden. The director said it was OK and I was so glad to do it for her. Now, I'm not sure if she realizes that it's hers today, but she smiles when she sees it and comments on it. And she always comments on the pretty flowers, isn't that a pretty color . . . aren't those yellow daylilies just gorgeous . . . look how beautiful and green that tree is . . . things like that, even when she's not actually outside she's observant about what's going on outside.

Mid-Level Activity in the Garden

Redirection and Relief from Stress and Agitation

Clearly, working in an assisted living facility is a stressful job. Effects of stress were often commented as problematic for both residents and staff members. As in the literature, the garden was mentioned as a place for "redirection" and stress relief. People with dementia often get agitated for various reasons. The following are such examples:

TABLE 2. Concepts from Interview with CNA

Concepts from interview with CNA

ability	resident conversation
agitation relief	resident freedom
boredom	resident preference
effectiveness depends on resident	resident physical ability
family visits outdoors	risk
frequency of garden use	risk of falling
garden as therapy	safety/fence
garden use	safety reasons
independent use	small number of users
monotony of interior	staff opinion of effects on residents
nurse staff "time"	without garden space
operations	staff perception
outdoor preference	staff use of garden
percentage of residents using garden	unable to describe
programs	walk outdoors more than indoors
psychological	walkers after meal
reason for not going out	walking
reminiscence	

TABLE 3. Themes Associated with "Gardens as a Therapeutic Benefit"

Experiences of observing resident behavior	*Themes*
Gardens are used as part of resident's therapy	General therapy benefit (nonspecific)
Better sleep after walking outside	Physical therapy
Actively plants tomatoes and tends the plants	Physical therapy/Autonomy
Better appetites after being outdoors	Physical benefits
Enjoys singing outside and music therapy	Psychological benefits
Goes outside and sits quietly/smiles/seems happy	Psychological benefits
Better attitude when returning from going outside	Psychological therapy
Smokes outside	Enjoyment of life habit
Diversion activity if delusional	Psychological benefits
More receptive to indoor activities after going out	Psychological/Physical
Less "sundowning" when they go out	Psychological/Physical
Reminds them of their former homes and lives	Reminiscence therapy
Keeps them in touch with nature and "reality"	Reminiscence therapy
Talks about flower types and colors	Mental benefits – recollection
Gives them something to talk about	Socialization
Sunbathing, relaxing and visiting	Normalization/Socialization
Cookouts and social gatherings are fun and they respond	

*LPN, Sunshine Center–*Some of them . . . when they get agitated and stuff . . . you know, you can ask them, "Would you like to go outside for a little while?" And for some of them it really cools them down. It calms them to be outside and away from whatever was agitating them. They see something different or feel the breeze against their skin and then they forget why they were upset. They have something else to focus on.

*Nurse, Sunshine Center–*Oh, oh, my gosh! There was a time when redirecting them to the outdoors was so helpful. I remember when nine-eleven happened . . . You know, it was very devastating . . . Very, very devastating. And I think it bothered them more than it bothered people our age. They relived World War II. They were reliving Pearl Harbor. They were going over the same stories about Pearl Harbor over and over. They were stuck . . . I finally shut the TV off. And we would go outside. And one day . . . we lit the candles that night, you know . . . across the nation. We all went outside, and lit the candles, and went out in the garden. So . . . um . . . yeah, in nursing care it can be very therapeutic to use the outdoor space . . . especially in alleviating their stress.

Nurse, Sunshine Center–We had a resident who refused to eat, and she wanted to be outside. She would like to lie on the grass and pick flowers.

We had a really bad day once and she really hadn't eaten all day and it was dinnertime. She still wasn't eating so I said, "Let's go outside." We went outside and sat in the gazebo and I took her dinner there. We sat out there and talked about the different trees and picked up a few leaves and she calmed down enough to agree to eat. The fact that it (the outdoor space) might help not medicate somebody, that it means putting someone in a better mood when you're not in the mood to eat . . . that means feeling better about themselves and eating . . . that's pretty beneficial. And you know, you go on and forget your troubles. It takes you outside, it takes you in another dimension of life. There's a real world out there beyond the walls.

Sitting Outdoors

During both interviews and observations, sitting outdoors was one of the most frequently recurring activities. All but one interview mentioned 'sitting outdoors' when describing how the space was used. Sitting outdoors allows the resident a chance to get fresh air and offers a change of scenery and atmosphere. With residents spending so much time indoors in the 'temperature-controlled' building, a place to get away from confinement, feel the breeze and sit quietly to rejuvenate is beneficial. (Helen, 1998; Hoover, 1995; Kaplan, 1973, 1998; Ulrich, 1979, 1981, 1984).

On several occasions I observed family members sitting quietly and visiting with residents just outside the doors of the facility, usually under the canopy at Sunshine Center or under the porch cover at Garden View. This observation, along with comments from interviews confirmed that, "a healing garden is even more than a place to get out to; it is a sanctuary in which a basic drive to have contact with normal forces can be met." (Zeisel, 1999, p. 115).

There was a contrasting difference at Garden View. Going outdoors to sit was more of a "structured activity," at that location and was less spontaneous. In Garden View, I noticed that staff was required to take residents out only with supervision, as their doors were kept permanently locked and alarmed. This was not the case at Sunshine Center, where residents had free access to the outdoor space. Garden View had a more developed "garden" space, and a more established perennial garden, including looping walking paths, benches and gazebo. However, the residents were not allowed to go out freely and sit due to building code regulations.

Angela, LPN–I think they enjoy being outdoors and . . . sitting outdoors. I think anything growing, that's alive and growing is therapeutic to anyone. And it brings back memories for them. If they were flower people or outdoor people, or had flower gardens . . . or garden gardens (vegetables) and so forth. It brings back memories. Many of them it might bring back memories from childhood and they'll talk about it.

A connection to routine can also be found in sitting outdoors. On five separate occasions I observed two gentlemen walking to a bench and sitting together. They had this ritual of walking quietly together and sitting on the same bench each morning. No talking occurred, but they would sit for fifteen minutes or so, look up at the sky or down and the ground for a few moments, bask in the sun a little, then get up and walk back inside to the common area. An example of an account from staff regarding sitting outdoors:

> *Sally, LPN (Garden View)*–On a nice day like today, we can take them out there to see the flowers and to sit outside and just enjoy them. And then there are a few residents that we know they love flowers. They used to like gardening (before) and used to like growing things and stuff. It's like . . . when you take them outside it kind of jazzes them and revitalizes them, you know. So you take them out there . . . if it's their thing. You know, we try to identify the one thing that they really like. And when they get that one thing, it usually just brightens their day.

Smoking

While conducting behavior mapping, I noticed staff smoking out in the garden space several times. This research was conducted in the Midwest, where smoking is still socially acceptable. Smoking in long term care facilities has been almost eliminated, but it still remains the right of employees and visitors to have a place to smoke outside the walls of the facility. Not all comments about the garden were positive. Some staff members saw the garden as "simply a place to smoke."

> *Donna, CNA*–There's only so many designated spaces where we can go to smoke a cigarette. . . . I'm a smoker, so I have to go outside the employee breakroom, and there's no shade over there. So on a day like this . . . (it was 95° F), I like to use the gazebo in the garden space. It's shady and far enough away from any of the exit doors in the Pods, but I don't smoke in front of the residents.

> *Renee, Activity Staff*–I usually take my breaks inside. I don't go outside . . . because I'm not a smoker. It's a nice garden space, so you would think I'd want to go outside, but I don't, because I don't smoke. Other employees use it because they go out there to smoke.

Many staff members referred to "walking" as one of the main reasons for using the outdoor/garden space. This is consistent with the literature. It is sometimes referred to as non-purposeful activity, or "wandering" and that the walking is happening due to agitation.

> Wandering is often without an agenda and is aimless or exploratory. Pacing is ambulation (independent or in a wheelchair), often repetitious movement, with a self-perceived agenda . . . sometimes wandering and pacing behavior can be a 'negative behavior' and often it can be a 'supportive behavior' (Helen, 1998, p. 220).

However, several staff members talk about the distinctive activity of purposeful walking with residents outside in the garden and how it also affected the residents' moods. This is also consistent with the literature that explains the health benefits, not only physically, but psychologically, of walking and gardening as good exercise which promotes wellness (Mace and Rabins, 1981, 1991, 1999; Helen, 1998; Wilcox, 2001).

When the question was asked, "What happens in the garden or outdoor space? The following statements regarding walking are representative of many of the comments made by both staff and family members,

> *Marilyn, CNA*–We walk them. Well, depending on the weather, we try to walk them at least twice a week around the garden they have out there. Sometimes . . . I know in Pod One, (Pod One being the highest functioning of the three pods), when the residents come back they're more . . . um, happy. You notice a difference in them. You know, it might not be very drastic, but there's something noticed that's different. They're not as they were before they went walking outside.

Other Physical Activities

One of the nurses summed up nicely the 'other activity' response that was representative of the majority of staff interviewed,

> *Angela, LPN*–Sometimes we play golf out there. We've done other things besides walking . . . Because no, ours (outdoor area for her unit), is not walkable . . . They're supposed to put up a gazebo out there like on the other side. (Pod 2). And they're supposed to fix the ground . . . the ground is kind of two-terraced and bumpy. They're supposed to raise that and put a walkway out there and they haven't done it yet. It would be nice if it was more like the one on the other side. (Referring to Pods Two and Three). I have taken my residents over there (from Pod One) before and we've walked around over there. They like it. I mean, not every one

of them. But many of them do. We've also played "toss the ball" and a small version of "baseball" that they can manage.

Music Therapy

It was observed that though music was a "passive" activity, the space that the music was happening in was the garden space as opposed to it occurring indoors. Because the residents who were outdoors were in the late stage of Alzheimer's disease, and many in hospice, this therapy being supported in the garden for the population is mid-level activity based on the responses of the residents. Music therapy catered to the disease's later stages by providing elements that stimulated (but not overly stimulated) residents. Use of the garden space as the therapeutic medium to deliver the stimulation is supported in research by Hoover (Stevens, 1995).

Social Activities

At times, facilities host special activities such as picnics or family gatherings to provide entertainment that is not part of the daily "activity" program. These activities are often related to holidays or spring and summer celebrations and use of the courtyards are promoted. Several staff members mentioned social activities, and below are two accounts:

> *Nursing Staff, Garden View*–Well, I've seen some of the residents in Pod Two go out there. And what they normally do there is to go out and have a picnic type of thing. Drinks and ice cream, snacks and that type of thing. And I've seen some family members joining the group. I think this is a very good courtyard.

Rituals

Staff members discussed how sometimes we forget where these residents "had lives before coming here." One CMA had a story to share about one of the residents from Florida who lived in a home with a back yard that included a pool for many years. This particular resident had a habit (ritual) in the spring and summer of sunbathing. Rituals are connected to reminiscence and can be a way of connecting people with dementia to their past, providing an important therapeutic goal of "retaining ties with something familiar" (Cohen and Weisman, 1991, p. 58).

The action of sitting was identified as a 'low-level' garden activity, but some staff and family members referred to "sitting" as a "ritual" of going out into the garden every day (or every visit in the case of family) to meditate or have quiet time. A staff member replied:

> *William, Sunshine Center—*Yes, quiet time, like at break time . . . mmm hmm . . . I do use the garden for when I'm by myself. You know . . . the garden . . . in general, garden is life. Garden is . . . Is life! I don't know how to explain (laughs) . . . It's so therapeutic to me. You reflect. You know, it gives you a little time for your meditation, you see . . . it is very positive. To give them . . . some space. The topography here is very good. Nursing home is kind of . . . you know . . . confined and institutional . . . you see the differences between here and there. Here there is so much more freedom. And the staff has so much more freedom by having a nice large yard to walk around in.

The activity creates a therapeutic environment for the staff members who are often working in a very stressful environment. Likewise, several staff members mentioned going out and sitting with residents as one of their "daily rituals."

High Level Activity

Picking Flowers, Planting and Physically Gardening

Actual use of the garden by "gardening" by planting flowers and seeds, picking flowers and working in the dirt is the highest form of garden and outdoor activity, or "self-actualization" of the garden space. Statements were made by staff and family when referring to physically gardening. The following statement illustrates both physical and psychological effects of the outdoor spaces.

> *Tom, CNA—*You know, we have flowers, plants outside. And here (in this house), like, Sam . . . Some days when he remembers, he says, "Oh, it's time now, I want to go take care of my flowers." He'll say something like that. And once outside, he'll say, "It's time, you know, to water," or something like that. He's aware that gardening is part of his life and enjoys it.

Staff supported gardening in the spring and summer in weather that was considered "safe" for the residents. As noted in the former accounts, most staff members commented about the weather being an issue in this part of the country.

Several staff and family members had a lot to say about how they interpreted the psychological as well as physical effectiveness of gardening on the residents:

Social Worker–I think because gardening it keeps their senses alive. Dementia folks cannot learn new things for the most part, unless you are extraordinarily repetitive. But, by any kind of physical therapy, and gardening is one of those, we can help maintain where they are at right now. In other words, if you had a broken hip, and you went to a physical therapist and he got you as well as you could be, but you still had a limp, if you went for a walk every day, you probably would always have a limp but you'd be able to walk. Whereas, if you didn't walk every day, you would become chair-bound. And, so the therapy of the garden is the same way. You keep your mind and body more alert. You remember perhaps names of flowers, and keep that memory instead of losing it. Every day I'm going to tell you, "Oh what a beautiful rose, did you ever grow roses?" And so, I'm just reminding you every day. And the beautiful smells that come from the garden, and color identification that they may forget without the garden. So, I think it's just *one* part of their therapy, but it's a necessary part in my opinion.

Other Themes and Comments

Weather Concerns

Because the sites are in the Midwest, discussion of the weather came up in almost every conversation. Weather was an issue during fieldwork. During the first week, doors were locked because the temperature was averaging over 90 degrees. This limited access for residents to the garden. During the second week, cooler weather and wind deterred residents from using the garden.

Facilities and Operations Management

Due to building code regulations, residents in Garden View could not use the garden unassisted since the doors leading to the garden were locked and alarmed. Therefore, much of the data processed from behavior mapping and fieldnotes indicated that the garden spaces were empty much of the time. Despite the positive comments from the staff regarding the garden and it's benefits, resident access was limited not only to the doors being locked, but because they were locked, when staff had the time to take them. This was a sore subject amongst staff.

Sunshine Center had a similar garden space design in that it was also surrounded by a wooden fence to keep residents inside the facility. However, the important difference was in access. Residents could freely go outdoors unassisted without the alarm engaging. The only time the doors were locked was during inclimate weather, for the safety of the residents. At those times, the residents comings and goings were monitored to minimize risk.

Most comments regarding the garden spaces were positive, however, there were some conflicting statements about the actual opinions regarding the 'use' of the garden space. A few of the staff members either did not notice much use of the space, or they were not outdoorsy-types and didn't like going outdoors themselves. Their replies indicate disparity in the findings, which must be mentioned in qualitative research (Cresswell, 2003). An example of such a report was:

> *Bart, CNA–They try to get through the door, but they don't really* know where they're going. They're not trying to get outside . . . they're just trying to get out.

Since there were conflicting reports and comments about the garden not being used and perceived as not being of particular value to everyone, the following question was asked, "Do you think it would be any different for the residents if they didn't have the outdoor area here? What do you think it would be like if it was just the building without the additional outdoor space?" Most frequent responses indicated that absence of garden spaces and outdoor access would be a problem for both residents and their family members.

CONCLUSION

Garden View and Sunshine Center provide exemplary outdoor spaces for their residents. The administration in both facilities understands that the outdoor space is essential to the wellbeing of their residents and recognizes the need brought forth by their clients, the primary caregivers and family members. Since there are no regulations or requirements for the outdoor spaces in dementia care facilities, the fact that such nice garden spaces are offered to the residents says much about the caring nature of the management of the two facilities. However, the results of the post-occupancy evaluation showed how improvements can continue to be made within the existing spaces. John Zeisel, in *Inquiry by Design* (1981), describes design development as "a spiral metaphor" that reflects the pattern of thinking that designers go through when solving a design problem. Backtracking through the process to revise or alter previous design decisions and to repeat previous design activities with a shifted focus, together with the simultaneous movement of backtracking, repetition, and linking the cycles of imaging, presenting, and testing brings the designer closer to an application to a built solution (Zeisel, 1981, pp. 14-18).

Using Robert Kumlin's (1995) architectural programming conceptual framework as a guide, along with analysis of the research from architects, family and staff, the following recommendations for improvements to the existing garden spaces were proposed:

Issue: Therapeutic gardens for people in special care units with dementia

Objective: The garden design should reflect the understanding of the disease symptoms of dementia and progression of the disease and support the population that inhabits the space (residents, staff and visitors).

Concept: Safety, comfort and clear paths to encourage garden use as therapeutic support which complements the activity and therapy happening inside the building.

Consider the following improvements to the existing facilities:

- Provide a few outdoor handrails for residents in the garden space so that those who have an unsteady gait have something to hold onto while walking. Residents have a habit of using the handrails or walkers indoors, and a continuation of that design element and physical support would allow them to be more confident going outdoors.
- Provide the courtyards with more shade (awning or umbrellas could assist) since the sun and glare are barriers to use.
- A solarium or conservatory can act as an extension of the outdoors since the residents often complain of being cold, or the weather being 'too windy' even in the summertime. This could be located off of a common living or dining area. Such a feature could assist with heating in the winter and provide a place for horticultural therapy.
- Provide a walking path with less glare. Adding color to the concrete would be better. It gets too bright for the residents.
- Additional shade trees could assist with the glare issue. More shade trees would be inviting to use the outdoor space.
- Plant more flowers with bright colors. Residents notice bright yellow and red flowers and enjoy a variety of color. When they notice the flowers it cues them to go outdoors or cues conversation.
- Provide a small spot (preferably waist-high) where residents can "get their hands dirty." Residents discuss working in the soil and often talk about wishing they could plant something like they used to do. Such a provision enhances physical therapy.
- The dog house in Pods 2 and 3 at Garden View confused residents. Some residents were afraid during walks that a dog would come out. Moving

this 'reminiscence' item to Pod 1 would allow residents who have higher functioning abilities to appreciate it. The dog is located in Pod 1, therefore it is appropriate to move the doghouse there. Another problem with the dog and use of the Pod 1 grassy area was lack of a place for the dog to relieve himself.

- Additionally, residents in Pod 2 commented that, "we don't get mail," so the mail boxes are acting as purely decorative elements. Moving them to Pod 1 and integrating an activity with them would lessen confusion.
- Providing fall *and* spring plant material so that there is "seasonal interest" increases time awareness and cues conversation.
- Planting non-toxic plant materials.

Reflections on the Notion of Gardens in Special Care Units

The results do not offer all the answers to the questions regarding the effects of therapeutic gardens, but it is possible, through collaboration, to initiate a conversation about the process. A multidisciplinary approach involving designers, medical staff, administrators, family members, social workers, physical therapists, etc., as a team can enhance the benefits of the outdoor spaces. Each member can then contribute towards a comprehensive therapeutic intervention that enhances quality of life for residents. There is no 'prototype' for therapeutic garden design that will fit the needs of every special care unit. However, once landscape architects develop a collaborative relationship with health care professionals, they can begin to define the role of the garden in health care today. Dementia care facilities have a special needs population with corresponding special requirements for design. Until the late stages of dementia, however, residents are often able to participate in using an outdoor space. As one nurse mentioned, "getting residents involved in the design process would allow them to take ownership."

The majority of residents living in special care units require assistance with various activities of daily living which primarily happens on the 'inside' of the building. The findings in this study suggest that some activities could be taken outdoors (such as physical therapy, meals and music therapy) to complement some of the more medically-related therapies residents receive. Such a complementary and integrative approach in incorporating the garden space as an important aspect of living in the facility would benefit not only the residents, but the staff and family members as well. The garden additionally becomes a 'coping mechanism' for family members to seek respite and staff members to seek diversion.

Due to the unrelenting effects of chronic illnesses such as dementia, it is not surprising that integrative and complementary medicine has gained popularity in recent years. 'Alternative medicine' is a term that has been used to suggest a separate paradigm for a miscellaneous group of unconventional treatments by practitioners, both medical and nonmedical, who use a holistic approach to patient care. Other terms such as 'complementary' and 'integrative' have been suggested, which includes examples of therapies such as acupuncture, aromatherapy, massage and physical therapy. It is estimated that at least one half of all patients seek cures by such methods, and HMO's and third party payers are beginning to reimburse for such unconventional therapy (Ulett, 2001). Findings show important benefits from complementary therapies to people suffering from chronic diseases (Ulett, 2001; Weil, 2002; Ornish, 1995; Yancey, 2001).

Based on this study, I believe that therapeutic gardens should be considered in this body of 'integrative' treatments used to complement the special care unit of the dementia care facility. Such an approach can even be taken into the nursing home once administrators and health care providers can see how the garden space is essential to the wellbeing of resident's care. Residents without a garden space to look out onto or walk into miss out on a vital component of nature, sunshine and fresh air, an opportunity to socialize and even the opportunity to 'get their hands dirty,' which may result in reminiscence and maintenance of physical and mental abilities. As one of the staff members noted, "garden and outdoor space symbolizes life."

Until a cure is found for Alzheimer's disease and other forms of dementia, a more holistic approach to therapy, including therapeutic gardens, can improve the quality of the environment by incorporating nature into the equation. I suggest therapeutic gardens as a new building standard in nursing homes. If Medicare, Medicaid and private insurances reimbursed facilities for providing such garden spaces, the potential might be that they become a standard in the long-term care housing industry. Based on what is happening in the demand for outdoor spaces and gardens in assisted living facilities, the evolution of getting away from the standard medical model seems plausible.

In addition, landscape architects can contribute to improving the quality of life of people living with dementia by understanding the clinical aspects of diseases so that they can properly design outdoor spaces for them. In this way landscape architects will be able to engage in conversation with the medical community to provide alternative solutions for healthy environments. Likewise, facility managers and owners should be prepared to live with the consequences of negative environment and behavior reactions as a result of ignoring valuable advice. If it is the goal of the medical doctor to "do no harm" then the built environment should follow this lead by providing an essential element–the garden that complements the interior space.

The garden is a metaphor for life. Just as the soil rejuvenates the plant and supports its growth through the plant life cycle, the design of the garden supports the resident with dementia through their human cycle, connecting them to the reality of their own mortality in a non-threatening and natural way.

REFERENCES

Abeles, P.R., Gift, H.C., & Ory, M.G. (1994). *Aging and quality of life.* New York: Springer Publishing Co.

Alzheimer's Association. (2006). Alzheimer's Disease Statistics. Chicago, IL. Informational fact sheet. http://www.alz.org.

American Horticulture Therapy Association. http://www. ahta.org.

ASLA Seminar. (2001). *"Therapeutic Environments: New Developments in Canada and the US."* On-line seminar. Participant. Robert Hoover, Virginia Burt and Vince Healy, guest speakers.

Barker, R. (1968). *Ecological Psychology.* Stanford, CA: Stanford University Press.

Barker, R. & Wright, H. (1978). *Habitats, Environments and Human Behavior.* San Francisco: Jossey-Boss.

Brannon, D. & Smyer, M.A. (1994). *Good work and good care in nursing homes.* Generations, 18(3), 34-38.

Brawley, E. C. (1997). *Designing for Alzheimer's disease: Strategies for creating better environments.* New York: Wiley.

_____ (2002). *Therapeutic Gardens for Individuals with Alzheimer's Disease.* Alzheimer's Care Quarterly 3(1): 7-11. Aspen Publishers, Inc.

_____ (2002). The Relationship Between Alzheimer's Disease & Design. In *The Center for Health Design.* Retrieved April 10, 2002, from AEsclepius Online Newsletter. http://www.healthdesign.org/brawley.html.

Calkins, M. P. (1988). *Design for Dementia: Planning Environments for the Elderly and the Confused.* National Health Publishing.

_____ (1989). *"Designing Cues for Wanderers"* In *Architecture.* October, pp. 117-118.

Carstens, D. Y. (1998). *"Outdoor Spaces in Housing for the Elderly"* In *People Places,* second edition, C. Cooper Marcus and C. Francis, editors. New York: Van Nostrand Reinhold.

Carpman, J., Grant, M., and Simmons, D. (1986). *Design that Cares: Planning, Health Facilities for Patients and Visitors.* American Hospital Publishing, Inc.

Chambers, N. (1995). *Enhanced Therapeutic Outcomes: Therapeutic Horticulture Gardens.* Journal of Healthcare Design. vol. 7, pp. 169-174.

Chaudhury, H. (2002). "Place-Biosketch as a Tool in Caring for Residents with Dementia" In *Alzheimer's Care Quarterly.* 3(1): 42-45.

Clark, P. & Bowling, A. (1989). *Observational study of quality of life in NHS nursing homes and a long stay ward for the elderly.* Aging and Society, 9, 123-148.

Cohen, G. D. (1998). *Anxiety in Alzheimer's disease: theoretical and clinical perspectives.* Journal of Geriatric Psychiatry. 31(2): 103-115.

Cohen, U. and Day, K. (1993). *Contemporary Environments for People with Dementia*. Baltimore, Maryland: The John Hopkins University Press.

Cohen, U. and Weisman, G. (1991). *Holding on to Home*. Baltimore, MD: Johns Hopkins University Press.

Coons, D. (1991). *Specialized Dementia Care Units*. Baltimore, MD: Johns Hopkins University Press.

Cooper Marcus, C. (1978). "Remembrance of landscapes past." In *Landscape*. 22(3): 35-43.

_____. (1992). "Environmental memories." In *Place Attachment*, ed. I. Altman and S. M. Low. NY and London: Plenum Press.

Cooper Marcus, C. and C. Francis. (1998). *People Places*, New York: Van Nostrand, Reinhold.

Cooper Marcus, C. and Barnes, M. (1995). *Gardens in Healthcare Facilities: Uses, Therapeutic Benefits, and Design Recommendations*. Martinez, CA: The Center for Health Design.

_____. (1998). "Gardens in hospitals: their role in reducing stress and fostering human well-being." In *ASLA Annual Meeting Proceedings,* ed. D. L. Scheu, 53-56. Washington D.C.: The society.

_____. (1999). *Healing Gardens: Therapeutic Benefits and Design Recommendations*. New York: John Wiley & Sons, Inc.

Corbin, J. and Strauss, A. (1990). Grounded theory research: Procedures, canons, and evaluative criteria. *Qualitative Sociology*, 13(1), 3-21.

Coyne, R.K., and Clack, R.J. (1981). *Environmental Assessment and Design: A New Tool for the Applied Behavioral Scientist*. New York: Praeger Publishers.

Cresswell, J.W. (1998). *Qualitative Inquiry and Research Design: Choosing among five traditions*. Sage Publications.

Cummings, J., (1999). *Practical Alzheimer's Disease Management: A Comparative Review of New Compounds, Diagnosis, Treatment, and Outcomes Assessment*. Postgraduate Medicine; A Special Report. May 1999.

Dannenmaier, M. (1995). *Healing Gardens*. In *Landscape Architecture*, January.

Day, K., Carreon D., and Stump, C. (2000). "The therapeutic design of environments for people with dementia: A review of the empirical research." In *The Gerontologist*. 40(4): 397-416.

DeBaggio, T. (2002). *Losing My Mind: An Intimate Look at Life with Alzheimer's*. New York: The Free Press.

Doherty, E., ed. (1989). *New Images: Quality of life in a long term care facility*. Denver: Colorado Gerontological Society.

Ebel, S. (1991). *Designing stage-specific horticultural therapy interventions for patients with Alzheimer's disease*. Journal of Therapeutic Horticulture. 6: 3-9.

Evans, L. (1996). *Healing Gardens*. In *Metropolis*. October, pp. 135-137.

Faletti, M.V. (1984). "Human factors research and functional environments for the aged." In I. Altman, M.P. Lawton and J.F. Wohlwill, eds. *Elderly People and the Environment*. New York: Plenum.

Flanagan, J.C. (1978). *A research approach to improving our quality of life*. American Psychology. 33: 138-147.

Francis, M. and Hester, R. (1990). *The Meaning of Gardens: Idea, Place and Action.* MIT Press.

Gerlach-Spriggs, N. (1999). "A healing vision." In *Landscape Architecture.* 89(4): 134-135.

Gerlach-Spriggs, N., Kaufman, R.E., & Warner, S.B.J. (1998). *Restorative Gardens: The Healing Landscape.* New Haven and London; Yale University Press.

Glaser, B., and Strauss, A. (1967). *The Discovery of Grounded Theory.* Chicago: Aldine.

Gubrium, J.F. (1992). *Qualitative research comes of age in gerontology.* In *The Gerontologist.* 32(5), 581-582.

_____ (1975). *Living and Dying in Murray Manor.* The University Press of Virginia.

Hammersley, M. (1992). *Deconstructing the Qualitative-Quantitative Divide,* in J. Brannen (ed.), Mixing Methods: Qualitative and Quantitative Research, Aldershot, Avebury.

Hartig, T., Mang, M., & Evans, G.W. (1991). "Restorative Effects of Natural Environment Experiences," *Environment and Behavior,* 23(1), 3-26.

Haas, K. and McCartney, R. (1996). "The Therapeutic Quality of Plants." In *Journal of Therapeutic Horticulture.* Vol. VIII.

Healy, V. (1987). *The Hospice Garden: Addressing the Patient Needs Through Landscape.* Harvard University.

Helen, C. R. (1998). *Alzheimer's disease: activity-focused care.* Butterworth-Heinemann.

Hill, J., Schirm, V. (1996). *Attitudes of nursing staff toward restraint use in long-term care.* Journal of Applied Gerontology, 15 (3), 314-324.

Horrigan, P. 1997. *"The Hospice Garden: Sustaining Wellness and Resolution."* ASLA Annual Meeting Proceedings, 1997.

Hoover, R.C. (1995). "Healing gardens and Alzheimer's disease." In *The American Journal of Alzheimer's Disease.* March/April.

Institute of Medicine. (1986). *Improving the quality of care in nursing homes.* Washington, DC; National Academic Press.

Kamp, D. (1996). "Healing Environments I: Restorative Gardens". In *Loeb Fellowship Forum.* Cambridge, MA. Spring/Summer. pp. 4-5.

Kaplan, M. (1994). "Use of sensory stimulation with Alzheimer's patients in a garden setting." In *People-plant relationships: setting research priorities,* ed. Joel Flagler and Raymond P. Poincelot. Binghamton, NY: Haworth Press.

Kaplan, R. (1973). "Some Psychological Benefits of Gardening". *Environment and Behavior.* Vol. 5(2): 145-152.

Kaplan, R. and Kaplan S. (1989). *The Experience of Nature: A Psychological Perspective.* Cambridge, MA: Cambridge University Press, 1989.

_____. (1982). *Humanscape: Environments for People.* Ann Arbor, Michigan.

Kaplan, S. (1995). "The restorative benefits of nature: toward an integrative framework." In *Journal of Environmental Psychology.* 15(3): 169-182.

Kaplan, R., Kaplan, S., and Ryan, R.L. (1998). *With People in Mind: Design and Management of Everyday Nature.* Washington, D.C., Covelo, California; Island Press.

Kitwood, T. (1997). *Dementia Reconsidered: The Person Comes First.* Scarborough; Open University Press.

Knopf, R.C. (1987). *Handbook of Environmental Psychology*, pp. 783-925.

Kuhn, Daniel (1999). *Alzheimer's Early Stages: First Steps for Family, Friends and Caregivers.* Hunter House, Inc. Publishers. 2nd edition, 2000.

Kumlin, R. (1995). *Architectural Programming: Creative Techniques for Design Professionals.* McGraw-Hill.

Lawton, M.P. (1991). "A multidimensional view of quality of life in frail elders." In J. E. Birren, J. Lubben, J.C. Rowe, & D.E. Deutchman (Eds.), *The concept and measurement of quality of life* (pp. 3-27). New York: Academic Press.

Lawton, M.P. (1997). *Assessing quality of life in Alzheimer's disease research.* Alzheimer's Disease and Associated Disorders. 11(6): 91-99.

_____(1998). Environment and Aging Theory Revisited. In R. J. Scheidt and P.G. Windley (Eds.) *Environment and Aging Theory.* Westport, Connecticut: Greenwood Press.

Lawton, M.P., Van Haitsma, K. & Klapper, J. (1996). *Observed affect in nursing home residents with Alzheimer's disease.* Journal of Gerontology; Psychological Sciences, 51B, P3-P14.

Lawton, M., Brody, E. & Sapersetien, A. (1989). *A controlled study of respite service for caregivers of Alzheimer's patients.* The Gerontologist, 29, 8-16.

Lawton, M.P. and Rubenstein. (2000). *Interventions in Dementia Care: Toward improving quality of life.* New York: Springer Publishing.

Lewin, K. (1936). *Principles of Topological Psychology.* New York: McGraw-Hill.

Lewis, C. A. (1996). *Green Nature/Human Nature: The Meaning of Plants in Our Lives.* Urbana and Chicago; University of Illinois Press.

Lovering, M.J. (1990). *Alzheimer's disease and outdoor space: Issues in environmental design.* The American Journal of Alzheimer's Care and Related Disorders & Research. May/June.

Mace, N. and Rabins, P. (1991). *The 36-Hour Day: A Family Guide to Caring for Persons with Alzheimer Disease, Related Dementing Illnesses, and Memory Loss in Later Life.* Johns Hopkins Press Health.

Maslow, A. (1954). *Motivation and Personality.* New York: Harper and Row.

_____. (1968). *Toward a Psychology of Being.* New York: D. Van Nostrand Company.

Mather, J.A., Nemecek, D., & Oliver, K. (1997). *"The effect of a walled garden on behavior of individuals with Alzheimer's."* American Journal of Alzheimer's Disease. November/December.

Maxwell, J. (1996). *Qualitative Research Design: An Interactive Approach.* Sage Publications.

Miles, M.B., & Huberman, A.M. (1984). *Qualitative data analysis: An expanded sourcebook* (2nd) ed. Thousand Oaks, CA: Sage.

Mooney, P.F. and Hoover, R.C. (1996). *"The Design of Restorative Landscapes for Alzheimer's Patients."* ASLA Annual Meeting Proceedings, 1996.

Mooney, P. and Nicell, P. (1992). "The importance of exterior environment for Alzheimer residents: effective care and risk management." In *Health Care Management Forum.* p. 8.

Munson, R. (2000). *Intervention and Reflection: Basic Issues in Medical Ethics.* Wadsworth.

National Nursing Home Survey. National Center for Health Statistics, 1985; p. 49.

Nelson, J. (1995). "The influence of environmental factors in incidents of disruptive behavior." In *Journal of Gerontological Nursing.* 21(5): 19-23.

Namazi, K.H., & Johnson, B. (1992). "Pertinent autonomy for residents with dementias; modification of the physical environment to enhance independence." *American Journal of Alzheimer Care and Related Disorders and Research.* 16-21.

Nollman, J. (1994). *Why We Garden: Cultivating a Sense of Place.* New York: Henry Holt.

Olds, A.R. (1985). Cited in Cooper Marcus, C. and Barnes, M., *Healing Gardens: Therapeutic Benefits and Design Recommendations.* John Wiley & Sons, 1999. p. 8.

Oliver, D. and Tureman, S. (1988). *The Human Factor in Nursing Home Care.*

Patton, M. (2002). *Qualitative Research & Evaluation Methods.* London, UK: Sage Publications

Petersen, R. (2002). *Mayo Clinic on Alzheimer's Disease.* New York.

Post, S. G. (1995). *Ethical Issues from Diagnosis to Dying: The Moral Challenge of Alzheimer Disease.* 2000. 2nd Edition. The Johns Hopkins University Press.

Purcell, A.T., Lamb, R.J., Peron, E.M, and Falchero, S. (1994). "Preference or preferences for landscape." In *Journal of Environmental Psychology.* 14: 159-209.

Rawlings, R. (1999). *Healing Gardens.* London.

Relf, D. Ed. (1992). *The Role of Horticulture in Human Well-Being and Social Development.* Portland, OR: Timber Press.

Rodgers, E. B. (2001). *Landscape Design: A Cultural and Architectural History.* New York: Harry N. Abrams, Inc.

Rubin, A. and Babbie, E. (1993). *Research methods for social work.* Pacific Grove, CA: Brooks/Cole Publishing Company.

Schoggen, M. (1978). *Ecological Psychology and Mental Retardation.* In G. Sackett (Ed.), *Observing Behavior. Volume One, Theory and applications in mental retardation.* Baltimore, Maryland: University Park Press.

Schwarz, B. (1996). *Nursing Home Design: Consequences of Employing the Medical Model.* New York: Garland Publishing.

Schwarz, B. et al. (2002). *Impact of Design Interventions in Nursing Home on Residents with Dementia, their Families and the Staff.* Institute on Aging and Environment, University of Wisconsin, Milwaukee.

Sebastian, K. I. (1999). *The Garden as an Environment for the Treatment of Alzheimer's Disease.* Master's Design Project, University of Massachusetts.

Shenk, D. (2001). *The Forgetting. Alzheimer's: Portrait of an Epidemic.* New York: Doubleday.

Shimer, P. (2002). *New Hope for People with Alzheimer's and Their Caregivers.* Prima Publishing.

Sommer, R. (1969). *Personal Space.* Englewood Cliffs, NJ: Prentice-Hall, Inc.

Steven, M.L., and Armstrong, H. (1995). "The congruent garden: The role of the domestic garden in satisfying fundamental human needs." In *International People-Plant Symposium,* July. Sydney, Australia.

Stevens, M. (1995). "Life in Fast-Forward Reverse." In *Landscape Architecture.* 85(1): 76-79.

Strauss, A. (1987). *Qualitative Analysis for Social Scientists*. New York: Cambridge University Press.

Strauss, A., and Corbin, J. (1990). *Basics of Qualitative Research: Grounded Theory Procedures and Techniques*. Newbury Park, CA: Sage.

_____. (1994). "Grounded theory methodology: An overview." In *Handbook of qualitative research*. Thousand Oaks, CA: Sage.

Taylor, G. and Cooper, G. (2001). "Anatomy of a Healing Garden." *Landscape Architect and Specifier News*, February 2001.

Thomas, W.H. (1994). *The Eden Alternative: Nature, Hope and Nursing Homes*. First printing: June, University of Missouri.

Thompson, W.J. (1998). "A question of healing." In *Landscape Architecture*. 88(4): 66-73, 89-92.

Tuan, Y.F. (1977). *Space and Place*. Minneapolis: University of Minnesota Press.

Tyson, M. (1989). *The Healing Landscape*. New York: McGraw-Hill.

_____. (2002). "Treatment Gardens: Naturally Mapped Environments and Independence." *Alzheimer's Care Quarterly* 3(1): 55-60. Aspen Publishers, Inc.

Tyson, M. (2002). Telephone Interview.

Ulrich, R.S. and Parsons, R. (1992). "Influences of Passive Experiences with Plants on Individual Well-Being and Health". In *The Role of Horticulture in Human Well-Being and Social Development: A National Symposium*, D. Relf, editor-in-chief. Portland Oregon: Timber Press.

Ulrich, R.S. (1979). "Effects of Interior Design on Wellness: Theory and Scientific Research." In *Journal of Health Care Design*.

_____. (1981). "Natural versus urban scenes, some psychophysiological effects." In *Environment and Behavior*. 13:523-556.

_____. (1993). "Biophilia, Biophobia, and Natural Landscapes." In *The Biophilia Hypothesis*. Island Press.

_____. (1984). "View through a window may influence recovery from surgery." In *Science*. April. v. 224, pp. 420-421.

US Dept. of Health and Human Services. (1998). *Alzheimer's Disease: estimates of prevalence in the United States*. Washington, DC: General Accounting Office; 1998. HEHS-98-16.

Warner, S.B. (1992). "The Human Side: A Brief History of Healing Gardens in Healthcare Settings." *Journal of Healthcare Design*, vol. 7, pp. 213-219.

_____. (1995). "Restorative Landscapes." Landscape Architecture. 85(1): 128.

_____. (1994). "The periodic rediscoveries of restorative gardens: 1100 to the present." In *The Healing Dimensions of People-Plant Relations: Proceedings of a Research Symposium;* eds. Mark Francis, Pat Lindsey, Jay Stone Lindsey. University of California at Davis.

Westphal, J. (1999). "More Hype than Healing? A status report on the therapeutic garden." *Landscape Architecture*. April.

Whitehouse, S., Varni, J.W., Seid, M., Cooper Marcus, C., Enserg, M.J., Jacobs, J.R. and Mehlenbeck, R.S. (2001). *Evaluating a children's hospital garden environment: Utilization and consumer satisfaction*. Journal of Environmental Psychology, vol. 21, pp. 301-314.

Wilson, E.O. (1984). *Biophilia*. Harvard University Press.

Zeisel, J. (1981). *Inquiry by Design: Tools for Environment-Behavior Research.* Belmont, California: Brooks/Cole Publishing Co.

Zeisel, J., Hyde, J., and Levkoff, S. (1994). "Best practices: An environment-behavior (E-B) model of physical design for special care units." In *Journal of Alzheimer's Disease* 9:4-21.

Zeisel, J. and Tyson, M. (1999). "Alzheimer's Treatment Gardens: Design Guidelines and Case Studies". In *Healing Gardens: Therapeutic Benefits and Design Recommendations.* C. Cooper Marcus and M. Barnes, editors. New York; Wiley.

doi:10.1300/J081v21n01_07

Wholistic Design in Dementia Care: Connection to Nature with PLANET

Garuth Eliot Chalfont

SUMMARY. Interdisciplinary evidence suggests that nature has a therapeutic role to play in dementia care, but designing a person's connection to nature within residential environments lacks a wholistic approach. This paper argues for design integration of nature into dementia care that is interdisciplinary and evidence-based, but one that is also informed by the daily acts of dwelling. To that end it proposes PLANET, a comprehensive checklist for investigating the potential for connection to nature for people living in dementia care environments. A brief review of the supporting literature on the benefits of nature is presented leading to the theoretical design and a description of the six domains: Person, Location, Architecture, Nature, Energy and Technology. Evidence is presented from people with dementia using nature in edge spaces of buildings to demonstrate the person-centered approach to the ongoing development of the tool. doi:10.1300/J081v21n01_08 *[Article copies available for a fee from The Haworth Document Delivery Service: 1-800-HAWORTH. E-mail address: <docdelivery@haworthpress.com> Website: <http://www.HaworthPress.com> © 2007 by The Haworth Press, Inc. All rights reserved.]*

Garuth Eliot Chalfont, PhD, ASLA, is Researcher, School of Architecture, University of Sheffield, Western Bank, Sheffield S10 2TN UK (E-mail: g.chalfont@sheffield.ac.uk).

[Haworth co-indexing entry note]: "Wholistic Design in Dementia Care: Connection to Nature with PLANET." Chalfont, Garuth Eliot. Co-published simultaneously in *Journal of Housing for the Elderly* (The Haworth Press, Inc.) Vol. 21, No. 1/2, 2007, pp. 153-177; and: *Outdoor Environments for People with Dementia* (ed: Susan Rodiek and Benyamin Schwarz) The Haworth Press, Inc., 2007, pp. 153-177. Single or multiple copies of this article are available for a fee from The Haworth Document Delivery Service [1-800-HAWORTH, 9:00 a.m. - 5:00 p.m. (EST). E-mail address: docdelivery@haworthpress.com].

Available online at http://jhe.haworthpress.com
doi:10.1300/J081v21n01_08

KEYWORDS. Dementia, residential care, nature, environment, edge space

INTRODUCTION

Nature-related activities are a normal part of life–looking out the window, pottering in the garden and walking in the countryside. Such basic pleasures are often unattainable for a person with dementia living in a care setting, which by design may exclude a wide range of natural, sensory experiences. Design professionals and care practitioners aim to construct 'living' environments in both senses of the word. This paper contributes to these efforts by arguing for a wholistic, interdisciplinary approach to integrating nature into dementia care environments. Such an approach would provide care environments that support both natural sensory stimulation and nature-based activities. To design, upgrade and improve such care environments would require a comprehensive checklist tool such as PLANET to investigate the potential for the environment to provide a connection to nature for the residents. This paper will first argue for a wholistic approach to designing nature into dementia care environments by presenting a brief review of the supporting literature as well as describing the theory supporting the tool. Data from observational studies of dementia care settings in the USA, the UK and Scandinavia are presented as they contributed to the early development of PLANET, which is then described with its six domains.

Need for a Wholistic Approach and a Comprehensive Checklist Tool

From published literature, practical knowledge and design expertise one can establish a basic checklist of the elements required for people to engage in the outdoors or to actively participate in nature-based activities. There are existing checklists for elements and characteristics of therapeutic landscapes, healthcare gardens and outdoor areas in long-term care environments. Although these are a helpful step towards improving environments, the provision of features alone does not ensure the garden will be used. There remains the great divide between indoors and outdoors, architecture and landscape architecture, designers and care providers, and managers and care staff which remains central to the chronic underutilisation of these spaces. It is these divisions which the approach and the tool described in this paper hope to address.

An extensive review of the evidence on the importance of nature for older people, and particularly for people with dementia, and on current nature-based treatment approaches was conducted to determine the range of elements and dynamics an environment must contain or support in order to provide a connection to nature. A brief sampling from that review which appears elsewhere (Chalfont, 2006) is presented below. What this survey of the literature revealed was a lack of ethnographic evidence of how people with dementia actually use and experience natural stimuli, in other words, their subjective experience which would give a more wholistic picture. Such an approach would require evidence gathered from people in the daily acts of dwelling–the moments throughout the day in which people habitually and routinely engage with nature, not just the specific nature-based activities we tend to think of in care provision, but the ways we as physiological beings maintain an ongoing sensory relationship with the natural world. With this evidence, in addition to interventional studies, a comprehensive checklist tool can then consider the broadest possible range of environmental elements providing the potential for connection to nature for people with dementia living in the building. To address this need for evidence, a study was designed to explore how people accomplish connection to nature on a daily basis–not just what physical elements existed, but what natural stimuli the environment contained and how people used or engaged with them. From this study (a sample of the data is presented in the following section) a set of six domains was constructed, hence the acronym PLANET. Within each domain a set of criteria began to be constructed with which a care environment could then be investigated for connection to nature for residents. Beyond the practical questions of how people accomplish connection to nature lies the more important consideration of why people use nature–why the mechanism of connection to nature is important and meaningful. This will be highlighted as it arose in the data presented below, but in-depth treatment of this topic is forthcoming (Chalfont, 2008) and beyond the scope of this paper.

LITERATURE REVIEW

Connection to nature is beneficial for individual health and wellbeing (Devlin, 1980; Kaplan, 1973, 2001; Lewis, 1996; Ulrich, 1984, 1999), within the home environment (Kaplan, 2001; Markus & Gray, 1973) and for older people (Devlin, 1980; Ottosson & Grahn, 2005; Tang & Brown, 2005; van Loon, 2004). Architectural design to incorporate nature begins with a synthesis of the program needs of the client and building users with the existing natural setting, resulting in the overall form and organization of interior and exterior spaces to accommodate functions and patterns of movement. Within this design process nature is brought into the building as a result of this overall attention to form (floor plan, building height, spatial arrangement, aspect, orientation, light penetration, surfaces, materials, ceiling and window height, building form, placement on the lot, etc.) (see Torrington, 2004), and through architectural features such as doors, skylights and fenestration. If the building is not configured organically to invite nature inside, then windows and doors become crucial in connection to the outside world. Furthermore, a well-designed building may be compromised by actual patterns of movement and with unintended usage (doors locked or blocked, height or location of furniture out of relationship to windows, schedule of room occupation, etc.) which will lower a person's connection to nature. Caregivers can compensate for interior spaces low in daylight, fresh air and views by modifying the environment or the time the resident spends there.

Beyond the architect's intention and the actions of family and professional caregivers, providing nature therapeutically for people with dementia differs in aims, methods and tools for accountability. Intervention studies concerning nature are of two basic kinds: physical treatment to the person (e.g., sensory stimulation with herbal compounds) or modifications to the environment (e.g., making a nature-enhanced area by enlarging lounge windows towards a view of the rabbits)–each with mixed results. Sensory stimulation studies lack evidence of positive lasting effect for people with dementia in terms of reduced agitation, aggression or other symptoms, although short term benefits occur (Baker et al., 2001; Ballard, O'Brien, Reichelt, & Perry, 2002). Intervention by environmental modification measures empirically the effect on a person's behavior. But the effects of nature are not easily isolated from those of the intervention itself. For instance, a controlled study of the Eden Alternative which introduced pets, plants and children into a nursing home observed (but did not report measurement) of qualitative improvement in staff and residents (Coleman et al., 2002).

Methods of providing connection to nature for people with dementia			
Approach	Actors	Examples	Assessment
Intervention by physical treatment to affect behavior or symptoms	Care or nursing staff Massage therapists	Aromatherapy, massage, Snoezelen and multi-sensory stimulation (MSS)	Quantitative & qualitative studies
Intervention by social activities or 'culture change' for therapeutic or rehabilitative effect	Horticultural therapists Social workers Volunteers Activity directors	Social & therapeutic horticulture (UK) gardening for dementia' Horticultural therapy (USA) Eden Alternative (pets & plants)	Participant counts Qualitative accounts
Design of the outdoor environment by using gardens or landscaping	Landscape architects Garden designers	Sensory gardens Alzheimer's gardens	POEs, User surveys
Design of buildings and design of the built environment	Architects & designers Builders & care providers	Daylighting to combat SAD Views to internal courtyards	POEs User surveys
Intervention by environmental modification to existing bldgs to affect behavior or symptoms	Architects & designers Builders Care providers	Enhanced environment Ward relocation	Quantitative & qualitative studies

While intervention studies must strive to factor out the positive effects of human contact, horticultural therapy activities on the other hand seek to increase human contact while engaging clients with nature. Such people-plant interactions benefit older people (Abbott, Cochran, & Clair, 1997; Mattson & Hilvert, 1976; Mooney & Milstein, 1994; van Loon, 2004) and are enjoyed by people with dementia, although lack of measured benefits often results in withdrawal of funding for nature-based activity programs, regardless of anecdotal success.

Residential design promotes the inclusion of plants, nature and gardens for older people (Pickles, 1999; Torrington, 1996) and gardens in particular for people with dementia (Chalfont, 2005; Cobley, 2002; Lovering, 1990; Pollock, 2001). Design guidance for including nature within residential environments is concerned with the availability of outdoor areas, circular paths, seating and raised planters, visibility from indoors and bringing the outdoors in (Brawley, 1997; Calkins, 1988; Cohen & Weisman, 1991; Dunlop, 1994; Weisman, Cohen, & Day, 1990). It is understood that environmental design affects people psychologically, for instance Seasonal Affective Disorder (SAD) links depressive symptoms to low levels of natural light. People with dementia are strongly affected by environment (Day, Carreon, & Stump, 2000; Lawton, 1990; Lawton, Liebowitz, & Charon, 1970; Lawton & Nahemow, 1973; Marshall, 1997) as they are less able to alter it themselves. Modifying dementia environments to include nature has shown positive effects. An enhanced environment was preferred by residents and families (Cohen-Mansfield & Werner, 1998) and the exterior environment and gardens (Mooney & Nicell, 1992), "beneficially affect(ed) behaviour and . . . .quality of life for such residents" (p. 26).

But natural environments are underused, as shown in studies of a walled garden (Mather, Nemecek, & Oliver, 1997), visits to an outdoor garden (Cohen-Mansfield & Werner, 1998) and use of wandering parks (Cohen-Mansfield & Werner, 1998, 1999). While the causes of under-use continue to be investigated, the benefits of nature for people with dementia are strongly endorsed in the dementia care literature with a call for putting nature back into life (Borrett, 1996; Judd, 1998; MacDonald, 2002). To do that wholistically means to integrate architecture and landscape, indoors and outdoors, to provide for independent actions on the part of the person with dementia as well as activities facilitated by care providers. Programming for nature in dementia care involves both sensory stimulation and nature-based activities.

THEORETICAL SUPPORT

From the dictionary 'nature' is defined as something organic, animate or climatic (water, animals, plants, breeze, stars, flowers, rain, wildlife, etc.).

Having a 'connection' to it means that nature is experienced physically by being accessible to the person's senses–natural stimuli are sniffed, heard, felt, seen or tasted. For nature to be sensed the environment surrounding the person must 'afford' it. Just as a chair affords sitting, standing on and hiding under (depending on your age), the availability of elements affords personal involvement with them (Gibson, 1968, 1986; Heft, 1999). Gibson's 'theory of affordances' supposes that the presence of nature in one's environment affords active and passive uses of it. Furthermore, there are two components to stimulus input: imposed (passively received) and obtained (actively gained). Therefore, one needs an environment that affords the opportunity to receive natural stimuli simply by being present and sensing (smelling, breathing, feeling the air on their face, the rain on their skin) as well as by actively seeking (reaching, touching, walking, moving the body and verbally asking for it).

Two Components of Receiving Stimulation (Gibson, 1968 p. 32)			
Components of stimulus input	Two ways to modify the stimulus input		Result
Imposed stimulation (forced on a passive observer)	Exploratory (investigative)	Moving the 'sensory' organs of the body	Accomplishes the pick up of stimulus information
Obtained stimulation (occurs through activity)	Performatory (executive)	Moving the 'motor' organs of the body	Accomplishes behaviour

Observations of Connection to Nature in 'Edge Spaces' of Dementia Care Settings

Research was conducted in 2001-2003 with residents and caregivers in two separate assisted living facilities in the United States, a specialist home for people with dementia in Scandinavia, and two residential care homes in the UK. This paper draws upon some of the data gathered during these site visits. As it was an exploratory study rather than an empirical one, details of the study sample are not given. Ethnographic observation of daily engagement with nature by the residents revealed the physical aspects of the built and natural environment that facilitated stimulation. Field notes from these observations, surveys of the built and natural environments and communication with residents contributed to the development of the checklist tool.

A particular type of space at the edge of the building, was used by the residents to connect to nature. In ecology, edge is a location where two different habitats meet. Between forest and field is a richly diverse habitat offering wildlife the benefits of both ecosystems. Likewise, the river bank and the beach are dynamic places that support an abundance of life dwelling at the water's edge. Architecturally, the edge space can be indoors (seat near a window or a bench in a lobby area) or outdoors (e.g. porches, balconies or entrances), and this paper contains both types. Edge spaces, due to their position against an exterior wall of the building, afford a person simultaneous qualities of indoors and outdoors–sensory stimulation from outdoors in terms of light, air and views, at the same time having the comfort, protection, privacy and physical support of being indoors. Edge spaces are defined by their essential criteria.

Essential Criteria	
INDOOR Edge Space	**OUTDOOR Edge Space**
An **indoor space**	An **outdoor space**
against an exterior wall of the building	against an exterior wall of the building
having a **window** or an **opening** to the outside	within **25 feet of the door** with a **view of the entrance**

For an in-depth comparative study in residential care homes in the UK which looked closely at the importance of nature for people with dementia, including a more in-depth treatment of the spatial typology of indoor and outdoor edge spaces, the uses people made of edge spaces and the contribution of nature to selfhood and identity construction through the use of introspection and metaphor, see Chalfont (2006). For more on the concepts and literature of edge space and for practical advice for building lively edge spaces in dementia care environments, see Chalfont and Rodiek (2005). Examples of people with dementia using edge spaces are given below with transcript data, floor plans and photographs. These observations were applied to the development of PLANET, as explained in the following section. The first edge space is in a Sunrise assisted living community in the United States.

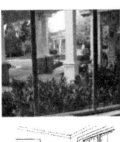

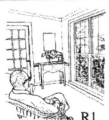
R1

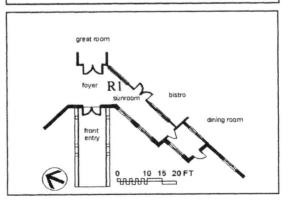

Edge Space 1:
Sunroom in an assisted living facility in the USA

great room

foyer R1
sunroom   bistro

dining room

front
entry

0   10 15 20 FT

Residents using this 'sentry' location by the front door had views of people coming and going from the home. (R1 and R2: Residents with dementia A: Author)

A: How do you know if it's windy?

R1:   *If I see a woman outside and her skirt's blowing. It's a rainy day, I saw somebody using an umbrella. . . . It's a busy road . . . a Volkswagen, don't see many of those anymore. I owned one myself, back in the years. My wife drove (it) mostly. But she left me and went to heaven.*

He turns to the woman (W:) sitting beside him and asks,

R1:   *Did your husband leave you too?*

W: Yes. He went to heaven too.

R1:   *Women do that you know.*

Use of wrist bracelets and door sensor technology allows outdoor access. If a resident goes outside, a staff member (S:) accompanies them until they are ready to come back in.

R1:   *I may go out. There may be enough light for a sneeze.*

S: He's going out for his sneeze . . . I'll stay with him.

A lady resident goes to the front door, pushes the button, stands in the doorway and takes six long, slow breaths. Shortly she is back inside doing her crossword puzzle.

R2:   *I like to be near the door sometimes.*

A: Are you getting fresh air?

R2:   *Yes, you need it. It's too hot in here for me. Most people like it.*

The edge space afforded this person an awareness of climatic conditions which prompted social interaction, reminiscence and introspection. It also allowed him to go out for a sneeze. The other person used the edge space to get some fresh air when she needed it. The second setting is a dementia care corridor of a residential care home in England, UK. People used natural stimuli for introspection and story-telling during social interaction. This dialogue occurred in a bedroom.

Edge Space 2: Bedroom in a residential care home in England, UK

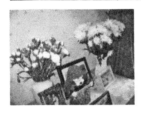 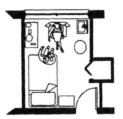 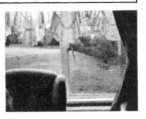

A: You've got some pretty flowers in your room.

R: *Yes, aren't they nice.*

A: Where did they come from?

R: *Uh, me husband brought me some over. I don't really (know), he'd have got 'em out of garden somewhere. Ah, they are nice. Got some nice flowers.*

A: Is that something you enjoy?

R: *What, flowers?*

A: Uh huh.

R: *I love flowers.*

A: What kind's your favorite?

R: *Well, I like any kind of flowers you know . . . Same as me husband, we both like flowers. But I don't do 'em so much now. And that's that! (laughs)*

This person has been a widow for some time, but having flowers nearby and talking about them afforded her the opportunity to speak about her husband in the present tense, which pleased her.

The following dialogue occurred in a dining room of the same care home.

Edge Space 3: Dining room in a residential care home in England, UK

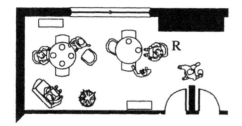
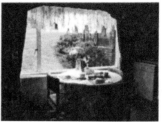

A: What can you see out the window?

R: *Not a lot . . . Can't see anything out of there . . . can't see any animals or anything.*

A: There was a bird a few minutes ago . . .

R: *Aye. Has he gone?*

A: I don't know . . . Do you remember what he looked like?

R: *Oh I do, a tan, dark colored bird.*

A: What was he doing?

R: *Just looking at us lot, thinking when are we going to throw him any grub. Did we give him something?*

A: I don't think we did.

R: *He'll think we're so many miserable boogers. Well he would, wouldn't he? Wouldn't you, if you were hungry and we didn't give you a bit of nought to eat? You'd think to your sen (self) you're a miserable sod, wouldn't you? And I would.*

(10 second pause) . . . *How much more have you to do?*

A: Today?

R: *Only today?*

A: Mmmm.

R: *I've more than today, I think. I think I have more than today to do.*

This person did have 'more than today to do', but she has recently passed away. Talking about nature was a starting point for her to address personal issues concerning her own mortality. The following dialogue occurred in a lounge of a second residential care home in the UK.

Edge Space 4: Lounge in a residential care home in England, UK

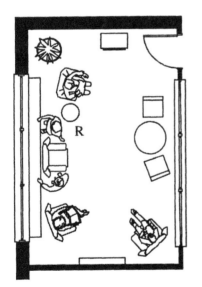
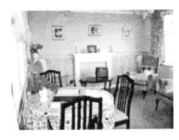
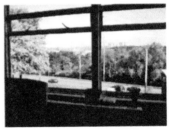

R: *I can see all the houses across there . . . and that road. There's all those people going to a bus . . . going to work . . . people . . . beautiful outside . . . Look at them cars all going up there . . . I can see the sunshine, beautiful isn't it? Well, to be able to look out and nosey, (laughs) out of the window.*

A: 'and nosey'. . . . What does that mean?

R: *Well . . . you know, you're looking round . . . houses.*

A: Looking round, at what?

R: *Don't know, anything that's going.*

Each of the conversations above contained some dialogue made possible because edge space afforded natural stimuli. Physical features of the building or the landscape, a piece of technology, an action on the part of a caregiver, the location of the person within the room or the location of the room within the building, or aspects of the person themselves facilitated sensory stimulation and social interaction. The last example comes from a group home for people with dementia in Scandinavia. The porch adjacent the dining room, kitchen and living room areas comprised the edge space where the residents engaged in routine nature-related activities, as witnessed by direct observation, relayed through caregiver accounts or evidenced by the artifacts within the environment. This edge space was routinely used for meals during warmer weather, was adjacent to planting beds, a clothes line, vegetable and herbs in planting boxes and a bird feeder–all of which showed evidence of regular use. The porch drew people outside because things need to be done–normal tasks such as wiping the furniture. Also, the close proximity of the porch to other houses afforded residents normal social exchanges, such as chatting with the next door neighbor.

Edge space 5: Porch and adjacent dining room in a group home in Scandinavia

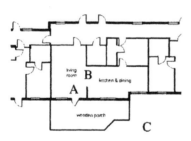

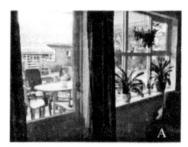

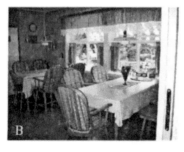

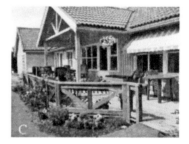

The dialogues and observations shown above, plus more conducted in other homes, were analysed along with building plans and photographs to determine functional characteristics that were either helpful or essential in contributing to the moment during which the person engaged with nature. Below is a short list of characteristics to illustrate how the findings were interpreted.

Examples of Functional Characteristics of Edge Spaces PLANET Would Check for:

1. Places for the person to sit:

    - with comfortable seating–available and positioned so viewing is possible
    - with sight lines higher than the windowsill
    - with a view containing foreground and distance
    - with places for another person to sit near enough to hold a conversation
    - with a nearby piece of furniture to set down a drink or personal belongings

2. Places for a person to stand:

    - near a window–available floor space close to the window, not blocked by furniture
    - with support–a windowsill, ledge or piece of furniture offering support while standing

3. Views through windows and doors that change as the person moves through the building
4. Views that contain people, houses, roads, traffic, trees, grass, neighbors and landmarks

Using this process of observing and analysing interactions, the checklist tool evolved. The six domains were determined and the individual questions were scripted within them–a process that has continued over the past 5 years as the checklist tool is trialled in more places. Simple yes/no questions in Person, Location, Architecture, Nature, Energy and Technology check not only for existing elements but for evidence of their use, based on observation in the home and conversations with residents, staff and family caregivers.

PLANET: POTENTIAL FOR CONNECTION TO NATURE IN DEMENTIA CARE ENVIRONMENTS

There are six domains for PLANET (Person, Location, Architecture, Nature, Energy and Technology). The domain of Person asks about the person's ability to engage with their surroundings in three ways–*physical, emotional and sensory.* Their *physical* ability includes mobility (sitting, standing, walking, using ramps & stairs), strength and flexibility. *Emotional* ability questions the person's fear of falling, their desire to move about and participate, and their alertness. *Sensory* ability checks for sight, hearing, smell and balance. The 17 questions are answered with a simple 1 or 0 by observing or engaging with the person. A low score in this domain reflects diminished capability on the part of the person, and perhaps also a level of dependence upon assistance from others, conditions that lower the person's self-directed, autonomous, bodily engagement with nature. These are the questions for the Person domain:

PERSON
SITTING: Able to stay sitting upright unaided
STANDING STILL: Able to stand still unaided
STANDING UP: Stands up from a sitting position unaided
WALKING CORRIDORS: Walks unaided or with handrail
WALKING RAMPS: Walks unaided or with handrail
WALKING STAIRS: Walks unaided or with handrail
STRENGTH & FLEXIBILITY–UPPER BODY: Movement possible unaided
STRENGTH & FLEXIBILITY–LOWER BODY Movement possible unaided
FEAR OF FALLING Not usually afraid of falling
DESIRE TO MOVE ABOUT: Usually wants to move about
DESIRE TO PARTICIPATE: Usually wants to participate
ALERTNESS & ENGAGEMENT AWAKE: Alert and engaged when awake
BEING AWAKE: Normally awake in the daytime
SIGHT: Could see a tree outside of a window
HEARING: Can hear well enough to converse
SMELL: Can smell a bouquet of flowers they are holding
BALANCE: Not having a problem with their balance

Location is measured in six ways: *Proximity, Frequency, Edge Spaces, View, Outdoor Area and Seating. Proximity* asks about the nearness of the person within a room to sunshine, daylight, fresh air, views and outdoor spaces. *Frequency* asks how often doors and windows are opened. *Edge Spaces* are building features or spaces such as a porch or balcony, rich in natural stimuli from outdoors but also offering comfort and safety. *View* is important for health and wellbeing (Hartig, Mang, & Evans, 1991; Leather, Pyrgas, Beale, & Lawrence, 1998; Ulrich, 1984; Verderber, 1986) and four components of view are checked: aspect, extent, content and depth. Outdoor Area asks if an area is within close proximity and meant for use by residents. If so, Seating scores the provision, location, visibility and choice within that outdoor area.

LOCATION
A window is visible from at least one seat
A window is visible from at least half of the seats
A window is visible from all the seats
Sunshine reaches at least one seat
Sunshine reaches at least half of the seats
Sunshine reaches all the seats
Daylight enters the room during the morning
Daylight enters the room during the afternoon
Daylight enters the room year round
At least one seat is near a window that opens
At least half of the seats are near windows that open
All the seats are near windows that open
If this is a ground floor, this room has a door to the outside
If this is an upper floor, this room has a door to a balcony, roof garden, etc.
Frequency–There is a door to the outside from this room and it is opened regularly or frequently
Frequency–There are windows in this room that are opened regularly or frequently
PORCH exists and is meant to be used by these residents and it has seating . . . and level access from this room
ENTRANCE exists that is meant to be used by these residents . . . and has seating
BALCONY exists that is meant to be used by these residents . . . and has seating
COVERED WALKWAY exists that is meant to be used by these residents . . . and has seating
MUDROOM or ENTRANCE PORCH exists . . . and it has seating
VIEW–Aspect–from any seat in the room you can see at least one compass direction
VIEW–Aspect–sitting in the room you can see more than one compass direction

VIEW–Extent–Standing at the largest window, to take in the view requires turning one's head
VIEW–Content–the view includes countryside or rural land
VIEW–Content–the view includes people & activities
VIEW–Content–the view includes landscaped areas or gardens
VIEW Content–includes transportation vehicles (cars, bicycles, buses or taxis etc)
VIEW Depth–view contains land or grounds within the property lines
VIEW Depth–view contains land or grounds that are outside the property lines
There is an OUTDOOR AREA within close proximity to this room that is meant to be used by the residents . . . and is visible from indoors
and SEATING is provided outdoors in a sunny place during the winter
and SEATING is provided outdoors in a shady place during the summer
and SEATING is provided adjacent to plantings
and SEATING is provided that is visible from indoors
and there is a choice of sunny or shady spots to sit outdoors
and moveable outdoor SEATING is provided for these residents

The domain of **Architecture** looks for features such as doors, windows and windowsills as well as the existence and use of *Outdoor Structures and Amenities* such as greenhouse, shed, clothesline, sports or recreation area or outdoor eating space. Questions *about* doors and *windows* reflect frequency and control of their use by the residents as well as quantity, direction they face and adjustability. *Windowsills* are judged as being wide enough, sunny, suitable for plants and if they appear to be in use.

ARCHITECTURE
GLAZING–This room is a glass enclosed room or conservatory
GLAZING–This room has skylights or a glass ceiling (only one glazing question is true)
DOORS–Quantity–This room has at least one outside door
DOORS–Control–Residents regularly open and close the doors to this room
DOORS–Permeability–in this room is an outside door with a window in it
WINDOWS–Quantity–there are 3 or more separate windows in this room
WINDOWS–Quantity–there is a large picture window (it may have multiple panes)
WINDOWS–Juxtaposition–the windows in this room are on more than one wall

WINDOWS–Control–Residents regularly open and close the windows in this room

WINDOWS–Control–Residents regularly open or close the curtains or shades

WINDOWS–Aspect–There is a south-facing window in this room

WINDOWS–Complexity–Windows on the same wall open in at least two directions

WINDOWS–Panes & Complexity–This room has a bay window

WINDOW SILLS are being personalised with plants or decorative or domestic items

WINDOW SILLS are being personalised by the resident(s)

WINDOW SILLS are wide and sunny enough for growing plants

WINDOW SILLS are being used for growing plants by resident(s)

GAZEBO (platform with roof) or ARBOR (overhead structure) exists onsite

GAZEBO or ARBOR has SEATING in it

GAZEBO or ARBOR is meant to be used (and is used) by these residents

GREENHOUSE exists on site

GREENHOUSE exists on site, is meant tobe used and is used by these residents

SHED exists on site (protected space for DIY projects out of doors; space for sitting and tinkering . . . .)

SUMMERHOUSE exists on site (small structure, used in the warmer months with seating and windows)

SUMMERHOUSE exists on site, is meant for and is used by these residents

CLOTHES LINE exists on site

CLOTHES LINE exists on site and is used by these residents

SPORTS OR RECREATION AREA–Game courts, shuffle board, bowling green . . . exists onsite or locally

SPORTS OR RECREATION AREA exists and is used by these residents

FOOD AREA–Barbeque, picnic, or outdoor eating space exists

FOOD AREA–exists and is used by/for these residents

The domain of *Nature* investigates the elements of the natural world that are physically present in the setting. Questions include plant materials and their diversity, vitality, ability to create habitat, provide sensory stimulation and have practical uses. Nature domain also includes structures and shelters that encourage the presence of nature (nesting boxes, a trellis or a wall for climbing plants), cosmic forces (stars and moon visible?), weather (rain audible and visible from inside?), local ecosystems available nearby and use of plants indoors (living or artificial).

NATURE

DIVERSITY 1 Seasonal bedding plants, annuals or vegetables on or near the site

DIVERSITY 1 . . . and can be viewed from inside by the residents

DIVERSITY 2 Some large, mature shade trees exist on or near the site

DIVERSITY 2 . . . and can be viewed from inside by the residents

DIVERSITY 3 large, mature evergreen or conifer trees

DIVERSITY 3 . . . .and can be viewed from inside by the residents

DIVERSITY 4 Some large, mature shrubs exist on or near the site

DIVERSITY 4 . . . and can be viewed from inside by the residents

DIVERSITY 5 Flowering shrubs exist on or near the site

DIVERSITY 5 . . . and can be viewed from inside by the residents

DIVERSITY 6 Evergreen trees or shrubs grow on or near the site

DIVERSITY 7 Groundcover or vines grow on site or nearby

DIVERSITY 8 Herbaceous perennials grow on site or nearby

SENSORY Tactile plants grow on site

SENSORY Fragrant plants grow on site

SENSORY Species that move in the wind and make a rustling noise

HABITAT 1 Overgrown shrubs, wild unmaintained areas, brush piles, wood piles etc. on or near site

HABITAT 2 Berries, soft fruits or nut bushes for birds on site or nearby

HABITAT 3 Nesting places for birds (evergreen trees, ivy-covered trees, ivy on walls) on or near site

USE–Species exist that are being used here for eating, cooking or herbs

USE–Species exist that are being used inside the home for decorating, crafts or cut flowers

STRUCTURES–(site perimeter) A Wall or Fence is colonised with vines/moss and wildlife usage is evident

STRUCTURES (site perimeter) Wall or fence provides a warm, protected area (pleasant microclimate)

SHELTER–(site interior) A vertical structure (trellis or screen) creates sheltered spaces, colonised with plants

HABITAT Structures–there is a nesting box, feeding station or bat box

There is a Garden Sculpture or Artwork that residents helped create

Hanging baskets are present and being used

Window boxes present and being used

Garden Materials (compost, soil, plants) are available to residents

A Work Area with tools is available to the resident for outdoor projects

PATHS provide equal access even with changes in level

PATHS–surface conditions can be seen by these residents from indoors

COSMIC FORCES – Stars and Moon can be seen by these residents from indoors . . .

WEATHER–Rain is audible and visible on the windows by these residents

WEATHER–Rain is audible on the ground or on the plant foliage to the residents inside

ECOSYSTEMS–Most of these residents travel out to visit a natural environment once or twice a year

Real Live Plants and Cut Flowers are regularly found in the living areas of these residents

Silk artificial flowers or plants are found in the living areas of these residents

Energy is the most innovative of the domains because it attempts to score the presence of the life force–energy known as Chi. Energy seeks to quantify emotional response to a place (an unarticulated gut feeling) which has very clear implications in terms of attitudes towards a space and therefore frequency of use. A landscaped park that is overgrown and full of litter/rubbish both sends out and attracts negative energy–not a place an older person would gravitate towards. **Care & Maintenance** checks for positive inputs of human energy resulting in the look and feel of a place that is being cared for. Likewise, **People Interactions** questions whether people put their positive energy into the space. **Creativity** asks whether the person has danced, sang, played music or exercised in the area. (Positive energy becomes embedded in a place during celebration or group activity and the place becomes meaningful. A place that resonates with meaning attracts people into it and it continues to be used in this way, not unlike ritual places.) **Animals** checks for the presence of pets, wildlife or farm animals. Can residents feed the squirrels, hang a bird-feeder, keep a dog, visit a farm nearby or go for a dog sled ride or a hayride? Such questions also reflect on management, policy, the regulatory environment and societal expectations for older people.

ENERGY

CARE & MAINTENANCE–The outdoor areas appear to receive a leaf clean up and shrub pruning . . .

C & M–The outdoor areas receive seasonal plantings such as annuals, bedding plants or bulbs

C & M–The outdoor areas receive weekly care (mowing, sweeping, wiping furniture or litter pickup)

C & M–Materials such as topsoil, mulch, woodchips, compost, etc are delivered to the outdoor areas . . .

C & M–A gardener/landscaper works in the outdoor areas doing planting, mowing or pruning . . .

C & M–These residents have participated by watering plants outdoors

C & M–These residents have planted or gardened outdoors

PEOPLE–An interested Staff Person or Horticuoltural Therapist has worked with the residents outdoors . . .

PEOPLE–An interested Staff Person or Horticultural Therapist has worked with plants with the residents . . .

PEOPLE–A Physical Therapist or Occupational Therapist has worked with the residents outdoors this year

PEOPLE–A Social Worker, Psychotherapist or Counsellor has talked with a resident in the outdoor area

PEOPLE–A Volunteer, a Caregiver or other interested Staff Person takes care of plants indoors

PEOPLE–A Volunteer, a Caregiver or other interested Staff Person takes care of plants outdoors

PEOPLE–I know a resident who regularly uses the outdoors to visit with a partner or family member

PEOPLE–Volunteers or a local group regularly spend time with the residents outdoors

PEOPLE–A local school group regularly spends time with the residents outdoors

PEOPLE–An outdoor area is useful for private conversations between residents and visitors

CREATIVE ENERGY–The residents have danced, played music, sang or exercised outdoors

CREATIVE ENERGY–They have danced, played music, drummed, sang or exercised in a group outdoors

ANIMALS–The residents can keep a pet or the home has a pet

ANIMALS–The Residents can let their dog out during the day

ANIMALS–The Residents can take their pet or the home's pet for a walk daily

ANIMALS–Pat dogs or other visiting pets came this year

WILDLIFE–Residents can hang a birdfeeder on or outside their window

WILDLIFE–Residents can put birdfeeders in the outdoor area

WILDLIFE–Residents can put nuts out for the squirrels, feed ducks, etc.

Farm & Domestic Animals live nearby–Residents can see or can visit

These residents live with a bird, hamster, rabbit or fish in a tank

The final domain of **Technology** with 15 questions checks for the availability of assistive technology or adaptations to enable a person to connect with nature. Examples would be the use of a wrist bracelet and a door sensor system, to allow a person to come and go freely, and to feel secure that if they run into difficulty a staff person is aware of their location. Other technology includes automatic door openers, elevators, nightlighting of outdoor areas, pumps for water features, specially adapted hand tools, mechanically adjusted hanging baskets and passive alarms at the perimeters of the property. (Technology questions are not listed as few devices are seldom found). Overall the checklist gives an indication of the potential for connection to nature based on observations and affordances. A short 25 question Checklist for Caregivers, drawn from the questions listed above, helps a caregiver determine the potential connection to nature in a care facility before a loved one moves in (available at www.chalfontdesign.com).

CONCLUSION

Although nature is known to benefit people with dementia and a range of methods are used to bring nature to the resident as part of the care they receive, integrating a connection to nature into both care practice and building design is not often achieved, which at times may result in nature deprivation for people with dementia living within the homes. For example, Cutler and Kane (2005) reported that of 1,068 nursing home residents 32.2% responded they went outdoors less than once a month (p. 37). This paper called for a wholistic approach to providing a connection to nature by investigating the potential inherent in the person and their built, natural and social environment. A checklist tool has been proposed which can be completed by a person with no specialist skills or training based simply on observations and discussion within the care setting. Investigating environments in this way contributes to design that is interdisciplinary and informed by the daily acts of dwelling, not an idealised intention (build it and they will come) of how people will use the space, which actually never occurs. This statement from the same study by Cutler and Kane supports this approach:

> Beautiful outdoor spaces were built, often with community support, but it was unrealistic to think that residents could make use of the spaces, either independently because of their distance from resident rooms or with the assistance of staff because of the time required to assist residents to the space. (Cutler & Kane, 2005, p. 43)

Furthermore, edge spaces can maximise the integration between indoors and outdoors, providing people with tools that afford connection to nature as well as to the wider social world:

... the most used outdoor spaces and indoor window spaces were those that either had a view of or were located in a setting of real life activity. (ibid.)

After the checklist tool was presented, findings from five edge spaces were given. Residents showed a range of psychosocial uses of edge space, including expressions of humor and ethical reasoning, emotional resilience, character, heart, spirit and concern for others. From these facilitated social interactions were derived the functional characteristics the spaces required if sensory stimulation was to be afforded. The domains of PLANET continue to be developed through observations within care environments and during conversations with residents, insuring that the voices of people with dementia be heard (Goldsmith, 1996) and that their needs are addressed in the design of the physical, natural and social space. There remains the great divide between indoors and outdoors, architecture and landscape architecture, designers and care providers, managers and staff and family caregivers which seems central to the chronic underutilisation of nature in dementia care environments. It is these divisions which the approach and the tool described herein attempt to address. Our home provides environmental support while we go about the daily task of living. By design, the built spaces within our home, and particularly within dementia care settings, can assist that task by affording us an essential connection to real life which includes the natural world.

REFERENCES

Abbott, G., Cochran, V., & Clair, A. A. (1997). Innovations in intergenerational programs for persons who are elderly: The role of horticultural therapy in a multidisciplinary approach. *Activities, Adaptation & Aging, 22*(1-2), 27-39.

Baker, R., Bell, S., Baker, E., Gibson, S., Holloway, J., Pearce, R., et al. (2001). A randomized controlled trial of the effects of multi-sensory stimulation (MSS) for people with dementia. *British Journal of Clinical Psychology, 40*, 81-96. doi: 10.1348/014466501163508

Ballard, C. G., O'Brien, J. T., Reichelt, K., & Perry, E. K. (2002). Aromatherapy as a safe and effective treatment for the management of agitation in severe dementia: The results of a double-blind, placebo-controlled trial with Melissa. *Journal of Clinical Psychiatry, 63*(7), 553-558.

Borrett, N. (1996). Our crucial connection with nature. *Journal of Dementia Care*, 22-23.

Brawley, E. C. (1997). *Designing for Alzheimer's disease: strategies for creating better care environments.* New York: John Wiley & Sons.

Calkins, M. P. (1988). *Design for Dementia: Planning Environments for the Elderly and the Confused.* Owings Mills, MD: Health Publishing.

Chalfont, G. E. (2006). *Connection to Nature at the Building Edge: Towards a Therapeutic Architecture for Dementia Care Environments.* PhD Thesis. University of Sheffield, Sheffield.

Chalfont, G. E. (2005). Creating enabling outdoor environments for residents, *Nursing and Residential Care* (Vol. 7, pp. 454-457).

Chalfont, G. E., & Rodiek, S. (2005). Building Edge: An ecological approach to research and design of environments for people with dementia. Alzheimer's Care Quarterly, *Special Issue–Environmental Innovations in Care, 6*(4), 341-348.

Chalfont, G. E. (2008). *Design for Nature in Dementia Care.* A Bradford Dementia Group Good Practice Guide. London: Jessica Kingsley Publishers.

Cobley, M. (2002). Using outdoor spaces for people with dementia–a carer's perspective. *Working with older people, 6*(2), 23-30.

Cohen, U., & Weisman, G. D. (1991). *Holding on to home: Designing environments for people with dementia.* Baltimore: Johns Hopkins University Press.

Cohen-Mansfield, J., & Werner, P. (1998). The effects of an enhanced environment on nursing home residents who pace. *Gerontologist, 38*(2), 199-208.

Cohen-Mansfield, J., & Werner, P. (1998). Visits to an outdoor garden: impact on behavior and mood of nursing home residents who pace. In B. Vellas & L. J. Fitten (Eds.), *Research and Practice in Alzheimer's Disease* (pp. 419-436). New York: Springer Publishing Company.

Cohen-Mansfield, J., & Werner, P. (1999). Outdoor wandering parks for persons with dementia: A survey of characteristics and use. *Alzheimer Disease & Associated Disorders, 13*(2), 109-117.

Coleman, M. T., Looney, S., O'Brien, J., Ziegler, C., Pastorino, C., & Turner, C. (2002). The Eden Alternative: Findings after 1 year of implementation. *Journal of Gerontology: MEDICAL SCIENCES, 57A*(7), M422-M427.

Cutler, L. J., & Kane, R. A. (2005). As great as all outdoors: A study of outdoor spaces as a neglected resource for nursing home residents. In S. Rodiek & B. Schwarz (Eds.), *The role of the outdoors in residential environments for Aging* (pp. 29-48). New York: Haworth Press. doi:10.1300/J081v19n03_03

Day, K., Carreon, D., & Stump, C. (2000). The therapeutic design of environments for people with dementia: A review of the empirical research. *Gerontologist, 40*(4), 397-416.

Devlin, A. S. (1980). Housing for the elderly: Cognitive considerations. *Environment and Behavior, 12(4), 451-466.*

Dunlop, A. (1994). Hard architecture and human scale designing for disorientation. Stirling: Dementia Services Development Centre.

Gibson, J. J. (1968). *The senses considered as perceptual systems.* London: George Allen & Unwin.

Gibson, J. J. (1986). *The Ecological Approach to Visual Perception.* Hillsdale, New Jersey: Lawrence Erlbaum Associates.

Goldsmith, M. (1996). *Hearing the Voice of People with Dementia: Opportunities and obstacles.* London: Jessica Kingsley Publishers.

Hartig, T., Mang, M., & Evans, G. (1991). Restorative effects of natural environmental experiences. *Environment and Behavior, 23*, 3-26.

Heft, H. (1999). Affordances of Children's Environments: A Functional Approach to Environmental Description. In J. L. Nasar & W. F. E. Preiser (Eds.), *Directions in Person-Environment Research and Practice* (pp. 43-69). Aldershot: Ashgate.

Judd, S. (1998). Building for dementia: A matter of design. In *Design for Dementia*. London: Journal of Dementia Care.

Kaplan, R. (1973). Some psychological benefits of gardening. *Environment and Behavior, 5*(2), 145-162.

Kaplan, R. (2001). The nature of the view from home: Psychological benefits. *Environment and Behavior, 33*(4), 507-542. doi: 10.1177/00139160121973115

Kitwood, T. (1997). *Dementia Reconsidered: The person comes first*. Buckingham: Open University Press.

Lawton, M. P. (1990). Residential environment and self-directedness among older people. *American Psychologist, 45*(5), 638-640.

Lawton, M. P., Liebowitz, B., & Charon, H. (1970). Physical structure and the behavior of senile patients following ward remodeling. *Aging and Human Development, 1*, 231-239.

Lawton, M. P., & Nahemow, L. (1973). Ecology and the aging process. In C. Eisdorfer & M. P. Lawton (Eds.), *Psychology of Adult Development and Aging* (pp. 619-674). Washington, D.C.: American Psychological Association.

Leather, P., Pyrgas, M., Beale, D., & Lawrence, C. (1998). Windows in the workplace: Sunlight, view and occupational stress. *Environment and Behavior, 30*(6), 739-762.

Lewis, C. A. (1996). Green Nature/Human Nature: The Meaning of Plants in Our Lives. Urbana & Chicago: University of Illinois Press.

Lovering, M. J. (1990). Alzheimer's disease and outdoor space: Issues in environmental design. *The American Journal of Alzheimer's Care and Related Disorders and Research, 5*(3), 33-40.

MacDonald, C. (2002). Back to the real sensory world our 'care' has taken away. *Journal of Dementia Care*, 33-36.

Markus, T. A., & Gray, A. (1973). *Windows in low rise, high density housing – the psychological significance of sunshine, daylight, view and visual privacy.* Paper presented at the 'Windows and their function in architectural design' conference, October.

Marshall, M. (1997). Therapeutic Design for People with Dementia. In S. Hunter (Ed.), *Dementia: Challenges and New Directions* (31 ed.). London: Jessica Kingsley.

Mather, J. A., Nemecek, D., & Oliver, K. (1997). The effect of a walled garden on behavior of individuals with Alzheimer's. *American Journal of Alzheimer's Disease, 12*(6), 252-257.

Mattson, R. H., & Hilvert, R. T. (1976). Psychological, social, physical and educational effects of horticultural therapy for geriatrics. *Hortscience*.

Mooney, P., & Nicell, P. L. (1992). The importance of exterior environment for Alzheimer residents: Effective care and risk management. *Healthcare Management Forum, 5*(2), 23-29.

Mooney, P. F., & Milstein, S. L. (1994). *Assessing the benefits of a therapeutic horticulture program for seniors in intermediate care.* Paper presented at the The Healing Dimensions of People-Plant Relations Conference.

Ottosson, J. and Grahn, P. (2005). Measures of restoration in geriatric care residences: The influence of nature on elderly people's power of concentration, blood pressure and pulse rate. In S. Rodiek & B. Schwarz (Eds.), *The role of the outdoors in residential environments for Aging* (pp. 227-256). New York: Haworth Press. doi:10.1300/J081v19n03_12

Pickles, J. (1999). *Housing for Varying Needs: a design guide. Part 2: Housing with Integral Support*. Edinburgh: The Stationery Office.

Pollock, A. (2001). *Designing gardens for people with dementia*. Stirling: Dementia Services Development Centre.

Tang, J. W. & Brown, R. D. (2005). The effect of viewing a landscape on physiological health of elderly women. In S. Rodiek & B. Schwarz (Eds.), *The role of the outdoors in residential environments for Aging* (pp. 187-202). New York: Haworth Press. doi:10.1300/J081v19n03_10

Torrington, J. (1996). *Care Homes for Older People: a briefing and design guide*. London: Chapman and Hall.

Torrington, J. (2004). *Upgrading buildings for older people*. London: RIBA Enterprises.

Ulrich, R. S. (1984). View through a window may influence recovery from surgery. *Science, 224*, 420-421.

Ulrich, R. S. (1999). Effects of Gardens on Health Outcomes: Theory and Research. In C. C. Marcus & M. Barnes (Eds.), *Healing Gardens: Therapeutic Benefits and Design Recommendations* (pp. 27-86). New York: John Wiley & Sons.

van Loon, M. (2004). Grey and green in the Netherlands: Research supporting the value of nature-based activities for elderly people. *GrowthPoint* (99), 6-7.

Verderber, S. (1986). Dimensions of person-window transactions in the hospital environment. *Environment and Behavior, 18*(4), 450-466.

Weisman, G., Cohen, U., & Day, K. (1990). *Programming and design for dementia: Development of a 50 person residential environment*. Milwaukee: Center for Architecture and Urban Planning Research.

doi:10.1300/J081v21n01_08

Alzheimer's Garden Audit Tool

Clare Cooper Marcus

SUMMARY. Increasing numbers of dementia units are being built, many with attached outdoor space. Some are successful in providing for users' needs; others less so. The Alzheimer's Garden Audit Tool (AGAT) provides a relatively simple evaluative framework for assessing whether a garden incorporates those design elements and qualities that are necessary for a successful dementia care garden. The rationale for including items on this checklist-tool is explained. The possible uses are discussed. The tool is presented in its relatively preliminary state in the hope that people will use it and send their comments to the author for modification and improvement. doi:10.1300/J081v21n01_09 *[Article copies available for a fee from The Haworth Document Delivery Service: 1-800-HAWORTH. E-mail address: <docdelivery@haworthpress.com> Website: <http://www.HaworthPress.com> © 2007 by The Haworth Press, Inc. All rights reserved.]*

KEYWORDS. Alzheimer's, dementia gardens, design assessment, outdoors, frail elderly, long-term care

Clare Cooper Marcus is Professor Emerita in the Departments of Architecture and Landscape Architecture, University of California, Berkeley, and Principal of Healing Landscapes, Berkeley, CA.

Address correspondence to: Healing Landscapes, 2721 Stuart Street, Berkeley, CA 94705 (E-mail: clare@mygarden.com).

[Haworth co-indexing entry note]: "Alzheimer's Garden Audit Tool." Cooper Marcus, Clare. Co-published simultaneously in *Journal of Housing for the Elderly* (The Haworth Press, Inc.) Vol. 21, No. 1/2, 2007, pp. 179-191; and: *Outdoor Environments for People with Dementia* (ed: Susan Rodiek and Benyamin Schwarz) The Haworth Press, Inc., 2007, pp. 179-191. Single or multiple copies of this article are available for a fee from The Haworth Document Delivery Service [1-800-HAWORTH, 9:00 a.m. - 5:00 p.m. (EST). E-mail address: docdelivery@haworthpress.com].

INTRODUCTION

An aging population in North America has triggered the development of more and more dementia-care units, many with associated outdoor spaces. Empirical research and less-formal observation studies suggest that these outdoor spaces are sometimes very successful in meeting the needs of residents and caregivers, sometimes quite unsuccessful. (Grant, 2003; Galbraith and Westphal, 2004; Mahan, 2004; Cooper Marcus, 2005) The less successful examples fall into three categories: those that were designed with apparently little regard for what is known about the use of the outdoors by Alzheimer's patients; those that were thoughtfully designed but which are rendered "off limits" to residents due to staff policy (doors kept locked, etc.); and those that have some good qualities but also contain problems or omissions which make it difficult for caregivers to encourage uses they want to promote.

Since the installation and maintenance of an outdoor area entails considerable budgetary outlay, it is important that the design of such spaces and their relationship to adjacent building(s) meet the needs of users to the greatest extent possible. Some research suggests that when dementia patients have access to the outdoors, they sleep better and need less medication (Galbraith and Westphal, 2004; Gold, 2004). Hence, it is critical that this essential component of the environment of dementia care receive serious attention. The overall objective of the Alzheimer's Garden Audit Tool (AGAT) is to facilitate the assessment of a garden design in terms of how well it serves the needs of users with Alzheimer's and other forms of dementia. While it would be desirable to conduct a full-scale post-occupancy evaluation of a dementia garden one wishes to evaluate, time, budget and lack of the necessary skills generally render this unfeasible. Such studies, few in number, have mostly been carried out by academics (Galbraith and Westphal, 2004; Grant, 2003). Of course, we need many more such studies, but in the meantime, the AGAT provides a relatively simple evaluative tool which enables a designer or non-designer to assess how well a particular outdoor space is functioning for its users (residents, visitors, caregivers) without the expense of a complete post-occupancy evaluation.

The Structure of the AGAT and How it Might Be Used

This tool could be used in a variety of ways, for example as:

1. A checklist for staff and policymakers interested in learning more about creating higher-quality outdoor environments for people with Alzheimer's disease.
2. The basis of an evidence-based program (or brief) for a new or renovated garden.

3. A reference tool for landscape architects and other designers working to design or re-design quality outdoor space for those with Alzheimer's disease.
4. A checklist to enable administrators of an existing facility to determine which specific elements of the outdoor space need improvement.
5. A reference tool for funding agencies promoting high-quality outdoor space in Alzheimer's facilities.
6. A research instrument to study the implications of outdoor environmental quality on the quality of life of residents in an Alzheimer's facility.
7. A teaching tool to raise the consciousness of design students regarding the needs of this patient-population.

Unlike other environmental assessment tools recently published–for example, POEMS (Preschool Outdoor Environment Measurement Scale); TESS-2 + (Therapeutic Environment Screening Scale); and PEAP (Professional Environmental Assessment Protocol)–AGAT is very much a work in progress. It has not yet been widely tested and is published here to encourage others to use it and contribute to its development.

However, like the tools cited above, the specific design elements being evaluated (which the user employs as a checklist) are culled from existing research and observation as to which specific features of the environment are important for this particular user-group (for example from Tyson and Zeisel, 1999; Grant, 2003; Mahan, 2004; Galbraith and Westphal, 2004; Cooper Marcus, 2005; Hoover, 1995; Lovering, 1990).

The checklist is divided into seven sections, moving from Location and Entry to the Garden, to Layout and Pathways, Planting, Seating, Overall Design and Details, to Maintenance and Amenities. Each of seventy-four items is scored on a four-point scale. Users of the checklist are asked to give a score of "0" if a feature is absent (e.g., there is no entry patio), or if a suggested quality is missing (e.g., a homelike, familiar milieu). A score of "1" indicates that the provision of an element or quality is only "poor to fair"; "2" if it is "moderately good, could be improved"; or "3" if it is "very successful." Obviously, if a number of independent assessors score a particular item as "0" or "1," for example, that is an area of the design that needs to be considered for improvement.

Of course the answers to questions on any assessment tool or checklist are somewhat subjective. It is possible that a professional designer, a staff member, or a family member might score items differently. Hence, future work on this tool will entail comparing how different evaluators relate to the scoring system. That designers as a group tend to score items in very similar, if not identical ways is suggested by the experience of the author with earlier attempts at checklist tools.

Pilot-Testing AGAT and Other Assessment Tools

The first attempt by this author at formulating an assessment tool for healthcare outdoor space was a pilot format tested out at a large acute care hospital in Albuquerque, New Mexico with assistance and input from Marni Barnes and Naomi Sachs (both landscape architects) in 2002. An improved iteration of this tool was tested out at a large acute care hospital in Miami, Florida in 2003 with assistance and input from landscape architect Connie Roy-Fisher.

At an ASLA (American Society of Landscape Architects) conference in 2004, thirty members of the Therapeutic Garden Professional Group pilot-tested a revised and improved acute care hospital garden design checklist at a garden at St. Rose Hospital in Salt Lake City. In 2005, twenty-five students (mostly landscape architects) in the Chicago Botanic Garden's Therapeutic Garden Design Certificate Program pilot-tested at Shriner's Children's Hospital a checklist specifically created to assess the appropriateness of designs for children's hospital outdoor space.

The AGAT was pilot tested in the summer of 2005 by thirteen participants attending a multi-disciplinary symposium on healing landscapes in Portland, Oregon. The information gleaned was less useful than other tests as it was carried out at an Alzheimer's garden in a public park, whereas this checklist is intended for use in evaluating the outdoor space attached to a residential or day-use building. In all these cases, all pilot-tested by designers, overall inter-observer reliability was strong (85% or better). Where a few specific questions elicited varying responses, it was because of ambiguity of wording.

Sources of AGAT Checklist Items

The specific items in this checklist are derived from several sources. Some items relate to research on how the physical environment impacts all older adults. For example, research indicates that all aging eyes (not just those of patients with dementia) have a problem dealing with glare, hence the checklist includes a question on non-reflective path surfaces. Similarly, the frail-elderly, whether suffering from dementia or not, are more likely to use the outdoors if there are places to rest at frequent intervals, hence a question suggesting the need for seating approximately every fifteen feet along major pathways.

Some items in the checklist refer more specifically to what we know about cognitive changes in dementia patients. For example, one item on the checklist asks about the provision of features that might evoke early memories for residents (depending on location, cultural background, etc.). Another raises the issue of a garden structure, such as an arbor, trellis or pergola, which may cast slatted shadows on the ground which can be misinterpreted by residents as "troughs" or changes in depth, causing stumbling or avoidance.

A third group of checklist items refers to important garden elements which make it easier for staff at a dementia unit, or one for the frail elderly, to schedule programmed activities in the garden, such as a shaded patio just outside the main entry to the garden large enough to accommodate tables, chairs, and wheelchairs; and a clear destination point, such as a gazebo or seating arbor that can also be used for scheduled events.

A fourth group of items are based on general design knowledge regarding successful garden design. These do not specifically relate to Alzheimer's patients nor to their caregivers. These are included since observation of dementia-care gardens suggests they are often overlooked. These include providing sufficient shade, a high ratio of green to hard surfaces, plants selected for seasonal interest, seating options, night lighting, and so on. Finally and importantly, suggestions for the format, wording and content of the AGAT were solicited from a number of experts in Alzheimer's garden design (John Paul Carman, Teresia Hazen, Emi Kiyoto, and Susan Rodiek) and the checklist went through a number of iterations.

The AGAT appears as the Appendix. All comments are welcome. Please send to Clare Cooper Marcus at clare@mygarden.com.

REFERENCES

Cooper Marcus, C. (2005). No Ordinary Garden: Alzheimer's and other patients find refuge in a Michigan dementia-care facility. *Landscape Architecture.* 95 (3), 26-39.

Galbraith, J. and Westphal, J. (2004). Therapeutic Garden Design: Martin Luther Alzheimer Garden. *Proceedings of ASLA conference, Salt Lake City.*

Gold, M.F. (2004). Designs for extended living. *Provider,* November, 18-33.

Grant, C. (2003). Factors Influencing the Use of Outdoor Space by Residents with Dementia in Long-Term Care Facilities. PhD dissertation, Department of Architecture, Georgia Institute of Technology.

Hoover, R. (1995). Healing Gardens and Alzheimer's Disease. *The American Journal of Alzheimer's Care and Related Disorders and Research.* March-April, 1-9.

Lovering, M. J. (1990). Alzheimer's Disease and Outdoor Space. *The American Journal of Alzheimer's Care and Related Disorders and Research.* May-June, 33-40.

Mahan, C. (2004). Lessons Learned: Post Occupancy Evaluation of Eight Dementia Facilities. *Proceedings of ASLA conference, Salt Lake City.*

Mooney, P. and Nicell, P. L. (1992). The Importance of Exterior Environment for Risk Management. *Healthcare Management Forum,* 5 (2), 23-29.

Regnier, V. (1993). *Assisted Living for the Aged and Frail: Innovations in Design, Management and Financing.* New York: Columbia University Press.

Tyson, M. and Zeisel, J. (1999). Alzheimer's Treatment Gardens. In C. Cooper Marcus and M. Barnes (Eds.) *Healing Gardens: Therapeutic Benefits and Design Recommendations.* (437-504) New York: John Wiley & Sons.

doi:10.1300/J081v21n01_09

APPENDIX

Name of Auditor _____

Date _____

Therapeutic Garden Audit
for Alzheimer's Facility

Name of Garden: _____

Location of Garden: _____

Scoring System:

0	=	Feature not present (e.g., no entry patio)
		Quality missing (e.g., not familiar, homelike)
1	=	Poor to fair
2	=	Moderately good, could be improved
3	=	Very successful
NA	=	Not applicable

Score garden according to each of the following issues and
add notes as appropriate.

A. LOCATION AND ENTRY TO GARDEN

Score:

1. Visibly accessible from inside building so that residents can see the garden when going about their daily activities inside.

Score:

2. Door to garden is easy to find.

3. Door into garden is easy to operate.

4. Door is usually unlocked.

5. Threshold of entry door is flat and smooth.

☐ 6. Provision of shaded entry patio with seating just outside the door for those who want to come outdoors but cannot venture further.

☐ 7. Attractive garden view from entry patio since this space may get used more than garden itself.

☐ 8. Entry patio is large enough to accommodate several people in wheelchairs, together with tables and chairs for programmed group activities.

☐ 9. In regions with significant bug problems in summer, entry patio is screened and lit at night.

Score:

☐ 10. Location of entry patio/screened porch to receive late afternoon sun, thus avoiding long shadows that accompany increased agitation at that time of day ("sundowning").

☐ 11. Provision of a conservatory or solarium with plants, birds in cages, etc., looking over garden where residents can enjoy a semi-outdoor experience year-round. Bright, natural light beneficial to health.

☐ 12. A single entry door to garden, designed as a "landmark" so that those using garden can easily see where they have to return to get back indoors.

☐ 13. The whole garden can be viewed from inside the building by staff going about their daily activities or from a nurse's station (if there is one).

B. LAYOUT AND PATHWAYS

☐ 14. The layout of the garden is easy to see and understand to minimize confusion for those who are not functioning well.

☐ 15. Provision of a simple looped, circular or figure-of-eight pathway system with no dead ends or confusing choices whether to turn left or right to return home.

☐ 16. A simple, clear garden layout with one or two destination points, since Alzheimer's residents experience disorientation, or short-term memory loss as it relates specifically to a sense of physical location, and can become easily disoriented and agitated in unfamiliar settings.

APPENDIX
(continued)

Score:

17. Appropriate destination points, such as a gazebo, seating arbor, or large shade tree, that can be used for programmed activities.

18. Provision of a level pathway system including exit from building and patio, since residents may exhibit lack of coordination and balance (apraxia) but are still impelled to move without apparent goal or purpose (wandering behavior).

19. Handrail along all or part of pathway system for those with balance problems.

20. Non-reflective path surface since aging eyes have a hard time dealing with glare. Tinted concrete is good solution.

21. Appropriateness of pathway surfaces for wheelchairs, walkers, reclining geri chairs, shuffling feet of the frail elder, etc. Brushed concrete or asphalt provide appropriate traction.

22. Consistent pathway color, since an Alzheimer's resident reacts to contrasting ground plane colors as if there were a change in depth ("visual cliffing," an example of agnosia, or the inability to understand and use sensory information).

Score:

23. Raised edges to pathways to prevent wheelchair user from rolling into planted area.

24. Pathways wide enough for two wheelchairs to pass (at least six feet).

25. Provision of "markers" or landmarks along the pathway to assist in spatial orientation and allow staff or family members to measure how far a patient can walk.

C. PLANTING

26. High ratio of green to hard surfaces in garden — ideally around 70:30.

27. Provision of a flat lawn area large enough for an informal grouping of movable chairs, a game of croquet, etc., or for young residents to sit or lie on.

28. Provides a great diversity of plants selected for seasonal interest, sensory variety, shade qualities, screening, wildlife habitats, etc.

29. Vegetation introduced in a variety of ways: raised beds, vine-covered arbors and trellises, perennial borders, tubs of annuals, trees, hedges, etc.

Score:

30. Provision of a rich multisensory experience (vision, touch, hearing, smell) to activate the senses.

31. An area specifically designed for supervised gardening activity program (raised beds, potting shed, tool shed, various large containers, gathering area, access to drinking fountain, close to building entry, etc.).

32. Garden receives at least half a day of sun in order for plantings to flourish.

33. Avoidance of toxic plants in gardens for late-stage Alzheimer's patients, since people tend to revert to infancy and put everything in their mouth at this stage in the disease.

34. Avoidance of trees whose fruit or leaves could cause slipping/trip hazards on pathways.

35. Plants are maintained so that walkways are clear of hazards such as branches too low, shrubs "spilling" onto hardscape, etc.

36. Provision of plants popular during youth of residents for potential to promote reminiscing (e.g., roses and lilac in New England).

Score:

D. SEATING

37. Avoidance of plant shapes, structure, shadows, statues, etc. that might trigger delusions since Alzheimer's patients may perceive things that don't exist, and become agitated.

APPENDIX
(continued)

38. Seating options available for person alone or couple.

39. Seating available for groups larger than two to sit and easily converse.

40. Appropriate seating design (e.g., with back and arms for ease of pushing up from a seated position).

41. Comfort of seating material (wood, fabric or hard plastic preferable; steel, aluminum or concrete, least preferable).

42. A bench or chairs for two in a niche that gives the illusion of privacy, since this may encourage social interaction.

43. Choice of seating in sun/shade throughout most of day/year.

Score:

44. Seating at relatively frequent intervals along main paths; every 15 feet is necessary for those who are quite frail, and to encourage those who pace or wander excessively to take a rest.

45. Near view from most seats is attractive/interesting (varied plant materials by color, leaf shape, height, etc.; variety of objects that might be interesting to look at—bird feeder, bird bath, sculpture, etc.).

46. Some moveable seating available; easily moved, but still sturdy enough to prevent tipping.

E. OVERALL DESIGN AND DETAILS

47. Provision of features that might evoke memories for residents. Depending on location, cultural background, etc., these might include a garden shed, mail box, vegetable garden, barbecue, bicycle or small piece of farm equipment (fixed to ground).

48. Small scale design changes so that a person moving slowly would have a variety of visual experiences (enclosed/open, sunny/shaded, varied plant materials, etc.).

49. Avoidance of any garden structure (arbor, trellis, pergola) which might cast slatted shadows which can be misinterpreted as "troughs" or changes in depth.

Score:

50. Potential to observe wildlife (e.g., plants that attract birds, butterflies; bird feeder, bird bath, etc.).

51. Incorporates a bubbling fountain where moving water can be watched and listened to; or a simple water-wall where water can be touched.

52. The extent to which this outdoor space might allow a resident, visitor or staff member to experience an environment in complete contrast to the building interior.

53. The extent to which this outdoor space offers users the opportunity to make *choices* (other than walking routes, which can cause confusion), thus allowing residents a sense of control (e.g., choice of seating arrangements, variety of sub-spaces, etc.).

54. The extent to which this outdoor space is nurturing, calming, familiar, and homelike, not an "artistic statement" or "envelope-pushing" design that might be unfamiliar or jarring to residents.

55. Educational/interpretive material that might be of interest to visitors or residents (e.g., plant labels, plan of garden, etc.).

Score:

56. Garden is very attractive, well maintained, and rich with amenities (gazebo, glider, bird bath, flower beds) so that family members might be encouraged to visit more often, and take their relative outdoors.

57. Lighting so that space can be used for walking, sitting, etc. on warm evenings; or viewed from inside when dark

58. Opportunity for staff to find a place to take a break or eat a brown-bag lunch where they might feel truly "away" from their work, and out of sight of residents.

APPENDIX
(continued)

| | 59. | Appropriateness of space to local climate |

| | 60. | Appropriateness of space to local culture (e.g., using local plants, construction materials, decorative images). |

| | 61. | Degree of privacy from resident rooms/windows looking out onto space. |

| | 62. | Degree of privacy for those inside rooms adjacent to garden. |

Score:

| | 63. | Building edge encloses garden as much as possible, so that the degree to which garden has to be fenced is minimized. |

| | 64. | Boundaries of space provide complete enclosure with trees and tall shrubs screening view of fences or walls and forming a permanent attractive framework to the garden. |

| | 65. | Gate into garden for maintenance staff, and/or serving as an emergency exit is subtly disguised with planting. |

| | 66. | Outdoor space is free from intrusions of unpleasant/incongruent sounds (e.g., traffic, loading dock, loud air conditioners, etc.). |

G. MAINTENANCE AND AMENITIES

| | 67. | Maintenance quality of built features, furnishings and landscape. |

| | 68. | Maintenance quality of plant materials (plant health). |

| | 69. | Availability of litter receptacles and (where appropriate) ash trays. |

Score:

☐ 70. Maintenance quality of litter pick-up.

☐ 71. Availability of phone or communication device (in weather proof box) for emergencies.

☐ 72. Availability of nearby toilets with signage to same in garden.

☐ 73. Provision of a specific outdoor smoking area in this garden or elsewhere.

☐ 74. Storage facility for maintenance staff.

Additional features, design elements, qualities that you think should be added to this audit tool:

With thanks to the following for comments on an earlier draft:
John Paul Carman, Teresia Hazen, Emi Kiyoto, Susan Rodiek

PART II

Therapeutic Effects
of an Outdoor Activity Program
on Nursing Home Residents with Dementia

Bettye Rose Connell
Jon A. Sanford
Donna Lewis

ABSTRACT. *Objective*: The purpose of this one-year pilot study was to obtain preliminary information on the effects of an outdoor activity program, in comparison to an indoor activity program, on sleep and behavior in nursing home residents with dementia. Structured activity programs have been shown to improve dementia-related behavior problems, and there are some indications that improved behavior is associated with improved sleep. Previous research has shown that sleep disturbance is common in nursing home residents, and that limited exposure to light bright enough to entrain circadian rhythms contributes to their sleep problems. Thus, we expected to see improvements in behavior in both the outdoor and indoor activity groups, but improvements in sleep in the outdoor activity group only.

Methodology: A two-group (outdoor program, indoor program) two phase (baseline, intervention) design was used. Subjects were random-

Bettye Rose Connell, PhD, Jon A. Sanford, MArch, and Donna Lewis, RN, GNP, are affiliated with Atlanta VA Medical Center.

Please note this article was authored by 3 federal government employees as part of their official duties: therefore it is a "work of the federal government."

[Haworth co-indexing entry note]: "Therapeutic Effects of an Outdoor Activity Program on Nursing Home Residents with Dementia." Connell, Bettye Rose, Jon A. Sanford, and Donna Lewis. Co-published simultaneously in *Journal of Housing for the Elderly* (The Haworth Press, Inc.) Vol. 21, No. 3/4, 2007, pp. 195-209; and: *Outdoor Environments for People with Dementia* (ed: Susan Rodiek and Benyamin Schwarz) The Haworth Press, Inc., 2007, pp. 195-209. Single or multiple copies of this article are available for a fee from The Haworth Document Delivery Service [1-800-HAWORTH, 9:00 a.m. - 5:00 p.m. (EST). E-mail address: docdelivery@haworthpress.com].

Available online at http://jhe.haworthpress.com
doi:10.1300/J081v21n03_10

ized to the outdoor or indoor program groups. Sleep and behavior disturbance were assessed over a 10-day period at baseline (usual activity conditions, which were expected to include little or no time spent outdoors) and at intervention (daily structured activity program offered outdoors or indoors). Sleep was assessed with wrist actigraphs with photocells, which also allowed for monitoring of light exposure. Behavior disturbance was assessed with the Cohen-Mansfield Agitation Inventory. Both activity programs were offered Monday-Friday over a 2 week period, included similar content and were offered by research project staff. The analytical approach emphasized primary changes between baseline and intervention measures of sleep and behavioral symptoms in the two activity groups. Because this was a pilot study, the significance level was set a priori at $p < 0.10$.

Findings: The outdoor activity group experienced significant improvements in maximum sleep duration. Both groups showed significant improvements in total sleep minutes. There also was a significant improvement in verbal agitation in the outdoor activity group. doi:10.1300/J081v21n03_10 *[Article copies available for a fee from The Haworth Document Delivery Service: 1-800-HAWORTH. E-mail address: <docdelivery@haworthpress.com> Website: <http://www.HaworthPress.com>]*

KEYWORDS. Dementia, sleep, behavior problems, activity program, outdoor, nursing home

BACKGROUND

Planned outdoor spaces are a common feature of long-term care facilities. Popularized as part of dementia special care unit initiatives in the 1980s and 1990s, planned outdoor spaces are generally assumed to be clinically important. However, there is little empirical evidence to support these expectations.

Poor sleep and behavior disturbances are prevalent among nursing home (NH) residents with dementia, and negatively impact their independence and quality of life (QOL) (Ancoli-Israel, Klauber, Jones, Kripke, et al., 1997b; Beck, Rossby & Baldwin, 1991; Bliwise, 1996; Jackson, Spector & Rabins, 1997). Non-pharmacological strategies are needed to improve sleep and dementia-related behavior disturbance in this population. Previous research suggests that spending time outdoors, engaged in meaningful activity, may positively impact sleep and behavior disturbances.

Sleep

Numerous studies report that NH residents' sleep is highly fragmented, as characterized by short periods of sleep throughout the day and night, frequent awakenings, and difficulty falling back to sleep, despite long periods of time spent in bed (Alessi, Yoon, Schnelle, Al-Samarrai, et al., 1999, Alessi, et al., 1997b; Bliwise, et al., 1995; Cohen-Mansfield, Werner & Freedman, 1995; Mishima, Hishikawa & Okwa, 1998). During the day, they are often drowsy and frequently observed asleep, in and out of bed. Some research suggests increased sleep disturbance is to be expected with advanced dementia (Bliwise, Hughes, McMahon & Kutner, 1995). Other research suggests that poor sleep and daytime drowsiness among NH residents can be attributed to insufficient and/or inappropriate physical and mental stimulation and structure during the day to keep residents awake and engaged, as well as nighttime NH environments (e.g., noisy equipment, staff talking loudly in halls) and care regimens (e.g., inconsistent or non-existent bedtime routines, 2 hour wet checks) that are not conducive to sleep (Alessi, et al., 1999; Cohen-Mansfield, et al., 1995; Ouslander, Buxton, Al-Samarrai, Cruise, et al., 1998; Schnelle, Cruise, Alessi, Ludlow, et al., 1998).

Although it is clear that there are many factors that contribute to poor sleep in NH residents, a critical determinant of sleep is human circadian rhythms. A major determinant of human circadian rhythms is exposure to bright light (Czeisler, 1995; Duffy, Kronauer & Czeisler, 1996). There is observational data that most NH residents experience very limited bright light exposure (Ancoli-Israel, et al., 1997b), and that the light they receive is too weak for circadian entrainment. There is extensive evidence that suggests spending time outdoors may result in improved sleep as a result of increased exposure to sunlight (Campbell, Dawson & Anderson, 1993; Campbell, Terman, Lewy, Dijk, et al., 1995; Czeisler, 1995; Duffy, et al., 1996). Previous research using bright light therapy in NH populations has typically relied on light boxes, not sunlight, to deliver bright light. This usually involved having residents sit in front of light boxes, which exposed them to light in the range of 2,000 to 2,500 lux for a prescribed period of time (e.g., an hour). In these studies, a staff person often interacted with participants to ensure they stayed awake and faced the light source for the prescribed period. Overall, results have been promising, but mixed (Ancoli-Israel, et al., 1997b; Ancoli-Israel, Martin, Kripke, Marler, et al., 2002; Kohsaka, Fukuda, Nobayashi, Honma, et al., 1998; Lyketos, Lindell Veiel, Baker & Steele, 1999; Mishima, et al., 1998). However, staff interactions to ensure compliance with the bright light intervention may introduce an unmeasured social component that influences study results

Dementia-Related Behavior Disturbance

In addition to cognitive losses that affect memory, persons with dementia often experience behavior changes and disturbances. More aggressive types of behavior disturbance have been estimated to occur in less than one-fourth of those with dementia, with less aggressive behaviors, such as verbal agitation, estimated to occur in over 90% of those with dementia (Cohen-Mansfield & Werner, 1997; Jackson, Druugovish, Fretwell, Spector, et al., 1989; Sloane, Mitchell, Preisser, Phillips, et al., 1998). A large number of correlates of behavioral symptoms of dementia have been reported, including cognitive status, dependence in activities of daily living, age, sleep disorders, over- and under-stimulation, and depression (Beck, et al., 1991; Cohen-Mansfield & Werner, 1997; Jackson, et al., 1989; Jackson, et al., 1997; Sloane, et al., 1998). Several explanations for dementia-related behavior disturbances have been advanced. Catastrophic episodes and other extreme forms of behavior disturbance may result from a combination of greater sensitivity to environmental stimulation and an inability to cope with or escape these stressors (Hall & Buckwalter, 1986). Another view is that behavior disturbances are a manifestation of unmet needs, such as hunger, pain, fear, disorientation, boredom, frustration, lack of autonomy and privacy, etc. (Algase, Beck, Kolanowski, Whall, et al., 1996). Structured activity programming that addresses unmet psycho-social needs and is geared to participants' preserved cognitive abilities has generally been effective in reducing behavior disturbance (Algase, et al., 1996; Beck, Vogelpohl, Rasin, Ururu, et al., 2005; Richards, Beck, O'Sullivan, Shue, 2005). A limited number of studies have examined the effect of bright light therapy on agitation (Lovell, Ancoli-Israel, Gervirtz, 1995). However, results have been mixed.

There is some evidence that sleep and behavior disturbances are related. One study reported that disruptive vocalizers were more likely to have poor sleep (Cariaga, Burgio, Flynn, Martin, 1991), and another found that less pacing and fewer repeated requests for attention were associated with improved sleep efficiency (time asleep:time in bed) (Cohen-Mnasfield, et al., 1995). Research also has linked behavior disturbance and depression (Kunik, Snow-Turek, Iqbal, Molinari, et al., 1999).

Build It and They Will Come?

Planned outdoor spaces for individuals with dementia were initially conceived as a restraint-free, staffing-neutral means of managing exiting behavior, one type of dementia-related behavior disturbance, and providing safe access to the outdoors for residents with dementia. It was expected that the presence of outdoor space would attract residents with dementia and be associated with less exiting behavior, even in the absence of outdoor activity programming. However, when access to outdoor space was provided, those with a history of exiting neither started using the outdoor space nor stopped exiting the unit (Connell, Sanford, Megrew & Engel, 1997). In addition, our preliminary research and that of others (Cohen-Mansfield & Werner, 1997) suggest that self-initiated outdoor space use by most NH residents with dementia, including those with no history of exiting, is quite limited. In other words, a "build it and they will come" approach does not appear to be sufficient to ensure residents with dementia will use available outdoor spaces on their own.

Early thinking about the design of outdoor spaces for residents with dementia addressed a number of user characteristics likely to impact use, including dementia-related cognitive deficits as well as age- and disease-related sensory and neuro-muscular deficits prevalent in long-term care populations. As a result, it is now common to find outdoor spaces that, for example, are readily accessible, both physically and visually, from indoor locations frequently used by residents and staff, are appealing to multiple senses, and support a variety of active and passive activities. However, people with dementia also often have problems in planning and carrying out activities, and these deficits likely influence their ability to access and use outdoor space independently. For example, using outdoor space independently would entail a resident initiating, and carrying out some or all of the following in roughly this order: deciding to go outdoors, getting the appropriate clothes on for current weather and temperature, wayfinding to the outdoor space without getting lost, forgetting the intended destination or being distracted from the task, locating any needed activity tools or props, and staying engaged in the activity. In contrast, outdoor space use by residents with dementia is far more likely to occur if structured activities programming is provided and staff are available to assist residents in going outdoors, offer activities that are meaningful to them, and provided them with the appropriate level of assistance to keep them engaged.

This Study

In this study, a two-phase (baseline, intervention), two-group (outdoor activity program, indoor activity program) design was used to obtain preliminary data on the effect of bright light exposure during participation in a structured activity program on sleep and behavior disturbance in NH residents with dementia. We hypothesized that an outdoor activity group (bright light exposure and structured activity program) would experience improvements in sleep, but that an indoor activity group, offered only the structured activity program, would not, and that both groups would experience improvements in behavior disturbance.

Activity programming content was planned with a horticultural focus, such as planting pots with seasonal materials and making decorative ornaments for the garden, one's room, or to give as gifts. Other activities, such as singing and telling jokes, were added to respond to participants' interests and abilities. In general, programming was the same to the extent feasible for both groups. Additionally, both the outdoor and indoor programs were offered in small groups of 4-6 persons, at a similar time of day (immediately before or after lunch, respectively) and for the same duration (10 days). Daily programs in both groups were approximately 1 hour in length. Thus, those in the outdoor activity group also received 1 hour of bright light exposure daily during the intervention phase. The outdoor program was offered at an existing outdoor space, directly accessible from the facility dining room, and the indoor program was offered at an activity space on the facility's living units.

This activity programming was delivered by a masters-prepared geriatric nurse practitioner and a certified nursing assistant with previous research experience with nursing home residents. These study staff also actively encouraged residents to attend activity programs, and assisted them in preparing for and traveling to and from both activity locations. During activities, appropriate levels of assistance were provided to foster participation.

The activity programs that were part of the study were offered in addition to activity programs offered routinely in the NH by the recreational therapy program. However, routine programming was not limited to residents with dementia, tailored to their abilities, or offered in small groups.

METHODOLOGY

Site and Sample

Subjects were recruited from a single NH. Inclusion criteria were: age ≥ 65; presence of dementia; not bedridden; no eye disease that would make bright light uncomfortable or block light exposure; expected to be in the NH for the duration of the study period; able to comprehend study procedures, risks, and benefits or appropriate surrogate available to provide informed consent on resident's behalf; and cleared by the medical director for participation. Among the 32 residents who met eligibility requirements, 24 (75%) were consented: 6 declined and 2 died prior to consenting. Four consented subjects began, but did not complete, the study. The final sample consisted of 20 residents, 10 per activity group, or 83% of those who were consented and began baseline.

Variables and Measures

Sleep status was monitored between 7 PM and 7 AM for 10 days at baseline and 10 days at intervention. Sleep was assessed with wrist actigraphs with photocells, which also allowed for monitoring of light exposure, an intervention check. Wrist actigraphy has been used successfully in a number of studies assessing sleep in frail, demented nursing home residents (Alessi, et al., 1999; Ancoli-Israel, et al., 1997b; Ancoli-Israel, et al., 2002; Ouslander, et al., 1998; Richards, et al., 2005), and has been shown to be correlated with polysomnographic evaluations of sleep (Ancoli-Israel, Clopton, Kauber, Fell, et al., 1997a).

Dementia-related behavior disturbance was assessed with the Cohen-Mansfield Agitation Inventory (CMAI) (Cohen-Mansfield, Marx & Rosenthal, 1989). Primary care staff were interviewed by study staff to determine the frequency of 14 behaviors during the baseline and intervention periods.

Changes between baseline and intervention measures of sleep and behavior disturbance for the two activity program groups were assessed with paired t-tests. Because this was a pilot study, the significance level was set at p <0.10. Standardized effect sizes were calculated and are reported for significant findings and are interpreted relative to values on pre-intervention outcome measures (Cohen, 1988).

RESULTS

Sample Characteristics

The final sample consisted of 19 men and 1 woman. Their age ranged from 64 to 90 (79.7 ± 8.3). Five participants (25%) were African-American and 15 (75%) were Caucasian. The two activity groups were similar with regard to age, race, and education. Although the average length of stay (LOS) of the outdoor group was about 3 times longer than that of the indoor group (outdoor m/sd 1,546 ± 1,216 days; indoor m/sd 450 ± 371 days; p < .01), the average LOS in both groups was more than 1 year. The sample had multiple medical diagnoses with cardiovascular (n = 14 participants) and neurological (n = 18 participants) diagnoses the most prevalent. About one-fourth had mood disorders: none were bipolar or schizophrenic. The sample included mildly, moderately, and severely cognitively impaired individuals, as measured by the Mini-Mental State Exam (MMSE) (mean = 15.3 ± 8.4) (Folstein, Folstein & McHugh, 1975). Participants randomized to the outdoor group were more demented than those randomized to the indoor group (outdoor group mean MMSE = 11.70 ± 8.51, indoor group mean MMSE = 18.90 ± 6.90; p = .05).

Three-fourths of the participants were wheelchair users. More than half the participants in each group were "independent" or required "supervision only" for bed mobility and locomotion on and off the unit.

Participation in Activity Programs

The outdoor group participated an average of 8.6 (of 10) days of the intervention and the indoor group participated an average of 7.8 (of 10) days. The most common reason for non-participation was attendance at special activities offered during one week of the intervention by the Recreational Therapy program (11 person days). Other reasons for non-participation related to participants reporting not feeling well or not wanting to get out of bed (7 person days), clinical appointments (6 person days), and refusal (5 person days). Although the activity program groups were nearly equal in number of days missed for clinical reasons and refusal (4 for indoor group, 5 for outdoor group), the indoor group missed 5 times more days than did the outdoor group due to competing events (9 and 2 person days, respectively) and due to not feeling well or not wanting to get out of bed (6 and 1 person days, respectively). These data suggest activities held outdoors are especially appealing to residents, even when content is the same as that offered indoors.

Bright Light Exposure

During baseline, there was no difference (p = .990) in the average maximum light exposure of participants randomized to the outdoor and indoor intervention groups, indicating equivalence at baseline between the two groups. For the outdoor group, average maximum light exposure was significantly higher during intervention than during baseline (p = .000), indicating a significant increase in bright light exposure during the period subjects participated in outdoor programming. In contrast, the indoor group's bright light exposure did not change significantly from baseline to intervention.

Sleep

Sleep was monitored for a total of 234,000 person minutes. Three summary sleep measures were used in analyses: *frequency of wakes* (average number of wakes per night, standardized over a 10 hour night to account for differences in numbers of minutes monitored post initial sleep onset within and across participants), *maximum sleep duration* (average time, in minutes, of longest sleep period each night), and *total sleep minutes* (average total minutes of sleep per night).

A conservative approach was used in determining the *frequency of wakes*: wrist activity indicative of an awakening was classified as a wake only when it followed 10 or more minutes of wrist activity indicative of sleep. Over 2,000 wakes were identified. The outdoor activity group experienced an average of 5.02 ± 2.53 wakes per 10 hour night during baseline (Table 1). Wakes declined to 3.80 ± 2.49 per 10 hour night during intervention. This decline in wakes (p = 0.11) approached the significance level set for the pilot study ($p < 0.10$). In the indoor group, there was no significant change in number of wakes from baseline to intervention (6.18 ± 1.99 wakes *vs.* 5.37 ± 2.08 wakes).

The outdoor activity group's average *maximum sleep duration* improved significantly from baseline (274 ± 169 minutes) to intervention (345 ± 210 minutes) (p = .08). The indoor group's longest sleep period also increased from baseline (226 ± 71 minutes) to intervention (272.44 ± 153), but the change was not significant. The standardized effect size (SES) for *maximum sleep duration* was .37, which is generally accepted as a small effect size (Cohen, 1998). However, when effect size was examined as a percentile standing of the average outdoor group subject at baseline relative to the average outdoor group subject at intervention (Cohen, 1998), the average maximum sleep duration at intervention exceeded that of 66% of the group before the outdoor activity program began.

Total minutes of sleep during intervention increased significantly in both groups. The SES for the change in total sleep for the outdoor activity group is .29, which indicates that the mean of the group's total sleep minutes at intervention was at the 62nd percentile of the group's baseline mean. The indoor ac-

TABLE 1. Sleep of Outdoor and Indoor Groups at Baseline & Intervention

Sleep Variables[1]	Outdoor Activity Group (n=10)		Indoor Activity Group (n=10)	
	Baseline	Intervention	Baseline	Intervention
	Mean (SD)	Mean (SD)	Mean (SD)	Mean (SD)
Frequency of wakes (no.)	5.02 (2.53)	3.80 (2.49)	6.18 (1.99)	5.37 (2.08)
Maximum. sleep duration (min.)	274.42 (169.46)	345.31 (210.29)*	226.83 (70.45)	272.44 (152.83)
Total sleep minutes	441.33 (181.76)	492.93 (179.05)*	416.73 (50.72)	477.39 (101.62)*

[1] Based on wrist actigraphy.
* $p < .10$`

tivity group's intervention total sleep mean was at the 76th percentile of their baseline mean.

Dementia-Related Behavior Disturbance

CMAI ratings were used to construct 3 subscale scores: aggression, physical agitation, and verbal agitation. Verbal agitation occurred most frequently in both groups at baseline (Table 2).

In the outdoor group, the frequency of aggression, physical agitation, and verbal agitation decreased from baseline to intervention. The decline in frequency of verbal agitation in the outdoor group was significant ($p = .01$). The effect size for the baseline to intervention verbal agitation scores was .91. This large effect (Cohen, 1998) for change in verbal agitation indicates that the score of the average subject at intervention was lower than the verbal agitation scores of 82% of the same group before the outdoor activity program began. In the indoor group, the frequency of aggression and verbal agitation also decreased from baseline to intervention, and physical agitation increased. However, none of the changes in behavior disturbance in the indoor group were significant.

DISCUSSION

The study sample experienced many of the sleep problems reported in the literature. Their average maximum sleep periods ranged from nearly 4 to nearly 6 hours long, which represented 54% to 70% of the total 7 to 8 hours of

TABLE 2. Behavior Disturbance in Indoor and Outdoor Groups at Baseline & Intervention.[1]

	Outdoor Activity Group		Indoor Activity Group	
	Baseline	Intervention	Baseline	Intervention
	Mean (SD)	Mean (SD)	Mean (SD)	Mean (SD)
Aggression	6.50 (2.92)	5.90 (2.23)	6.30 (2.91)	5.40 (2.88)
Physical Agitation	7.70 (3.30)	7.10 (3.07)	6.00 (2.31)	6.50 (1.90)
Verbal Agitation)	9.60 (3.03)	7.10 (2.42)**	8.60 (4.22)	7.80 (3.94)

[1] Based on primary care nurse ratings using the Cohen-Mansfield Agitation Inventory. Lower scores indicate less frequent occurrence of behavioral symptoms.
** $p < .05$

sleep they averaged per night. The 7 to 8 hours of sleep that these subjects averaged were often obtained over a 10 to 12 hour period between 7PM and 7 AM with the time they attempted to sleep broken up by a large number of wakes. Finally, the subjects' sleep was highly variable from person-to-person and night-to-night.

During intervention, the outdoor group's sleep improved on two of three sleep measures. Their average maximum sleep period improved by over an hour, and their average total minutes of sleep improved by about 50 minutes. Although the effect sizes associated with these changes are small, they, none-the-less, may represent changes that are important for daytime functioning and quality of life in this population. The improvement in total minutes of sleep in the indoor group was unexpected. However, one recent study (Richards, et al., 2005) has suggested that activity programs tailored to the needs of persons with dementia may have a positive effect on sleep.

This sample as a whole experienced low rates of all three types of behavior disturbance at baseline, resulting in limited room for improvement as a result of the intervention. The statistically significant improvement in verbal agitation in the outdoor activity group may represent clinically important changes that can affect the quality of life of residents. Because of the way the CMAI is scored, a 1 point reduction can represent, for example, a decrease in the frequency of a single problem behavior from "one or more times a day" to only "several times a week." The improvement in verbal agitation is consistent with other studies other studies that have reported an improvement in behavior problems following activity programs that respond to participant preserved abilities and interests. Given the similarity of the outdoor and indoor activity programs, the failure to obtain a significant improvement in behavior disturbance in the indoor group is difficult to explain.

The results of this pilot study suggest that structured activity programs that capitalize on the availability of planned outdoor space to provide bright light exposure may help to improve sleep and behavior in NH residents with dementia. However, the study had a number of limitations that we would like to acknowledge.

The census of the participating NH and the study sample were predominately male, in contrast to the prevalence of women in most NHs. Although gender often is not a significant predictor of sleep or most types of behavior problems in nursing home samples, future studies should seek a more gender-balanced sample, and examine the effects of gender analytically.

There also were differences between the characteristics of the outdoor and indoor activity groups that should be recognized. The outdoor group had resided in the NH longer than had the indoor group. However, the mean LOS of both groups was greater than a year, and it is unlikely that the difference in the mean LOS between the study groups is related to study results. In future studies with larger samples, LOS could be controlled analytically. The outdoor group also was more severely demented than was the indoor group. As suggested previously, increased dementia severity and poorer sleep often go hand-in–hand. Here, for example, the frequency of wakes per 10 hour night were inversely correlated with MMSE scores in both groups during baseline and intervention. However, the implications of these differences for responsiveness to the intervention and the within group comparisons reported here are unclear. In larger trials, it is expected that dementia severity in study groups would be more similar, and sample size would allow for differences to be controlled analytically. Moreover, if the intervention assessed here proves efficacious in larger trials, an important follow-on issue is to determine how dementia severity impacts responsiveness.

The results of this pilot study are promising and warrant follow-up. However, several aspects of the design of future studies will need careful consideration. Some researchers may be tempted to design a study with an outdoor bright light only group in order to isolate the effect of bright light exposure from the social effects of at least partially individualized activities and interactions with staff. We agree it might be possible to successfully implement a study with such a group if the study sample were limited to persons with mild dementia (with few other health problems) who were able to be compliant with intervention procedures (e.g., timing and duration of time outdoors and staying awake during those times with little or no assistance from staff). However, in our experience it would be difficult, if not impossible, to include such a study group with participants who were more demented, sicker and frailer, as is often the case among NH residents. Moreover, it is unlikely that facility staff would clear many residents with these characteristics for participation unless they were to be accompanied outdoors and, at a minimum, observed from nearby. The staff interactions that are likely to be required to keep such residents stay awake and exposed to bright light may be difficult to distinguish from the social interaction component of some types of individualized activities, making it potentially misleading to consider these participants in a bright light only group.

One approach to future studies that builds on the reality of NH resident characteristics and routine activities programming is to consider a 3 group design consisting of a usual activity programming, enhanced activity programming offered indoors, and enhanced activity programming offered outdoors following a baseline of usual activity. In designing future studies, the additional of follow-up measurement periods would permit assessment of how long any improvements in sleep and behavior are maintained after the intervention ends. If the interventions are found to be efficacious, it also will be important to characterize those who responded to the interventions, such as in terms of dementia severity.

An additional consideration in the design of future studies is the activity program. Interventions are normally standardized, both in terms of content and delivery, to ensure it is consistently delivered in the same way across study sites and study staff. However, in the case of persons with dementia, delivering the same intervention in the identical way to all participants would disregard individual differences likely to be present in almost any group of residents with dementia and relevant to their participation. An alternative approach is to individualize the intervention within a framework of planned activities, with planned adaptations specified in advance for how activities are to be offered to individuals as a function of a participant's preserved cognitive ability, sensory impairment, and motor function (range of motion, grasp). For example, during a program to plant fall bulbs, one participant may only require "set-up" (planting pot, potting soil, trowel, and bulbs laid out on workspace where resident will sit) and verbal encouragement, but another may require that the research assistant hold the pot and verbally prompt each step while offering hands-on assistance at some steps. Thus, although both participants are engaged in the same program, the delivery is individualized based on an understanding of participant abilities and pre-planned differences in the delivery of the intervention.

ACKNOWLEDGEMENTS

This study was funded by the Rehabilitation Research Service, Department of Veterans Affairs, Project E2422-P. The authors would also like to thank Patricia Griffiths, PhD, for her assistance with statistical analysis and interpretation.

LITERATURE REFERENCES

Alessi C.A., Yoon, E.J., Schnelle. J.F., Al-Samarrai, N.R., & Cruise, P.A. 1999. A randomized trial of a combined physical activity and environmental intervention in nursing home residents: Do sleep and agitation improve? *JAGS*, *47*:784-791.

Algase, D.L., Beck, C., Kolanowski, A., Whall, A., Berent, S., Richards, K., & Beattie, E. 1996. Need-driven dementia-compromised behavior: An alternative view of disruptive behavior. *Am J Alzheimer's Disease*, *11*(6):10,12-19.

Ancoli-Israel, S., Clopton, P., Klauber, M.R., Fell, R., & Mason, W. 1997a. Use of wrist activity for monitoring sleep/wake in demented nursing home residents. *Sleep*, *20*:24-27.

Ancoli-Israel, S., Klauber, M.R., Jones, D.W., Kripke, D.F., Martin, J., Manson, W., Pat-Horenczyk, R., & Fell, R. 1997b.Variations in circadian rhythms of activity, sleep, and light exposure related to dementia in nursing home residents. *Sleep, 20*:18-23.

Ancoli-Israel, S., Martin, J.L., Kripke, D., Marler, M., & Klauber, M.R. 2002. Effect of light treatment on sleep and circadian rhythms in demented nursing home patients. *JAGS, 50*:282-289.

Beck, C., Rossby, L., & Baldwin, B. 1991. Correlates of disruptive behavior in cognitively impaired elderly nursing home residents. *Arch Psychiatric Nursing, 5*:282-291.

Beck, C.K., Vogelpohl, T.S., Rasin, J.H., Ururu, J.T., O'Sullivan, P., Walls, R., Phillips, R., & Baldwin, B. 2002. Effects of behavioral interventions on disruptive behavior and affect in demented nursing home residents. *Nursing Research, 51*(4): 219-228.

Bliwise, D. L., Hughes, M., McMahon, P.M., & Kutner, N. 1995. Observed sleep/ wakefulness and severity of dementia in a Alzheimer's disease special care unit. *J Gerontology, 50A*:M303-M306.

Bliwise, D.L. 1996. Sleep disorders. In W. E. Reichman & P.R. Katz, eds, *Psychiatric Care in Nursing Homes.* Oxford: Oxford University Press, 118-132.

Campbell, S.S., Dawson, D., & Anderson, M.W. 1993. Alleviation of sleep maintenance insomnia with timed exposure to bright light. *JAGS, 41*:829-836.

Campbell, S.S., Terman, M., Lewy, A.J., Dijk, D.J., Eastman, C.I., & Boulos, Z. 1995. Light treatment for sleep disorders: Consensus report. V. Age-related disturbances. *J Biol Rhythms, 10*(2):151-154.

Cariaga, J., Burgio, L., Flynn, W., & Martin, D. 1991. A controlled study of disruptive vocalizations among geriatric residents in nursing homes. *JAGS, 39*:501-507.

Cohen, J. 1988. *Statistical Power Analysis For The Behavioral Sciences* (2nd ed.). Hilladale, NJ: Lawrence Erlbaum.

Cohen-Mansfield, J., Marx, M., & Rosenthal, A. 1989. A description of agitation in a nursing home. *J Gerontology, 44*:M77-84.

Cohen-Mansfield, J., Werner, P., & Freedman, L. 1995. Sleep and agitation in agitated nursing home residents: An observational study. *Sleep 18*(8):674-60.

Cohen-Mansfield, J., &Werner, P. 1997. Management of verbally disruptive behaviors in nursing home residents. *J Gerontology, 52A*:M369-377.

Cohen-Mansfield, J., & Werner, P. 1999. Outdoor wandering parks for persons with dementia: A survey of characteristics and use. *Alz Dis Assoc Dis, 13*(2):109-17.

Connell, B. R., Sanford, J.A., Megrew, M.B., & Engel, P.A. 1997. Evaluation of Environmental Interventions for Exiting Behavior of Dementia Patients. *Gerontologist, 37*(S1):159.

Czeisler, C.A. 1995. The effect of light on the human circadian pacemaker. *Ciba Foundation Symposium, 183*:254-290.

Duffy, J.F., Kronauer, R.E., & Czeisler, C.A. 1996. Phase-shifting human circadian rhythms: influence of sleep timing, social contact and light exposure. *J Physiology, 495*(pt1):289-297.

Folstein, M. F., Folstein, S.E., & McHugh, P.R. 1975. "Mini-Mental State:" A practical method for grading the cognitive state of patients for the clinician. *J Psychiatric Res, 12*:189-198.

Hall, G.R., & Buckwalter, K.C. 1987. Progressively lowered stress thresholds: A conceptual model for care of adults with Alzheimer's disease. *Arch Psychiatric Nurs, 1*:399-406.

Jackson, M.E., Drugovich, M.L., Fretwell, M.D., Spector, W.D., Sternberg, J, & Rosenstein, R.B. 1989. Prevalence and correlates of disruptive behavior in the nursing home. *J Aging Health, 1*(3):349-369.

Jackson, M.E., Spector, W.D., & Rabins, P.V. 1997. Risk of behavior problems among nursing home residents in the United States. *J Aging Health, 9*(4):451-472.

Kohsaka, M., Fukuda, N., Kobayashi, R., Honma, H., Sakakibara, S., Koyama, E., Nakano, O., & Matsubara, H. 1998. Effects of short duration morning bright light therapy in healthy elderly. II: Sleep and motor activity. *Psychiatry Clin Neuroscience, 52*:252-253.

Kunik, M.E., Snow-Turek, A.L., Iqbal, N., Molinari, V.A., Orengo, C.A., Workman, R.H., Yudofsky, S.C. 1999. Contributions of psychosis and depression to behavioral disturbances in geropsychiatric inpatients with dementia. *J Gerontology, 54A*:M157-M161.

Lovell, B.B., Ancoli-Israel, S., & Gervirtz, R. 1995. The effect of bright light treatment on agitated behavior in institutional elderly. *Psychiatry Res, 57*:7-12.

Lyketsos, C.G., Lindell Veiel, L., Baker, A., & Steele, C. 1999. A randomized, controlled trial of bright light therapy for agitated behaviors in dementia patients residing in long-term care. *Int J Geriatric Psychiatry, 14*:520-525.

Mishima, K., Hishikawa, Y., & Okawa, M. 1998. Randomized, dim light controlled, cross-over test of morning bright light therapy for rest-activity rhythm disorders in patients with vascular dementia and dementia of Alzheimer's type. *Chronobiol Int, 15*:647-654.

Ouslander, J.G., Buxton, W.G., Al-Samarrai, N.R., Cruise, P.A., Alessi, C, & Schnelle, J.F. 1998. Nighttime urinary incontinence and sleep disruption among nursing home residents. *JAGS, 46*:463-466.

Richards, K.C., Beck, C.K., O'Sullivan, P.S., & Shue, V.M. 2005. Effect of individualized social activity on sleep in nursing home residents with dementia. *JAGS, 53*:1510-1517.

Schnelle, J.F., Cruise, P.A., Alessi, C.A., Ludlow, K., Al-Samarrai, N.R., & Ouslander, J.G. 1998. Sleep hygiene in physically dependent nursing home residents: Behavioral and environmental intervention implications. *Sleep, 21*:515-523.

Sloane, P.D., Mitchell, C.M., Preisser, J.S., Phillips, C., Commander, C, Burker, E. 1998. Environmental correlates of resident agitation in Alzheimer's disease special care units. *JAGS, 46*:862-869.

doi:10.1300/J081v21n03_10

Effect of Increased Time Spent Outdoors on Individuals with Dementia Residing in Nursing Homes

Margaret Calkins
Joseph G. Szmerekovsky
Stacey Biddle

SUMMARY. There is growing evidence that exposure to bright light may improve circadian rhythms in individuals with dementia residing in shared residential settings. The vast majority of this research uses electric bright light boxes. However, the outdoor environment not only provides exposure to bright light but to natural elements which have been shown to have a restorative effect across a broad range of situations. Previous research that sought to explore the impact of time spent outdoors on sleep and/or agitation in individuals with dementia was hampered by low time spent outdoors. This project, conducted in three nursing homes (n = 17), used actigraphy, validated proxy measures of sleep and agitation and direct observation to explore the impact of increased time outdoors on sleep and agitation. The repeated measures design assessed residents with dementia under four conditions: winter/no activity, winter/inside activity, summer/no activity and summer/outside activity. Re-

Margaret Calkins, PhD, is President, IDEAAS Inc. and Board Chair, IDEAS Institute, 8055 Chardon Road, Kirtland, OH 44094-9580 (E-mail: mcalkins@IDEAS ConsultingInc.com)

Joseph G. Szmerekovsky, PhD, is Assistant Professor of Management, Marketing and Finance, North Dakota State University, Fargo, ND.

Stacey Biddle, COTA/L, is Research Associate, IDEAS Institute, Kirtland, OH.

[Haworth co-indexing entry note]: "Effect of Increased Time Spent Outdoors on Individuals with Dementia Residing in Nursing Homes." Calkins, Margaret, Joseph G. Szmerekovsky, and Stacey Biddle. Co-published simultaneously in *Journal of Housing for the Elderly* (The Haworth Press, Inc.) Vol. 21, No. 3/4, 2007, pp. 211-228; and: *Outdoor Environments for People with Dementia* (ed: Susan Rodiek and Benyamin Schwarz) The Haworth Press, Inc., 2007, pp. 211-228. Single or multiple copies of this article are available for a fee from The Haworth Document Delivery Service [1-800-HAWORTH, 9:00 a.m. - 5:00 p.m. (EST). E-mail address: docdelivery@haworthpress.com].

Available online at http://jhe.haworthpress.com
doi:10.1300/J081v21n03_11

211

sults suggest that increased time spent outdoors resulted in a modest improvement in sleep, and mixed or immeasurable impact on agitation. doi:10.1300/J081v21n03_11 *[Article copies available for a fee from The Haworth Document Delivery Service: 1-800-HAWORTH. E-mail address: <docdelivery@haworthpress.com> Website: <http://www.HaworthPress.com> © 2007 by The Haworth Press, Inc. All rights reserved.]*

KEYWORDS. Dementia, agitation, sleep, actigraphy, outdoors

Scientists estimate that to up 4 million people suffer from Alzheimer's disease in the United States, and the prevalence doubles every 5 years (U.S. Dept. of Health, 2002). There are approximately 360,000 new cases diagnosed every year, and these numbers will increase as the percentage of the population that is over 65 increases (National Institute on Aging, 1999). The changes that accompany Alzheimer's disease and related dementias [referred to as dementia in this article] are profound, beginning with memory loss, loss of executive function and higher level skills and deteriorating to the point that the person with dementia is incapable of even the most basic personal care, and no longer recognizes her or his closest relatives and friends. There are a number of consequences or behavioral correlates of dementia that are of significant concern to caregivers and, hence, also the research community. Agitation is the most commonly described behavior, affecting an estimated 70-90% of Alzheimer's patients (U.S., 1996). While efforts to determine the cause and develop effective medical treatments and cures are underway, there is a marked need for developing effective non-pharmacological treatments to help the individuals who are currently afflicted with this devastating disease.

One of the most comprehensive treatments has been the creation, largely over the past 20 years, of treatment settings specifically designed and operated to support the changing needs of people with dementia. Commonly referred to as Special Care Units, or SCUs, these settings have dramatically increased in numbers over the past decade. In 1987, the Office of Technology Assessment was able to identify 110 SCUs, although they acknowledge the number might have been closer to 500 (U.S. Department of Health and Human Services, 1987), p. 256). In contrast, a decade later, the National Institute on Aging (National Institute on Aging, 1999) estimated that nearly one in four nursing homes had at least one organized dementia care wing, unit or program, for a total of approximately 4,210 such units. This number does not include units or facilities that are not licensed nursing homes, such as assisted living, which also provide care and services for people with dementia. With the growth in the numbers of SCUs has been a concurrent rise in interest in understanding the efficacy of these units.

To this end, great strides have been made in understanding what constitutes a supportive environment for people with dementia (M. Calkins, 2001; M. P. Calkins, 1988; Cohen & Weisman, 1991) (Zeisel, Hyde, & Levkoff, 1994). At this time, however, these principles have been almost exclusively applied to interior environments. Yet many references, including many of the same references listed above, refer to the benefits of having access to outdoor spaces (E. Brawley, 1997); (M. P. Calkins, 1988)1996; (Cohen & Weisman, 1991) (Hoover, 1995) (Lovering, 1990) (Regnier, 1997). "Positive outdoor spaces can provide variety in the life of people with dementia, offering a choice of familiar opportunities for socialization and privacy, for physical activities, and for contemplation within a safe controlled environment" (Cohen & Weisman, 1991), p. 74).

There is substantial empirical evidence that access to nature-both physical access to natural settings and visual access to natural scenes-has significant, demonstrable, positive clinical health outcomes. Results range from improved recovery from surgery (Ulrich, 1984; Ulrich, Lunden, & Eltinge, 1993), lowered pain of burn patients (Miller, Hickman, & Lemasters, 1992), enhanced recovery from stress, as measured by lowered blood pressure, muscle tension, skin conductance and self-reported feelings (Hartig & Evans, 1993; Parsons, 1998; Ulrich et al., 1991), reduced depression (Genhart, 1993; Wileman, 2001) and improved sleep (Campbell, 1993; Partonen, 1994). Unfortunately, empirical scientific research on the impact of outdoor spaces-or time spent outdoors-for people with dementia is limited. One exception is a longitudinal study by Mooney and Nicell (1992) which found that the use of exterior environments reduced incidents of aggressive behavior, and contributed significantly to a risk management program.

This study was guided by two bodies of work. This first, which is relatively small, suggests that increased time spent outdoors can reduce agitation in individuals with dementia. Research by (Mather, Nemecek, & Oliver, 1997) suggests that individuals who spent more time outdoors expressed less disruptive behavior. They theorized that gardens or outdoor space can reduce the sense of confinement of a secure environment, giving residents the opportunity to move more widely and experience less frustration, wandering and agitation. Similarly, (Mooney, 1992) conducted a longitudinal study in 5 dementia care facilities, and found that the facilities with outdoor spaces adjacent to the unit had less agitation and disruptive behavior than the facilities with no outdoor space. They suggest that increased space for walking (freedom of movement, opportunities to avoid crowding, noise or too much stimulation) can "reduce frustrations and anxiety that characterize all dementias" (p. 24).

The second body of work relates to the impact of light on circadian rhythms and sleep quality. There is significant evidence of disrupted sleep patterns in

TABLE 1. Study design and timeline

Site 1	A B			C D		
Site 2		A B			C D	
Site 3			A B			C D
Timeline	Jan	Feb.	March	April	May	June

people with Alzheimer's Disease, which are most severe in long-term care residents, who have excessively low overall light exposure (Satlin, Volicer, Ross, Herz, & Campbell, 1992; van Someren, 1996). Melatonin is the hormone primarily associated with signaling circadian rhythms, and daylight is known to enhance melatonin levels, which decrease in general with age and are markedly decreased in individuals with dementia (E. Brawley, 2006). Numerous studies suggest a 1-2 hour exposure to bright light results in an improvement in sleep, measured either subjectively (usually by nursing staff) or objectively by actigraphy (S. M. Ancoli-Israel, JL; Gehrman, P; Shochat, T; Corey-Bloom, J; Marler, M; Nolan, S; & Levi, L., 2003; S. M. Ancoli-Israel, JL; Kripke, DF.; Marler, M; & Klauber, MR, 2002). This research is typically conducted with "bright light" devices, which has two significant practical limitations as an intervention. First, it is not necessarily an easy task to get people with moderate to advanced dementia to sit in front of a light box for one to two hours. Second, light boxes are not inexpensive ($250-$400 each). However, several pilot projects (e.g., Connell, 1998) the involved studying people with dementia who spent time outdoors had been identified in which naturally occurring outdoor activity levels were so low that virtually no data could be collected. Thus, some intervention might be necessary to get people to spend time outdoors.

The project described here was an exploratory pilot project to investigate a number of issues related to increasing time spent outdoors by individuals with dementia residing in nursing homes. There were two goals of the study: to examine the impact of increased time spent outdoors on sleep and agitation and explore a variety of methodological issues in preparation for a larger study. We hypothesized that increased time spent outdoors would improve the quality of sleep and decrease agitation. The study was conducted in three non-profit nursing homes in the mid-west. The study was designed as a pre-post quasi-experimental design, where residents served as their own control and, to the extent possible, some confounding variables were held constant.

Study Design: The study was constrained by several factors. First, it was considered unethical to restrict residents' access to outdoors if they wanted to go out. So we conducted observations during winter months when residents were less likely to go outside, and in summer months when spending time outside was more likely. Second, given previous studies which found naturally occurring time spent outdoors to be very low, individualized and small group activities (which could be conducted inside or outside) were planned as an incentive to get residents ourside for at least 30 minutes. In order to assure that it was time spent outdoors, not the activity, that impacted the results, there were 4 conditions or waves of data: A) winter/no activity, B) winter/inside activity, C) summer/no activity and D) summer/outside activity. A,B, and C can all serve as comparisons for D, which was considered the experimental condition. For waves A and C, data was collected for one week, while for waves B & D, data was collected for 2 weeks, recognizing that we would not be able to get people to participate in the planned activity every day.

STUDY SAMPLE

Study Sites: Three nursing homes, each with a significant number of residents having dementia, participated in the study. Two of the three sites had dementia specific units with directly adjacent outdoor courtyards for the exclusive use of residents of that unit, while the third facility did not segregate residents with dementia, and had a courtyard that all residents were free to utilize. The different building configurations were chosen to reflect what exists (both SCUs and integrated units). The three courtyards varied only slightly in terms of the extent to which they were predominantly concrete patio with raised planters, a combination of concrete, ground plantings and raised planters or primarily grass and garden areas with small concrete pads.

Participants: Inclusion criteria consisted of a diagnosis of dementia but still communicative (able to make wants and needs known and able to answer at least yes/no questions on a regular basis, as determined by the charge nurse/ unit director), self-ambulatory independently or with assistive technology, a resident of the facility for at least 3 months prior to the start of the study and expected to be in residence for the duration of the study, able to spend time outdoors (no light sensitive conditions or medications) and either a history of poor sleep patterns and/or a history of aggressive behavior (as determined by charge nurse/unit director). Letters were sent by the facility to family members of residents who met the inclusion criteria, describing the study and asking for consent for the research team to invite their resident to participate. Each resident for whom consent had been provided was approached by the Research Associate (RA) or Principal Investigator (PI), had the study described, and was invited to participate. Of the 18 participants recruited (6 from each site, determined by the number of actigraphy devices able to be purchased), 17 completed the study. One resident was dropped from the project during the first week for refusing to wear (i.e., taking off and hiding) the actigraphy device. Of the residents who completed the study, fifteen were female, and 2 were male; 15 were Caucasian (one of Russian descent), one African American and one Hispanic. Residents had an average MMSE score of 10.5 (range 0-21). Staff data were provided by 32 staff (30 female, 2 male; 14 Caucasian, 16 African American and two Hispanic).

Measures: There were several measures used. Sleep was assessed with the Actilume-L devces manufacturered by Mini-Mitter, which has been well validated against polysomnography. The actilume-L, which is the size of a man's watch and is worn on the wrist, uses an accelerometer to measure movement, and have have been shown in previous studies to be comparable to polysomography, which is considered the gold standard of sleep evaluation research (Ouslander, 2006). These actilumes were also equipped with light meters, which provided information about the amount of light each resident was exposed to. In addition, night shift staff completed a version of the Pittsburgh Sleep Quality Index (PSQ) (Smyth, 1999), modified for daily use. The PSQI is a well validated instrument for the measurement of subjective sleep quality which provides a global score of sleep quality. It was modified to be completed by staff (as opposed to self report) and included 9 questions.

Data on behaviors was collected using the Cohen-Mansifeld Agitation Inventory Short Form (CMAI), also modified for daily use. The CMAI is a series of 14 questions where staff rate the presence and frequency of behaviors typically considered disruptive or indicatinve of distress, such as call out, pacing, repritive motions and physical aggreesion. Day and evening shift staff were asked to complete data after every shift, and the research assistant (RA) observed the residents for every 20 minutes for 4 hours every day (stratified over morning, mid-day, afternoon and early evening time periods). The RA's CMAI form was modified to include Lawton et al's Facial Affect Rating Scale. This scale uses facial expressions to evaluate the mood of the residents into one of 6 categories (pleasure, anxiety, anger, sadness, alertness and no affect).

RESULTS

As an exploratory study, we were interested in a number of different sets of results. Preliminarily, we sought to explore whether residents did indeed spend more time outside during the summer than winter months, and whether this occurred naturally (condition C) or required an intervention (condition D, summer with outside activity). This can be answered by the actilume data on exposure to light. More significantly, we were interested in whether increased time spent outdoors would impact sleep as assesded by the actilume (referred to a "sleep" in the tables or the staff-completed PSQ), or agitation as assessed by staff-completed CMAI or RA-completed CMAI or facial affect ratings.

Seasonal weather conditions made the analyses more complicated. The city where the study was held experienced unseasonably warm weather during the spring, when residents were in the "indoor" activity phase. It was not appropriate/ethical to ask residents not to go outdoors if they chose to do so, which many did, which made data analysis more difficult. Further, the weather in June was quite cold and wet, making it difficult to get residents outside for activities, and the temperature was over 90°F in July, leaving only a short window of time each morning when it was safe to bring residents outside.

To test whether or not residents spent more time outdoors in the summer months, randomized block analysis was used to determine if there was a significant change in average light level among the four conditions. Blocking was done both by resident and by facility to account for different behavior among individuals at different times of the year. This blocking controlled for differences across individuals and across facilities so that the difference between base-line, control and experimental conditions could be identified. The design included four treatments corresponding to the four conditions: A (winter, no activity), B (winter, inside activity), C (summer, no activity) and D (summer, outside activity). Since average light level and sleep efficiency exhibited non-homogenous variance across treatments (due to the unanticipated weather conditions), Tamhane's T2 test was used to test for significant changes across treatments. This test uses pairwise comparisons similar to a t-test but does not require the assumption of equal variances. In addition, since Resident 14 refused to participate in the experimental conditions, data from that resident was not used in these tests. Of the six comparisons performed

TABLE 2. Average light levels across three conditions

D (Summer, outside activity) versus Other Conditions	Average Light Level in Lux	Estimated Difference	Significance
A (winter, no activity)	33.386	179.018	0.000
B (winter, inside activity)	91.137	121.267	0.025
C (summer, no activity)	85.130	127.274	0.006

with average light levels only three were significant. The average light levels (measured in Lux), estimated differences and significance levels for the three significant comparisons appear in Table 2.

From Table 2 we see that the average light level residents experienced during the experimental condition (D-summer, outside activity) when people were hypothesized to be spending the most time outside (212.404 lux) was signficiantly higher than in any of the other conditions. However, the light levels do not differ significantly between conditions A, B and C, suggesting that residents tended to remain inside during the these three conditions. These results suggest that the Actilume data is sufficient for identifying whether or not changes to outcome data (sleep and behavior) was due to change in exposure to higher light levels/spending time outdoors.

The second set of results relates to the impact of light on sleep and agitation levels. Initially, three sets of analyses were performed. First, analysis was performed to determine the results which would be achieved if only the Actilume data were gathered for the experiment (on light and sleep). Regression analysis was used to determine if there was any correlation between the average light levels and sleep efficiency (i.e., falling asleep soon after going to bed and staying asleep) recorded by the Actilume system and randomized block analysis was used to determine if there is a significant change in sleep efficiency between the four conditions. Second, analysis was performed to determine if the data from the Actilume system was representative of the data collected by the staff and the RA. For these purposes regression analysis was again used. Third, randomized block analysis was used to determine if there is any significant difference in the average facial expressions between the control and experimental data collected by the RA. Because of the weather-related challenges, the decision was made to also conduct a fourth set of analyses by actual time spent outdoors, as assessed by the Actilumes. The light data was coded so individuals were scored as high (10 or more minutes outside within a 24 hour period), moderate (3.5 to 9.5 minutes outside), or low (having 3 or less minutes outside). For these purposes residents were assumed to be outside if the recorded light level was at least 2000 lux. Randomized block analysis was then used to test for significant improvements in resident behavior during times of high, moderate and low light exposure.

Twenty-one different regression models were tested to check for correlation between average light levels and sleep efficiency. One used the data from all residents adjusting only for average differences in individual resident sleep efficiency, three others each used data from only one facility adjusting only for average differences in individual resident sleep efficiency and the final seventeen each used data from only one of the residents. Of the twenty-one analyses only two showed a significant correlation between average light level and

TABLE 3. Correlation between average light levels and sleep efficiency

Model	Coefficient	Significance
Resident 10	-0.07022	0.016
Resident 13	-0.04172	0.012

sleep efficiency at the .05 level. These were the model using only Resident 10's data and the model using only Resident 13's data. Correlations and significance levels for these models appear in Table 3.

Table 3 reveals that Resident 10 experienced a .07 decrease in sleep efficiency for each unit of increase in average light level and Resident 13 experienced a .04 decrease in sleep efficiency for each unit of increase in average light level. This negative correlation is unexpected; but can potentially be explained by Resident 10's protective wrist cover which often covered the Actilume device and Resident 13's tendency to sleep throughout the day.

Randomized block analysis similar to that reported for light levels in Table 2 was used to determine if sleep efficiency changed significantly based on condition. Of the six comparisons performed with sleep efficiency none were significant. The lack of significance for differences in sleep efficiency suggests that though the Actilume data captured the change in light exposure (as identified by Table 2) it did not capture any improvements in resident patterns of sleep resulting from the increased light exposure.

One-hundred twelve different regression models were tested to check for correlation between the Actilume data and the data collected by facility staff and the RA. Twenty-eight models used the CMAI data collected by the day shift with fourteen of these comparing average light levels to the fourteen questions and the other fourteen comparing sleep efficiency to the fourteen questions. Fifty-six other models were the same analysis using the evening shift CMAI data and the RA data. An additional twelve models compared average light levels and sleep efficiency to the facial affect data collected by the RA. The final sixteen models compared average light levels and sleep efficiency to the eight PSQ questions answered by the night shift staff. All regression models used the data from all residents adjusting for average differences in individual residents' responses.

Of the twenty-eight day shift models only one showed a significant correlation between the Actilume data and the staff responses at the .05 level. The coefficient, significance level and R-square value for this model appear in Table 4.

The model indicates that for each 1% increase in sleep efficiency residents were 0.137% less likely to exhibit inappropriate dress or disrobing during the

TABLE 4. Correlation between Actiwatch data and day shift staff ratings of residents

Model	Coefficient of Sleep	Significance	R-square
CMAI: Inappropriate Dress	-0.00137	0.017	0.302

day as indicated by a positive response to CMAI question regarding inappropriate dressing on the day shift form. This suggests that resident disrobing during the day may be related to residents sleeping poorly at night. However, the low R-square value of 0.302 indicates that sleep efficiency only accounted for 30.2% of the variation in inappropriate dress or disrobing. Hence, the sleep efficiency data collected by the Actilume system can not be used exclusively to explain the staff data.

Of the twenty-eight evening shift models none of the average light level models were found to be significant and only three of the sleep efficiency models showed a significant correlation at the .05 level. Table 5 shows the coefficients, significance levels and R-square values for these models.

Surprisingly, all three models indicate an approximate 0.2% increase in negative behaviors (aggressive behaviors/self-abuse, inappropriate handling of objects and screaming) for each 1% increase in sleep efficiency. This positive relationship may suggest that the negative behaviors are a product of the residents feeling sufficiently rested before the night is over. Again however, low R-square values indicate that sleep efficiency explains less than one-third of the variation in staff responses suggesting that the negative behaviors are heavily affected by additional factors not included in the models which may also account for the positive relationship.

Of the sixteen night shift models none of the average light level models were found to be significant. However, five of the eight sleep efficiency models showed a significant correlation at the .05 level. Table 6 shows the coefficients, significance levels and R-square values for these models.

From the models we see that for each 1% increase in sleep efficiency there is a 0.6% less chance that residents woke up and remained awake for several hours, a 0.5% less chance that residents woke up and wanted to get out of bed, a 0.6 decrease in average restlessness, a 2 minute reduction in the time the residents got up and a 0.4% less chance that residents went back to bed. Though the relationship between sleep efficiency and staff data is as anticipated this time, low R-square values still indicate that sleep efficiency explains only a small amount of the variation in staff data and alone is not sufficient to replace the PSQI data.

TABLE 5. Correlation between Actiwatch data and evening shift staff ratings of residents

Model	Coefficient of Sleep	Significance	R-square
CMAI: Aggressive Behavior	0.00222	0.026	0.061
CMAI: Inappropriate Handling of Objects	0.00247	0.024	0.32
CMAI: Screaming	0.00237	0.039	0.122

TABLE 6. Correlation of sleep rated by the PSQI and Actiwatch

Model	Coefficient of Sleep	Significance	R-square
PSQI: Trouble Returning to Sleep	-0.00609	0.000	0.241
PSQI: Wants Out of Bed	-0.00502	0.011	0.183
PSQI: Overall Restlessness	-0.00625	0.031	0.265
PSQI: Wake-up Time	-2.034	0.001	0.226
PSQI: Goes Back to Bed	-0.00395	0.042	0.167

Of the twenty-eight RA models corresponding to the fourteen CMAI questions only one of the average light level models and three of the sleep efficiency models showed a significant correlation at the .05 level. The coefficients, significance levels and R-square values for these models can be found in Table 7.

From the first model we see that for each unit increase in average light level instances of screaming decrease .002%. From the other models we see that for each 1% increase in sleep efficiency there is a 0.05% less chance that residents engage in destroying property, a 0.015% less chance that residents engage in aggressive or self abusive behavior and a 0.2% less chance that residents constantly request attention. Though the relationships are as expected the models still suffer from low R-square values indicating that only a small amount of the variation is explained.

Of the twelve RA models corresponding to the facial affect ratings only one showed a significant correlation at the .05 level. The coefficient, significance level and R-square value for this model appear in Table 8.

From the model we see that for each 1% increase in sleep efficiency anxiety decreased .003 in rating. Though the R-square value here is the best so far, sleep efficiency still explains less than half of the variation in anxiety levels.

TABLE 7. Correlations between sleep or light and behaviors

Model	Coefficient of Light or Sleep	Significance	R-square
CMAI: Screaming and Light	-0.00002235	0.043	0.071
CMAI: Grabbing/Destroying Property and Sleep	-0.000483	0.023	0.055
CMAI: Aggressive Behavior and Sleep	-0.000152	0.026	0.014
CMAI: Request for Attention and Sleep	-0.00186	0.000	0.138

TABLE 8. Correlations between sleep and affect

Model	Coefficient of Sleep	Significance	R-square
Anxiety and Sleep	-0.00317	0.023	0.475

Six randomized block designs were used to determine if residents exhibited improved facial affect ratings during the summer with activity condition as opposed to the winter with activity condition. The individual residents corresponded to the blocks in the design and the condition (summer or winter) corresponded to the treatment levels. For each facial affect average rating during winter conditions, average rating during summer conditions, estimated effect of summer conditions (after adjusting by individual residents) and significance level appear in Table 9.

From the table we see that during the experiment average Pleasure, Anxiety and No Emotion ratings increased significantly by 0.122, 0.187 and 0.104 respectively. This indicates that the experiment resulted in increased levels of both pleasure (possibly from the experience of going outside) and anxiety (possibly from the change of routine of the additional activities) for the residents. Though the changes in Anger, Sadness and Alertness were not significant, the estimated effects indicate that the ratings improved, with Anger and Sadness ratings decreasing 0.131 and 0.00981 respectively and Alertness ratings increasing 0.0424. The lack of significance for these changes is likely attributable to floor and ceiling effects. That is, Anger and Sadness ratings were low and Alertness was high in the winter conditions, hence there was not significant room for improvement in the ratings.

Finally, fifty-seven randomized block analyses were conducted to determine whether there was any correlation between daily exposure to light (Low, Medium and High) and staff and Research Assistant [RA] ratings of behavior. Thirty-seven of these correspond to comparing the fourteen questions on the

TABLE 9. Relationship between affect and light levels

Facial Affect	Average Winter with activity (condition B) Rating	Average Summer with activity (Condition D) Rating	Estimated Effect	Significance
Pleasure	0.36	0.49	0.122	0.000
Anxiety	0.49	0.69	0.187	0.000
Anger	0.08	0.06	-.0131	0.393
Sadness	.04	.03	-0.00981	0.496
Alertness	3.41	3.44	0.0424	0.412
No Emotion	3.13	3.23	.104	0.019

CMAI to the exposure to light during the day and evening shifts and the nine questions on the PSQI during the night shift while controlling for individual residents average scores on the CMAI and PSQI. Fourteen consider the same analysis with the CMAI using the RA data and six consider the same analysis but using the facial affect ratings from the RA. There were no significant correlations between day shift behavior ratings and exposure to light. Table 10 summarizes the significant relations.

For all significant results reported here, the results were only significant between the low light level (3 or less minutes) and the high light level (10 or more minutes), but not with the moderate light level (3.5-9.5 minutes). Evening shift staff reported residents with high light exposure exhibited greater requests for attention than residents with low light exposure and night shift staff reported that high light exposure was associated with an increased desire to get up and out of bed over low light exposure. They also reported an overall improvement in sleep behavior of residents with 10 + minutes of time outside over residents with 3 or fewer minutes of time outside. This increase of 0.209 on the average sleep was computed using 1 = slept soundly, 2 = slightly restless, and 3 = very restless. For the RA three of the fourteen behaviors on the CMAI showed significant decreases when residents had 10 or more minutes of time outside over when they had less than 3 minutes outside: grabbing, requests for attention, and strange noises. For facial affects, the RA indicated less alertness in residents that had received high light exposure compared to low light exposure.

An additional goal of the project was to determine if the Actilume would provide discernable data on agitation levels of residents. These analyses were not even run because the data from the staff related to time when behaviors assessed on the CMAI occurred were either missing or so general ("all shift") as

TABLE 10. Correlations between staff or RA behavior ratings and light levels

Shift or RA	Question	Difference between High and Low	Significance
Evening	CMAI:9	0.125	0.007
Night	PSQI:I5	0.171	0.012
Night	PSQI:I6	0.209	0.037
RA	CMAI:3	-0.0154	0.025
RA	CMAI:9	-0.0378	0.007
RA	CMAI:12	-0.0312	0.001
RA	Alertness	-0.0390	0.000

to be useless. Although this data was available from the RA, her observations were only for four hours per day and frequencies of agitated behaviors that were expressed physically (as opposed to verbally) were too infrequent. Further, visual scanning of the actigrams clearly showed high levels of movement (which is what would be indicative of agitation) at times when the resident was engaged in activities but not agitated (e.g., during meals or during certain hand-active activities such as bingo and exercise). There was no way to differentiate high readings from productive activity versus from agitation.

CONCLUSION

Overall, the results provide mild support our hypothesis that increased time spent outdoors would improve quality of sleep. Given the challenges of this pilot project, a 10% increase in sleep efficiency is an encouraging result. There were also several smaller but positive behavioral changes (less grabbing and fewer strange noises), and a few changes that are either contradictory (the RA noted less residents requests for attention during the day, but the evening shift noted more requests for attention) or open to interpretation about whether they are positive or negative (more likely to want to get out of bed). Given that spending time outdoors is an intervention that in many facilities does not need to cost more (assuming they have access to an outdoor space) and is associated with such positive sleep outcomes and modest behavioral outcomes, there is a clear need for further study in this area.

The evening shift reporting of residents increased requests for attention can be interpreted several ways. For staff, requests for attention represented an undesirable behavior during a period when they are trying to get residents to go the bed for the night. An alternative explanation would be that because these individuals are sleeping better, they don't want to go to bed as early–which could be viewed positively, but they need direction for something to do in the evening.

The disparity between the RA observations (with three significant behavior differences) and the day shift observations (no significant differences) is worth examining. There are two possible explanations. First, in addition to day shift not being very interested in completing the forms, they may not have given sufficient attention to rating the behaviors of residents. Alternatively, it was not possible to completely blind the RA to the purpose of the study, so consideration must also be given to the possibility that the RA was looking for improved behaviors in the outdoor condition. However, since a number of residents had high light exposure during the winter with activity condition, and the decision to drop the analysis by condition and replace it with analysis by high, moderate and low light level exposure was made after the data was completed, that would tend to mitigate this as an explanation.

Several useful methodological issues were addressed in this study, which will aid in the design of future projects. First, in general, the Actilume device was easily tolerated by most of the individuals in the project. Only 1 of 18 (5%) refused to wear the watch, and only 3 (15%) needed to be reminded several times why they were wearing the watch before they were comfortable wearing it. The watch bands were reasonably secure and were bright blue (in an attempt to make it look more like jewelry). Neither of the 2 male residents seemed upset by the blue color. Further exploration of watch band options should be considered. However, placement of the actigraphy device so that it accurately reads light levels was an ongoing issue. Many frail older individuals are often cold, even when the weather is warm. Thus they tend to wear long sleeved garments, which tend to cover the photocell of the actigraphy device. The RA repeatedly rolled sleeves back a little and encouraged residents not to cross their arms when they were outside. This level of oversight was not done when residents chose to spend time outdoors outside of the planned activity time, which may affect the quality of the light level readings.

Second, the staff at the facilities was not particularly reliable as a source of behavioral data. Significant efforts were made on an ongoing basis to get forms completed on a daily basis, and this project still ended with a significant amount of missing data. Consideration should be given to alternative methods for collecting this data.

Third, weather, when conducting a short pilot project outdoors, can be unpredictable and uncooperative. This should be less of an issue in a project of longer duration. The planned activity (which was the means to get people to spend time outdoors) had to be modified to be more individualize-based than group. To some extent, this impacted the amount of data the RA could collect, because she spent more time running a series of smaller group or individual activities, which meant fewer observations of residents who were not participating in the activity. Future projects should have separate individuals running the activities and doing behavior observations. Finally, the Actilume was not able to provide reliable data on agitation or stress levels–there was no way to differentiate between positive activities that involved hand motion and stress or agitation as expressed in wrist movement. Behavior observations by a trained researcher are likely to provide the most reliable and accurate data for agitation.

Overall, it does not appear that the Actilume data is effective in capturing all of the information contained in the staff data and RA data. It also appears that there are too many other factors involved for light levels and activity levels to capture everything that is going on. Based on the randomized block analysis using the facial affect rating data, there is evidence that residents showed both more pleasure and anxiety during summer than winter, and sleep did improve in people who spent more time outside. Experiments with residents that have broader ratings of facial affects could indicate if the experimental conditions can significantly improve Anger, Sadness and Alertness as well.

REFERENCES

Ancoli-Israel, S. M., JL; Gehrman, P; Shochat, T; Corey-Bloom, J; Marler, M; Nolan, S; & Levi, L. (2003). Effect of Light on Agitation in Institutionalized Patients with Severe Alzheimer Disease. *American Journal of Geriatric Psychiatry, 11*(2), 194-203.

Ancoli-Israel, S. M., JL; Kripke, DF.; Marler, M; & Klauber, MR. (2002). Effect of Light Treatment on Sleep and Circadian Rhythms in Demented Nursing Home Patients. *Journal of the American Geriatric Society, 50*(2), 282-289.

Brawley, E. (1997). Designing for Alzheimer's disease: Strategies for better care environments. New York: John Wiley and Sons.

Brawley, E. (2006). Design Innovations for Aging and Alzheimer's: Creating Caring Environments. Hoboken, NJ: John Wiley & Sons.

Calkins, M. (2001). Creating Successful Dementia Care Settings. (Vol. 1-4). Baltimore MD: Health Professions Press.

Calkins, M. P. (1988). Design for Dementia: Planning Environments for the Elderly and the Confused. Owings Mills, M.D.: National Health Publishing.

Campbell, S. S. D., Drew; & Anderson, Michael W. (1993). Alleviation of Sleep Maintenance Insomnia with Timed Exposure to Bright Light. *Journal of the American Geriatric Society, 41*(8), 829-836.

Cohen, U., & Weisman, J. (1991). Holding on to Home. Baltimore, M.D.: Johns Hopkins University Press.

Connell, B.R., Sanford, J.A., & Lewis, D. (in press). Therapeutic effects of an outdoor activity program on nursing home residents with dementia. *Journal of Housing for the Elderly ,21*(3/4).

Genhart, M. K., KA; Coursey, RD; Datiles, M; & Rosenthal, NE. (1993). Effects of Bright Light on Mood in Normal Elderly Women. *Psychiatry Research, 47*(1), 87-97.

Hartig, T., & Evans, G. (1993). Psychological foundations of nature experience. In T. Garling & R. Golledge (Eds.), Behavior and Environment: Psychological and Geographical Approaches (pp. 427-457). Amsterdam: Elsevier.

Hoover, R. C. (1995). Healing Gardens and Alzheimer's Disease. *The American Journal of Alzheimer's Disease*(March/April), 1-9.

Lovering, M. (1990). Alzheimer's disese and outdoor space: Issues in environmental design. *The American Journal of Alzheimer's Care and Related Disorders & Research, 5*(3), 33-40.

Mather, J. A., Nemecek, D., & Oliver, K. (1997). The Effect Of A Walled Garden On Behavior Of Individuals With Alzheimer's. *American Journal of Alzheimer's Disease, 12*(6), 252-157.

Miller, A., Hickman, L., & Lemasters, g. (1992). A distraction technique for control of burn pain. *Journal of Burn Care and Rehabilitation, 3*, 155-157.

Mooney, P., & Nicell, P. L. (1992). The Importance of Exterior Environment for Alzheimer Residents: Effective Care and Risk Management. *Healthcare Management FORUM, 5*(2), 23-29.

Ouslander, J., Connell, BR., Bliwise, DL., Endeshaw, Y., Griffiths, P., & Schnelle, JF. (2006). A nonpharmacological intervention to improve sleep in nursing home patients: Results of a controlled clinical trial. *Journal of the American Geriatrics Society, 54*(1), 38-47.

Parsons, R. T., Louis G.; Ulrich, Roger S.; Hebl, Michelle R. & Grossman-Alexander, Michele. (1998). The View From the Road: Implications for Stress Recovery and Immunization. *Journal of Environmental Psychology, 18*, 113-140.

Partonen, T. (1994). Effects of Morning Light Treatment on Subjective Sleepiness and Mood in Winter Depression. *Journal of Affective Disorders, 30*(2), 99-108.

Regnier, V. (1997). Design for Assisted Living. Contemporary Long Term Care, February, 50-56.

Satlin, A., Volicer, L., Ross, V., Herz, L., & Campbell, S. (1992). Bright Light Treatment of Behavioral and Sleep Disturbances in Patients With Alzheimer's Disease. *American Journal of Psychiatry, 149*(8), 1028-1032.

Smyth, C. (1999). The Pittsburgh Sleep Quality Index. *Journal of Gerontological Nursing, 25*(12), 10-11.

U.S. Dept. of Health, E., and Human Services / NIH. (2002). Alzheimer's Disease: Unraveling the Mystery (No. 02-3782). Washington DC: National Institute on Aging, National Institutes of Health.

U.S. Department of Health and Human Services. (1987). Losing a Million Minds: Confronting the Tragedy of Alzheimer's Disease and other dementias (Vol. # OTA-BA-323). Washington D.C.: U.S. Government Printing Office.

U.S., D. o. H. a. H. S. (1996). Alzheimer's Disease and Related Dementias: Acute and long-term care services: DHHS.

Ulrich, R. (1984). View through a window may influence recovery from surgery. *Science, 224,* 420-421.

Ulrich, R., Lunden, O., & Eltinge, J. (1993). Effects of exposure to nature and abstract pictures on patients recovering from heart surgery. Paper presented at the Thirty thrd Meeting of the Society of Psychophysiological Research, Rottach-Egren, Germany.

Ulrich, R., Simons, R., Losito, B., Fiorito, E., &, M. M., & Zelson, M. (1991). Stress recovery during expsoure to natural and urban environments. *Journal of Environmental Psychology, 11,* 201-230.

van Someren, E. H., EE; Lijzenga,C; Scheltens, P; deRooij, SE; Jonker,C; Pot, AM; Mirmiran,M & Swaab, DF. (1996). Circadian Rest-Activity Rhythm Disturbances in Alzheimer's Disease. *Biological Psychiatry, 40*(4), 259-270.

Wileman, S. E., JM; Andrew, JE; Howie, FL; Cameron, IM; McCormack, K & Naji, SA. (2001). Light Therapy For Seasonal Affective Disorder In Primary Care: Randomised Controlled Trial. *British Journal of Psychiatry, 178*(April 2001), 311-316.

Zeisel, J., Hyde, J., & Levkoff, S. (1994). Best practices: An environment-behavior model for Alzheimer special care units. *The American Journal of Alzheimer's Care and Related Disorders & Research, 9*(2), 4-21.

doi:10.1300/J081v21n03_11

Contact with Outdoor Greenery Can Support Competence Among People with Dementia

Erja Rappe
Päivi Topo

SUMMARY. Dementia disorders are increasing among populations all over the world due to growing life expectancy. Since dementia widely affects cognition, especially short-term memory and orientation, people with dementia are more dependent on provisions from their environment to act successfully than those without dementia. Green environments have been associated with reduced autonomic arousal leading to stress recovery and improved affective state. In this paper we introduce theories and empirical studies about healing and green environment, and present our findings on the impact of plants, and of seeing and being outdoors on the well-being of people with dementia in day care and in residential care. The first study is based on a survey of 65 nursing staff from ten residential care homes. The second study involved 123 people with dementia from two day care units and six residential care units. doi:10.1300/J081v21n03_12 [Article copies available for a fee from The Haworth Document Delivery Service: 1-800-HAWORTH. E-mail address: <docdelivery@haworthpress.com>

Erja Rappe, PhD, is Planning Officer, Department of Applied Biology, University of Helsinki, P. O. Box 27, FIN-00014 University of Helsinki, Finland, Europe (E-mail: erja.rappe@helsinki.fi). Päivi Topo, PhD, is Research Director, National Research and Development Centre for Welfare and Health, STAKES, P.O. Box 220, FIN-00531 Helsinki, Finland, Europe (E-mail: paivi.topo@stakes.fi).

[Haworth co-indexing entry note]: "Contact with Outdoor Greenery Can Support Competence Among People with Dementia." Rappe, Erja, and Päivi Topo. Co-published simultaneously in *Journal of Housing for the Elderly* (The Haworth Press, Inc.) Vol. 21, No. 3/4, 2007, pp. 229-248; and: *Outdoor Environments for People with Dementia* (ed: Susan Rodiek and Benyamin Schwarz) The Haworth Press, Inc., 2007, pp. 229-248. Single or multiple copies of this article are available for a fee from The Haworth Document Delivery Service [1-800-HAWORTH, 9:00 a.m. - 5:00 p.m. (EST). E-mail address: docdelivery@haworthpress.com].

Available online at http://jhe.haworthpress.com
doi:10.1300/J081v21n03_12

KEYWORDS. Dementia, green environment, plants, stress, competence, cognition, visiting outdoors

INTRODUCTION

Dementia Decreases Autonomy and Increases Dependence

The number of people with dementia is rapidly growing mainly due to ageing of the population and especially the increasing number of the oldest old. The risk of dementia increases in old age: 55% of people with dementia are aged over 80. Dementia syndrome is the major reason for moving to residential care and 80-90 percent of the residents have dementia illnesses in Finland (Noro et al., 2005).

Dementia is a syndrome caused by several diseases, for example Alzheimer's disease. The syndrome widely affects cognition and there are disturbances for example in short term memory, orientation and in judgment (ICD10). People with dementia also have a higher risk of depression. Although research interest in the etiology of dementia and in the development of pharmacological treatments is high, no curative treatment exists. Therefore, the emphasis is on nursing, on possibilities for maintaining functioning and on supporting the positive mood of the patients.

Difficulty in learning is often the first symptom of dementia, while physical functioning and recalling previously learned information are better preserved in the early stages of illness (Sulkava et al., 1994). Individuals with dementia are often confused because they have problems in orientating to place and time and in identifying objects and places (Zeisel & Tyson, 1999; Teresi et al., 2000). Therefore, the perception of familiar characteristics in the environment may result in a sense of comfort and feelings of control (Carman, 2002) as well as help in orientation.

Restlessness and agitated or aggressive behavior are common among people with dementia and it burdens caregivers, leading to restrictive care (Cohen-Mansfield, 2001; Kirkevold, 2005) and the use of sedative medicines that accelerate functional decline (Valla & Harrington, 1998). Sensory deprivation, boredom, and loneliness are common precursors to challenging behavior (Cohen-Mansfield, 2001).

In dementia illnesses, cognitive and functional abilities decrease progressively and individuals become more and more dependent on provisions from their environment (Sulkava et al., 1994). An environment that meets the needs of people with dementia may affect behavior positively and delay functional and cognitive declines (Valla & Harrington, 1998).

The aim of our paper is (i) to introduce theories about a healing environment and previous empirical studies on the green environment and well-being, (ii) to present our findings on the impact of plants on the well-being of people with dementia and on how nursing staff experience plants in the care environment, (iii) to describe our qualitative findings on well-being associated with visiting and seeing outdoors by people with dementia in day care and in residential care. At the end of the paper we discuss how to use green outdoor environments in maintaining the competence of people with dementia and how to improve the use of greenery in care environments.

Natural Knowledge Easy to Understand

Humans have strong ties to nature that are evidenced in physiological, psychological and emotional processes evoked by exposure to natural objects. Environments with plants as dominant elements have been found to engender therapeutic effects on people. So, there is reason to assume that contact with outdoor nature also provides some benefits for people with dementia.

Roger Ulrich (Ulrich, 1983; Ulrich et al., 1991) postulates in his psycho-evolutionary theory that acquiring a capacity for restorative response to certain natural settings gave major survival-related advantages to early humans. A high agreement across cultures in the positive responsiveness to nature supports the idea that modern humans might also have a prepared readiness to acquire restorative responses from unthreatening natural settings with particular characteristics, such as some spatial openness, and specific elements such as flowers (Ulrich et al., 1991; Ulrich, 1999). The theory suggests that the response to nature is initially preconscious and is evidenced by rapid onset of positive affective response to natural environments. The suggestion of a preconscious affective evaluation of environmental scenes was supported for example by results from Korpela et al. (2002). After a change towards a more positively-toned emotional state, exposure to nature decreases autonomic arousal as evidenced by positive changes in physiological activity levels. These changes are accompanied by sustained attention and a decrease in negative emotions. The physiological changes reducing autonomic arousal during stress recovery indicate that human response to nature has a parasympathetic nervous system component, especially during the initial minutes of recovery (Ulrich et al., 1991). The evidence of lower heart rate whilst seeing natural landscapes suggests that reduced autonomic arousal engenders less spatially selective attention and results in higher intake of environmental stimuli (Ulrich et al., 1991; Laumann et al., 2003).

Ulrich's theory has two major implications for people with dementia. First, it suggests that exposure to natural settings elicits autonomic responses, which can occur without recognition or conscious awareness of the elements of the settings (Ulrich et al., 1991). Therefore, even people with severe dementia are able to understand the natural cues of their environment without demanding conscious cognitive appraisals. Second, exposure to nature evokes rapid positive emotional changes that may alleviate the problems caused by confused and agitated mood or boredom as a result of loss of initiative or lack of stimulus in the indoor environment. Both reduced autonomic arousal leading to stress recovery and improved affective state are associated with positive health outcomes (van den Berg, 2005).

Being and Doing Outdoors

Dementia causes stress for the person affected throughout the progress of the syndrome. Experiencing the initial symptoms and receiving a diagnosis can be a very stressful (Heimonen, 2005). Later, when symptoms affect daily life more, the person faces disappointments and failures while witnessing a gradual loss of skills and abilities (Barnett, 2000). Awareness of the progressing syndrome is at some stage replaced by a different reality. Chaos is the word which was often used when people with mild or moderate dementia describe their daily life (DeBaggio, 2002). This stress can be increased by a care environment that lacks activity (Gubrium, 1997; Barnett, 2000). People with severe dementia may also find that kind of environment stressful since their own abilities to find meaningful and positive stimuli are impaired.

Ulrich et al. (1991, 1999) suggested that stress experiences could be alleviated by environments with conducive characteristics. According to his conceptual model, the key features for individuals in supportive, health-promoting environments are a sense of control, access to privacy, access to social support, possibilities for movement and exercise, and access to nature and to other positive distractions. These characteristics of an environment facilitate an individual's abilities to recover and cope with stress, which in turn results in improved health.

In dementia illness, functional ability and recalling previously learned information can be preserved in spite of the illness, therefore being available as resources through which contact with the outdoor environment can be maintained (Carman, 2002). Familiar activities that help to draw on memories of earlier life so as to keep residents involved in their lives (Zeisel & Tyson, 1999). Horticulture is one of the most common and enjoyed leisure pursuits of older adults (Hill & Relf, 1982; Sarola, 1994; Haas et al., 1998) and can be used to alleviate symptoms of dementia (Haas et al., 1998). In fact, gardening may prevent dementia: in a study of Fabrigoule et al. (1995) gardening was one of the activities associated with lower risk for dementia among older people in France. The authors suggested that the protective effect of gardening and other complex activities like knitting could be due to stimulation of cognitive functions.

According to Jarrot et al. (2002), therapeutic horticultural activities are appropriate for older adults with dementia since the activities are familiar and meaningful to most and provide opportunities for reminiscing as well as for exercising competence. In addition, horticultural activities are creative, result in tangible end-products, provide exercise for a wide range of physical and cognitive skills, and enhance social interaction. The continuity of familiar activities supporting a sense of competence and self-esteem may help in coping with a progressive loss of abilities. Plants provide sensory stimulation for all the senses through colours, structures, scents, tastes, forms and sometimes by sounds. Sensory stimulation is important for the elderly suffering from dementia since it can improve orientation, trigger memory, prevent emotional outbursts and facilitate connectedness in individuals with dementia (Haas et al., 1998; Carman, 2002).

Many design recommendations have been suggested for outdoor environments for patients suffering from dementia (e.g., Beckwith & Gilster, 1997; Ousset et al., 1998; Valla & Harrington; 1998, Zeisel & Tyson, 1999), but research findings that support the positive effects of particular designs are few. Some studies found that outdoor visits are associated with reduced aggression among people with dementia (Day et al., 2000; Cohen-Mansfield, 2001). What actually causes the recorded positive changes associated with outdoor walks is less clear since in most studies there are many changing variables such as social contact, increased autonomy, outdoor light, or fresh air, which may affect outcomes (Cohen-Mansfield, 2001). Privacy and personalization of space, residential character, and a comprehensible environment have been associated with both reduced aggressive and agitated behaviour and fewer psychological problems (Zeisel et al., 2003).

STUDY # 1 SURVEY OF DEMENTIA CARE STAFF

Aims

The aim of this study was to establish the role of plants in the well-being of the Finnish elderly individuals with dementia by gathering data with a questionnaire. The staff rather than patients was canvassed for information as the residents of the homes had such severe impairments that interviewing was impossible. The staff of the homes was asked what kind of observations and experiences they had regarding plants in residential care homes and whether they use plants in care work, and if they do, how. The questionnaire also inquired about their opinions on the effects of plants on the well-being of the residents and their work.

Subjects and Methods

The survey was conducted in ten residential care homes located in a city (Rappe & Lindén, 2004). The total number of staff in the homes, including deputies and students, was 85, of which 65 participated in the study. All participants were women; 33% were auxiliary nurses, 25% nurses, 20% home help assistants, social nurses or people having other education in health work, and 22% were people from other fields or students. The age distribution was as follows: 27% were aged 30 or younger, 36% between 31 and 45, and 37% were aged over 45. Gardening was a common hobby: 72% of staff respondents reported that they did gardening.

The number of residents in the homes ranged between 8 and 14 and the number of personnel between 6 and 10.The homes were non-institutional, home-like settings having numerous plants both outdoors and indoors. All the homes were single storied, which enabled easy access outdoors.

The questionnaire included both scaled responses and open-ended questions. The data from the scaled responses shown here were analyzed using descriptive statistics, cross tabulation and Chi-Square-test. Answers to open-ended questions were analyzed by qualitative content analysis and using a phenomenological approach.

Findings

According to nursing staff's opinions, plants in the homes promoted the well-being of the elderly with dementia. The health-related benefits the staff reported were derived from the positive impact on the physical environment caused by the plants and from horticultural or other activities associated with plants.

Physical Modifications to the Environment

Staff stated that plants created a pleasant, homelike environment. Both indoor and outdoor plants reduced noise and delineated spaces, thus providing havens. According to their observations plants were noted to increase humidity, remove pollutants and decrease dust in the air. These effects were reported previously by several experimental studies (Wolverton et al., 1989; Lohr, 1992; Lohr & Pearson-Mims, 1996).

Plants and the Well-Being of the Residents

The contribution of the plants to the psychological and social well-being of the residents was prominent according to the respondents (Table 1). The colors and scents of the plants stimulated the senses of the residents and activated their memories. Staff observed that it was not only familiar plants that residents were interested in, but also exotic, colorful flowers and berries that drew their attention. The characteristics of plants that accompany changes in the season helped residents to orientate themselves in time. Plants were also a source of positive emotions.

Plants contributed to social relationships as well and gave possibilities for rewarding activities (Table 1). Staff reported that gardening activities raised the self-esteem of the residents by providing feelings of success and accomplishment. Actions related to plants were often familiar to residents and enabled them use their skills in maintaining functional ability. The enhanced self-esteem and the feeling of competence supported the autonomy of the residents, thus alleviating feelings of inferiority.

Reported Problems with Plants

The problems staff reported concerning plants were mainly related to residents' actions. The nursing staff expressed that the main problem with plants was that the residents ate plants, berries and soil. In particular, the residents tended to eat and tear plants placed on the dining table. Although the plants were sometimes eaten, they reported no troubles with allergic reactions and poisoning, although there were several named poisonous plants in the homes such as *Nérium oleánder*, which is highly toxic. Residents suffering from disorders in perception sometimes trampled plants underfoot outdoors. In addi-

TABLE 1. The Associations of Plants with the Well-Being of Persons with Dementia: Staff Opinions, n = 65

Statement	Agree % of respondents
Familiar plants can evoke residents' memories.	98
Nursing of plants can maintain the residents' functional ability.	94
Plants can help residents to maintain their awareness of changing seasons.	84
Plants can help a resident to orient in space.	75
Residents are delighted when receiving plants.	97
Residents feel themselves needed when nursing plants.	97
Plants are a good topic of conversation between nursing personel and residents.	95
Residents are talking about plants among themselves.	60

tion, respondents indicated that the participation of the residents in gardening had some drawbacks. When the residents were weeding, they could not always distinguish a weed from a desirable plant. The residents might also root out the plants and move them from place to place without a reason. Sometimes the residents liked watering the flowers too much so that plants became too wet.

Use of Plants in Care Work

The attitudes of the staff towards plants were mainly positive and despite some problems plants caused, the staff did not identify reasons to restrict the presence of plants. It was noteworthy that of the respondents, 65% had used horticultural activities as therapy in care work although normally no horticultural therapy is included in the education of nursing staff in Finland. Those who did gardening as a hobby used horticulture more in care work than other groups ($\chi^2 = 8.74$, p = 0.003). Staff in the middle age group had used horticulture in care work more than staff in the younger and older age groups ($\chi^2 = 8.26$, p = 0.016).

The activities employed most often in care work were propagation, planting, watering, removing old flowers and leaves, raking leaves, tasting and smelling, picking flowers and harvesting. According to 86% of respondents, residents were interested in plants. This may indicate that individuals with dementia perceive plants as appealing. Plants were a good topic of conversation, increasing social interaction between residents and personnel, but also to some degree among the residents themselves. Personnel had moreover calmed down anxious and restless residents by drawing their attention to familiar plants. Plants were used in reminiscence and in validation therapy as well.

Although all but one of the respondents were of the opinion that plants belong in the care environment, the answers revealed a significant contradiction in the attitudes of the staff. On the one hand, they confirmed that horticultural actions promote the residents' well-being but on the other hand, some of the actions of residents were regarded by the staff as problematic, resulting in a mess or cutting down the aesthetic value of plants. It was regarded as negative if the residents were eager to pick flowers or break branches from shrubs or trees.

Although staff reported that plants added to the workload to some extent, they regarded plants as important features of the care environment. This positive attitude might result from their experiences of plants enhancing the atmosphere of the workplace. Research conducted in working environments established positive impacts of plants on the well-being of the workers (Lohr et al., 1996; Larsen et al., 1998; Fjeld, 2000). However, a lack of horticultural knowledge was felt to be a problem. Only 39% of the respondents felt that they know enough about specially adapted tools for gardening. Education about plants and adapted growing methods suitable for demented individuals was felt to be necessary.

Staff Recommendations for Plant Usage

The staff recommended that the plants should be beautiful and well-cared for in order to be therapeutic for persons with dementia; dead or suffering plants may aggravate their feelings of inferiority. They emphasized the use of a reasonable number of plants; indoor plants should not hamper one's moving or prevent one's possibilities to look out of windows. Poisonous plants should be avoided. Poisonous berries were of special concern. Thorny or sharp-leafed plants can cause skin injuries because the skin of the elderly is often thin and dry. Plants that frequently drop their flowers or leaves were not recommended. Plants should also tolerate harsh treatment and excessive watering. The respondents recommended using familiar, traditional plants. Foliage plants create a lush atmosphere and can be cleaned of dust with ease. Flowering plants delight with their colors and give topics for conversation. The respondents suggested that trees are important to elderly individuals with dementia, who should therefore be given the possibility to see them. Easily grown vegetables are enjoyed and can be used in cooking.

STUDY #2 OBSERVATIONAL STUDY OF DEMENTIA DAY CARE CLIENTS AND RESIDENTS WITH DEMENTIA

Aims

The overall aim of the larger project was to investigate the quality of dementia care from the clients' perspective (Sormunen et al., 2007). For this paper we analyzed the data on episodes when people with dementia were either visiting outdoors, trying to get outdoors or seeing greenery and talking about these issues. Our research questions were: how are well-being and experiences with green environments associated, and what impact does access to green environments have on the interaction?

Subjects and Methods

We carried out an observational study in eight care units, all providing care services for people with dementia. The inclusion criteria for the care units were a willingness to participate, four units should be for people with dementia only and four for both people with dementia and other people. Of these, two should provide day care only and six were residential care providers.

In the eight care units, all people with dementia for whom an ethical approval and informed consent had been received were observed for two days in 2003 and two more days again in 2004. In all the units, observations were done by two researchers on two subsequent days, six hours per day (Sormunen et al., 2007). A total of 123 people with dementia were observed. Before the observations, demographic and health data were collected on the participants (Table 2), showing that the participants in day care units were younger (mean 77 years) and that they were cognitively (Minimental Status Examination, MMSE by Folstein et al. 1975, mean 20) and physically more able (Katz et al., 1970, ADL mean 1,3) than the participants in residential care (age mean 84 years, MMSE mean 12, ADL mean 2,8), but there was a large variation in cognitive and physical functioning within each care unit. There were more women than men in both residential and day care units (for more details see Sormunen et al., 2007).

Observations were done at different times of the year but no data collection was done in the coldest period (January-February) or the warmest time of year (June-July). The method used was Dementia Care Mapping 7th (DCM) (Evaluating Dementia Care 1997) in combination with field notes. DCM was used for this paper to assess the well-being of the residents. Field notes included descriptions of the environment and episodes observed with the exact time and

TABLE 2. Sociodemographic Information About the Participants 2003-2004, %[1].

	Day care (n=73)	Residential care (n=50)
Age, years[2]		
60-69	14.0	6.9
70-79	46.0	13.9
80-89	38.0	50.0
90-104	2.0	29.2
MMSE[3]		
18-28, mild dementia	70.2	21.7
10-17, moderate dementia	27.7	39.1
0-9, severe dementia	2.1	39.1
ADL[4]		
1 (Independent)	76.0	7.1
2	22.0	22.9
3	2.0	51.4
4 (Dependent)	0	18.6

[1]Data collected when participating the study first time

[2] Data missing n=1

[3] Data missing n=7

[4] Data missing n=3

the names of the people with dementia. The observation notes were written by hand and were later typed into a Word document, where some sentences were completed.

In the following we report the findings of the qualitative deductive content analyses of the field notes (Dey, 1993). The Word document included over 541,000 words and they were analyzed by the AtlasTI program. For this paper all episodes concerning visiting outdoors or commenting on it and all comments on windows, views, doors and gates were extracted and analyzed. The episodes were coded according to their content and only those episodes involving doors leading to outdoors or staircases were included. During the total of 190 hours of observing, the field notes included descriptions of the following episodes: visiting outdoors or commenting on it (15 episodes), reminiscence of visiting outdoors (18), actually going outdoors or coming in (100), commenting on windows, views and indoor plants (68), commenting about going home or reminiscing about being outdoors at home (68), episodes concerning balconies (8), and episodes of locked doors and gates (38). In addition, 23 episodes were found which included comments about residents' feelings that they are locked in with no access outdoors.

Most episodes especially in residential care were short, for example *"Mr Niemi was confused and vocally intrusive when he approached the lunch table. He finished his lunch, stood up and looked through the window and walked to his room quietly"* Episodes where the participants actually were outdoors lasted much longer, 30 to 60 minutes. Many episodes included more than one of the themes listed above. The first analyses showed that there was a difference between the findings in the day care units and the residential care units: the episodes in residential care were shorter than in day care and mainly focused on window views, balconies, locked doors or gates, while in day care most episodes concerned actually going outdoors or coming in as well as reminiscing about visiting outdoors. As a result, the data from residential care and day care were analyzed separately.

Findings

Day Care: Visiting Outdoors is a Routine

Going outdoors was a daily routine in the day care units and the schedule for each day was organized to allow this: staff members, volunteers and students were all involved in going outdoors with the clients with mild to moderate dementia. The participants lived at home and going outdoors was often done when arriving at the centre or when leaving for home. These moments eased going outdoors because shoes and outdoor clothing needed to be changed only once, and it was easier to motivate even those participants with low initiative or low motivation. In addition, according to the caregivers, it is common that clients get restless before going home and taking them for a walk was seen to decrease worries associated with leaving the day care. The following is a citation from the field notes:

> *When going for a walk at the end of the day, Mr Koski with moderate dementia was taken home with a group of six clients and the caregiver. When turning to his house he waved his hand and smiled. The rest of the group walked a while and all clients were obviously enjoying the trip and some were joking with the caregiver. When returning to the centre two of the ladies were worried about whether the taxis were already waiting for them.*

In the other centre the staff took the clients for a walk one by one and the aim was to find time to concentrate on each client and ensure that the situation of each individual was known. In the day care units an individual client was typically met only once a week or even once every two weeks. Even those who were bashful while indoors became more interactive outside and also more involved with the group when coming in:

> *Mrs Virta with Alzheimer's disease and mild dementia has been silent the whole day. She was used to long strolls before getting problems in orientation and when she was taken for a walk she becomes far more talkative and looks happy and relaxed.*

Our qualitative observations were in accordance with previous studies: being outdoors seemed to stimulate all the senses, support well-being and encourage interaction of people with mild to moderate dementia. The next citation from the field notes describes how walking in a green park stimulated all senses including the sense of balance and the sense of touch, how the participants with dementia were able to use all their skills and abilities, how they showed more initiative and how walking in the green environment awoke memories. It can also be seen how the open space eased the psychosocial dynamics of the group and provided room to express negative or sad feelings without hurting anyone:

> *It was a sunny morning in early spring. The whole group of 4 men and 8 women with mild or moderate dementia and two caregivers (plus the two researchers) went for a long walk. The day care unit is next to a large park, lake and small woodland. We walked through the park to the lakeside where there was an old summer cottage, a sauna, a pier and*

some small boats on the bank still waiting to be transferred into the lake after the winter. We stayed together in a loose group, the clients chatted and talked and the caregivers gave feedback and encouraged the inter-action. Mr Seppä told me about a small boat he use to keep on the lake and after a while he started to talk about the wartime and how he had witnessed a man die next to him: 'That's something I have remembered all my life', he said very sadly. When we arrived at the centre, Mrs Mäki, Mrs Niemi and Mrs Saari stopped with the caregiver at a flowerbed. They talked about the plants and how it was time to clean the flowerbed for the summer. Mrs Niemi started to cut out old leaves from the fern and she obviously enjoyed the work. Mrs Mäki and Mrs Saari watched her working and reminisced about weeding and cleaning the garden during their life. After a while Mrs Mäki complained about how one of the men was swearing earlier on 'There should be some education'. Mrs Saari thought back to her late husband and how he had been violent. She said that life with him had been very hard but she stayed till the very end. When we came in everyone changed shoes. Mrs Niemi started to water the indoor plants. Caregiver: 'Are they dry?' Mrs Niemi: 'Not very but I always water them. It is my job'.

The green environment included permanent and stable elements, reminding them about different jobs and giving them a lot to talk about. Being outside to-gether and sharing memories–even dark ones–supported the identity and in-clusion of these people with mild to moderate dementia.

Residential Care: Access to Outdoors Through Windows

In the data gathered in the six residential care units, there were several epi-sodes in which the residents expressed anxiousness or confusion because of locked doors they were not able to open, for example:

Mr. Lampinen walks to the locked gate at the end of the living room of the unit. On the other side there is a small kitchen area and a hall with coats and a door to the staircase. He tries to open the gate and asks for help with it. He says that he wants to go home. The caregiver explains that it is impossible. He looks anxious even while the caregiver does her best to relax him by touching him gently and chatting. The episode is re-peated later a couple of times.

In contrast to the doors, which blocked the person's path, windows opened the indoor space and provided views to the outdoors and to green environ-ments. Through the windows the residents with moderate to severe dementia were connected to non-residential life: seeing people jogging, going to work, buses, trucks and cars on the roads and so on. By their own initiative, the residents commented on these views and talked about the weather they observed. Several episodes of relaxed sitting or standing next to the window were also observed, mainly among people with severe dementia. But there were also episodes when frustrated residents wanted to go outside but were not able to. In those moments windows or even balconies did not always work as a substitute. The next data extract is from one of the units were access outdoors was difficult if the person was not able to walk up or down stairs.

> *It is a beautiful day late in the winter; the sun is shining brightly and there is still plenty of snow. Mrs Kuusela with mild dementia is walking in the corridor with a walking aid and asks the caregiver if she could go out for a walk alone. The caregiver: "I wouldn't like you to do it. You can fall. What do you say if we go together tomorrow?" Mrs. Kuusela. "It is always the next day . . . " They decided to go outdoors tomorrow afternoon. The caregiver opens the door to the balcony for Mrs Kuusela, which was in the shade. She pops out for some minutes only."*

When the residents were going outside and when they came in they mainly expressed their well-being by words and gestures. Those moments also included interaction, and people with moderate to severe dementia either took the initiative or were clearly involved in such situations. The comments they made and their nonverbal expressions expressed that going outdoors was supporting their feeling of competence.

> *Mr Kallio with moderate dementia has just been outside with his visitor. He is taken to the dining room in the wheelchair. He smiles and asks the man next to him: "Have you been outside?" he continues: "I have been taken twice!"*

Being outdoors was a continuity of their lifelong habits. When people were coming and going outdoors it also created a more active atmosphere in the units which often were very quiet environments. Only one patient in a psycho-geriatric ward was repetitively expressing willingness to go outdoors and this was not eased by his daily walks outside.

In residential care, going outside was a daily routine in only one unit but visitors and sometimes also caregivers took the residents out in the other units. We also observed situations where the residents did not want to go outdoors. In such situations the residents were often just quickly asked if they were willing to go out and the further the dementia had progressed the more difficult it was for the resident to be able to react positively to such a sudden proposition.

Discussion & Conclusive Remarks

Nature and Well-Being of the People with Dementia

The results of our two studies briefly presented here indicate that access to outdoors may play a significant role in the quality of life among people with dementia, especially in residential care units. Experiences of nature seemed to have two-fold consequences for people with dementia: on the one hand seeing nature or being in it calmed them, but it also evoked memories and initiated activity and social interaction. Especially plants with their multisensory characteristics triggered memories and created associations in the mind.

Previous studies confirm that temporary escape from indoors to garden environments in institutional settings is associated with reduced stress levels and a better sense of control (Cooper Marcus & Barnes, 1995; Ulrich, 1999). In a study by Rappe et al. (2006), a high frequency of visiting an outdoor green environment and good self-rated health among residents of nursing care were strongly associated. The result indicates that even among old people with severe health impairments, visiting outdoors may promote a better perception of health. Moreover, it has been suggested that the positive affective effects of visiting the garden may be more pronounced among depressed old people than non-depressed (Rappe & Kivelä, 2005). Keeping in mind that in residential care a majority of the residents have some kind of dementia disorders and half are depressed (Noro et al., 2005), the impact of outdoor visits on the well-being of residents should be better recognized.

The physical environment has an impact on human behavior. An environment containing trees and flowers was found to enhance social well-being by reducing aggression (Kuo & Sullivan, 2001) and supporting social ties (Kweon et al., 1998). In a Swedish home for people with dementia, an increase in visits of relatives was recorded after establishment of a garden (Rappe, 2003). In particular, the younger relatives were more willing to visit their grandparents when they had the opportunity to spend time in the fresh air looking at flowers and drinking coffee together.

Outdoor social interaction is not so demanding for people with dementia since human attention is likely directed towards elements in the environment, and not towards the behavior of single individuals. In addition, the environment itself provides calming stimuli, reducing stress caused by social events. Our findings indicate that being outdoors also makes easier the expression of important memories, whether they are happy or dark; whether or not this is associated with the stress reducing elements of such environments needs to be further studied.

Enhanced Competence

According to our findings, outdoor visits in green environments can support the feeling of competence of people with dementia in several ways. In green environments, no demanding cognitive appraisals are needed to understand how to act successfully. The environment is easy to interpret even with a diminishing cognitive capability, because it provides abundant information and cues about time, place and purpose, helping orientation toward reality. In addition, green environments provide meaningful activities in which people with dementia are interested in engaging and can consolidate self-esteem. Cox et al. (2004) reported that a garden increased the pleasure of nursing-home residents with dementia, as measured by the Affect Rating Scale. They concluded that the residents derived pleasure from engaging spontaneously in gardening activities like watering and deadheading. Compared with a multisensory Snoezelen room, gardens tended to animate and engage the residents rather than relax and calm them. Gardens also positively affected the well-being of visitors and staff. A study by Gigliotti et al. (2004) reported higher levels of positive affect and engagement during horticultural therapy than traditional activities among people with dementia.

The Hindrances of Getting Outdoors

In our first study, easy physical access to outdoors areas promoted its daily use and our second study suggested that if the outdoors is difficult to access, the use is restricted. In a study by Rappe and Kivelä (2005), the residents mentioned slippery paths and snow in the winter, and cold and windy weather all year round as common hindrances. Maintaining paths in good condition, especially in winter, is of great importance. It is important to remove hindrances such as heavy doors and thresholds that prevent outdoor visits by people who are not independently mobile. Increasing the attractiveness and convenience of the outdoor environment may increase the frequency of outdoor visits. Both physically and mentally accessible, safe environments would encourage the elderly to go out independently without burdening the staff.

The elderly in long-term care report that the main reason for restrictions on outdoor visits is the difficulty in getting assistance for visits (Rappe & Kivelä, 2005). This may be a consequence of several factors, such as a low staff-client ratio, the care culture and care practices. For example, in the residential care units involved in our second study, the nurses changed uniforms before they entered the unit and they found that they needed to change all their clothes to go out with the residents, especially during cold periods of the year, which is about eight to nine months. After the first observations it was proposed that when the afternoon shift starts, some of those leaving or starting their work could take the residents out. The nurses agreed that the residents should be able to visit outdoors more often but found it difficult to change the routine and preferences in the unit. In addition, they complained that the residents should have warmer clothes and shoes and that they should be easier to put on.

In our second study presented here, two of the units were difficult to access for a walker or a wheelchair user. In these units the staff did not take the residents outdoors during the observations and they reported that going out would take too much of their time to allow them to meet the other basic needs of all the residents. The staff-client ratio in these units was low: 0.49 and 0.54. This qualitative finding shows how an unsuitable environment is an extra challenge in improving the quality of care and in fact how such an environment can promote care that is not person-centered.

Recommendations for Care Work

Our two studies presented here were in accordance with previous studies, in that contact with outdoor greenery can support the well-being of people with dementia (Cox et al., 2004; Gigliotti et al., 2004; Jarrot et al., 2002; Mckenzie et al., 2000). As our results show there can be a wide variance among the care units in recognizing the value of outdoor greenery for the well-being of the residents and in the frequency of visiting outdoors. To provide relaxing outdoor experiences and possibilities for exercise for people with dementia, establishing safe, fenced gardens may be one easy solution. For example, Sinnenas Trädgård (Garden for Senses) in Stockholm, Sweden, has proved to be a preferred place among the elderly with dementia since it has been designed to provide stimuli for all the senses and is accessible to people with physical and cognitive disorders (Rappe, 2003; http://www.stockholm.se/Extern/Templates/Page.aspx?id=90841) .

Staff and relatives that consider outdoor visits to be an important part of care which generates positive affects and good health effects for the elderly with dementia might be more motivated to provide more assistance in getting out. At least visual access to a green environment should be made available to the residents in institutional living, since seeing the plants may enhance the mood of the elderly and can help in the regulation of emotions. There is also a need to improve attitudes towards actions taken by people with dementia. The actions experienced as problematic by the staff can be therapeutic for the residents: e.g., by moving plants from place to place, a resident might be trying to achieve control over the environment. To promote a dementia care that is person-centered requires an improved understanding and acceptance of the reality and the needs of a person with dementia and an enhancing of his or her access to green environments.

REFERENCES

Barnett, E. (2000). *Including the person with dementia in designing and delivering care. 'I need to be me!'*. London and Philadelphia: Jessica Kingsley Publishers.

Beckwith, M. E., & Gilster. S. D. (1997). The paradise garden: A model garden design for those with Alzheimer's disease. In S. E. Wells (ed.). *Horticultural therapy and the older adult population* (pp. 3-16). New York: The Haworth Press, Inc.

Carman, J. (2002). Special-needs gardens for Alzheimer's residents. *Nursing Homes Long Term Care Management,* 51, 22-26.

Cohen-Mansfield, J. (2001). Nonpharmacologic interventions for inappropriate behaviours in dementia. *American Journal of Geriatric Psychiatry,* 9, 361-381.

Cooper Marcus, C., & Barnes, M. (1995). *Gardens in healthcare facilities: Uses, therapeutic benefits, and design recommendations.* The center for health design: University of California at Berkeley.

Cox, H., Burns, I., & Savage, S. (2004). Multisensory environments for leisure: Promoting well-being in nursing home residents with dementia. *Journal of Gerontological Nursing,* 30, 37-45.

Day, K., Carreon, D., & Stump, C. (2000). The therapeutic design of environments for people with dementia. *The Gerontologist,* 40, 397-416.

DeBaggio, T. (2002). *Losing my mind. An intimate look at life with Alzheimer's.* Waterville: Thorndike Press.

Dey, I. (1993). *Qualitative analysis. A user friendly guide for social scientists.* Routledge, London.

Evaluating dementia care. The DCM method. (1997). Bradford: University of Bradford.

Fabrigoule, C., Letenneur, L., Dartigues, J. F., Zarrouk, M., Commenges, D., & Barberger-Gateau, P. (1995). Social and leisure activities and risk of dementia: A prospective longitudinal study. *Journal of American Geriatric Society,* 43, 485-490.

Fjeld, T. (2000). The effect of interior planting on health and discomfort among workers and school children. *HortTechnology,* 10, 46-52.

Folstein, M. F., Folstein, S. E. & McHugh, P. R. (1975). 'Mini Mental State'. A practical method for grading the cognitive status of patients for the clinician. *Journal of Psychiatric Research,* 12, 189-198.

Gigliotti, C. M., Jarrott, S. E. & Yorgason, J. (2004). Harvesting health. Effects of three types of horticultural therapy activities for persons with dementia. *Dementia,* 3, 161-180.

Gubrium, J. G. (1997). *Living and dying at Murray Manor.* Charlottesville: University Press of Virginia.

Haas, K., Simson, S., & Stevenson, N. (1998). Older persons and horticulture therapy practice. In S. Simson & M. Strauss (eds.). *Horticulture as therapy. Principles and practice* (pp. 231-255). New York: The Food Product Press.

Heimonen, S-L. (2005). *Työikäisenä Alzheimerin tautiin sairastuneiden ja heidän puolisoidensa kokemukset sairauden alkuvaiheessa.* Studies in Education, Psychology and Social Research 263. Jyväskylä: University of Jyväskylä.

Hill, C., & Relf, D. (1982). Gardening as an outdoor activity in geriatric institutions. *Activites, Adaptations and Aging,* 3, 47-54.

ICD10 http://www3.who.int/icd/currentversion/fr-icd.htm. 26.6.2006

Jarrot, S., Kwack, H., & Relf, D. (2002). An observational assessment of a dementia-specific horticultural therapy program. *HortTechnology,* 12, 403-410.

Katz, S., Downs, T. D., Thomas, D., Cash, H. R. & Grotz, R. C. (1970). Progress in development of the index of ADL. *Gerontologist,* 20, 20-30.

Kirkevold, Ø. (2005). *Use of restraints in Norwegian nursing homes, focusing on persons with dementia.* Oslo: Faculty of Medicine, University of Oslo.

Korpela, K., Klemettilä, T., & Hietanen, J. (2002). Evidence for rapid affective evaluation of environmental scenes. *Environment and Behavior,* 34, 634-650.

Kuo, F. E., & Sullivan, W. C. (2001). Aggression and violence in the inner city. Effects of environment via mental fatigue. *Environment and Behavior,* 33, 543-571.

Kweon, B. S., Sullivan, W. C., & Wiley, A. (1998). Green common spaces and the social integration of inner-city older adults. *Environment and Behaviour,* 30, 832-858.

Larsen, L., Adams, J., Deal, B., Kweon, B.-S., & Tyler, E. (1998). Plants in the workplace. The effects of plant density on productivity, attitudes, and perceptions. *Environment and Behavior,* 30, 261-281.

Laumann, K., Gärling, T., & Stormark, K. M. (2003). Selective attention and heart rate responses to natural and urban environments. *Journal of Environmental Psychology,* 23, 125-134.

Lohr, V. (1992). The contribution of interior plants to relative humidity in an office. In D.Relf (ed.). *The role of horticulture in human well-being and social development* (pp. 117-119). Portland, Oregon: Timber Press.

Lohr, V., & Pearson-Mims, C. (1996). Particulate matter accumulation on horizontal surfaces in interiors. *Atmospheric Environment,* 30, 2565-2568.

Lohr, V. I., Pearson-Mims, C. H., & G. K. Goodwin, G. K. (1996). Interior plants may improve worker productivity and reduce stress in a windowless environment. *Journal of Environmental Horticulture,* 14, 97-100.

Mackenzie E., Agard, B., Portella, C., Mahangar, D., Barol, J. and Carson, L. 2000. Horticultural therapy in long-term care settings. *Journal of American Medical Directors Association* 1(2): 69-73.

Noro, A., Finne-Soveri, H.., Björgren, M., et al. (eds.) (2005). *Ikääntyneiden laitoshoidon laatu ja tuottavuus–RAI-järjestelmä vertailukehittämisessä* [Quality and Productivity in Institutional Care for Elderly Residents–Benchmarking with the RAI]. Helsinki: Stakes.

Ousset, P. J., Nourashemi, F., Albarede, J. L, & Vellas, P. M. (1998). Therapeutic gardens. *Archives of Gerontology and Geriatrics* 26 supplement, 6, 369-372.

Rappe, E. (2003). Kasvit ja vanhusten hyvinvointi. In E. Rappe, L. Lindén & T. Koivunen (eds.) *Puisto, puutarha ja hyvinvointi* (pp.117-127). Helsinki: Viherympäristöliitto.

Rappe, E. & Lindén, L. (2004).Plants in health care environments: Experiences of the nursing personnel in homes for people with dementia. *Acta Horticulturae* 639: 75-81.

Rappe, E., & Kivelä, S.-L. (2005). Effects of garden visits on long-term care residents as related to depression. *HortTechnology,* 15, 298-303.

Rappe, E., Kivelä, S.-L., & Rita, H. (2006).The effect of visiting outdoors green environment on self-rated health among the elderly in long-term care. *HortTechnology,* 16, 55-59.

Sarola, J. P. (1994). Asuinympäristön ja paikan merkitys vanhalle ihmiselle. In A. Uutela & J.-E. Ruth (eds.) *Muuttuva vanhuus* (pp. 116-131). Helsinki: Gaudeamus.

Sormunen, S. M. K, Topo, P. H., Eloniemi-Sulkava, U., Räikkönen, O. & Sarvimäki, A. (2007). Inappropriate treatment of people with dementia in residential and day care. *Aging and Mental Health,* in press.

Sulkava, R., Eloniemi, U., Erkinjuntti T., & Hervonen A. (1994). *Dementia.* 2nd edition. Jyväskylä: Gummerrus kirjapaino Oy.

Teresi, J. A., Holmes D., & Ory, M. G. (2000). The therapeutic design of environments for people with dementia. *The Gerontologist,* 40, 417-421.

Ulrich, R. S. (1983). Aesthetic and affective response to natural environment. In I. Altman & J. F. Wohlwill (eds.) *Human behavior and environment* vol. 6, Behavior and the natural environment (pp. 85-125).. New York: Plenum Press.

Ulrich, R. S. (1999). Effects of gardens on health outcomes: Theory and research. In C. Cooper Marcus and Barnes, M. (eds.). *Healing gardens.* New York, John Wiley & Sons, Inc. pp. 27-86.

Ulrich, R.S., Simons, R. F., Losito, B. D., Fiorito, E., Miles, M. A., & Zelson, M. (1991). Stress recovery during exposure to natural and urban environments. *Journal of Environmental Psychology,* 11, 201-230.

Valla, P., & Harrington, T. (1998). Designing for older people with cognitive and affective disorders. *Archives of Gerontology and Geriatrics,* 26 supplement, 1, 515-518.

van den Berg, A. E. (2005). *Health impacts of healing environments.* A review of evidence for benefits of nature, daylight, fresh air, and quiet in healthcare settings. Groningen: Foundation 200 years University Hospital Groningen.

Wolverton, B.C., Johnson, A., & Bounds, K. (1989). *Interior landscape plants for indoor air pollution abatement.* Final report, NASA, Stennis Space Center, MS.

Zeisel, J., & Tyson, M. M. (1999). Alzheimer's treatment gardens. In C. Cooper Marcus & M. Barnes (eds.). *Healing gardens* (pp. 437-504). New York: John Wiley & Sons, Inc.

Zeisel, J., Silverstein, N. M. Hyde, J., Levkoff, S., Lawton, M. P., & Holmes, W. (2003). Environmental correlates to behavioral health outcomes in Alzheimer's special care units. *The Gerontologist,* 43, 697-711.

doi:10.1300/J081v21n03_12

Gardens for People with Dementia: Increasing Access to the Natural Environment for Residents with Alzheimer's

Nancy J. Chapman
Teresia Hazen
Eunice Noell-Waggoner

SUMMARY. Although exposure to the natural environment has therapeutic benefits for nursing home residents and residents with dementia (Cohen-Mansfield & Werner, 1998; Lovering et al., 2002; Mooney & Nicell, 1992), many elders living in congregate facilities have limited access to the natural world. Long-term care facilities often do not incorporate the use of plants and natural settings into their daily activities due to limited knowledge, time, and funding. A twenty-two hour training

Nancy J. Chapman, PhD, is Professor Emerita, Nohad Toulan School of Urban Studies and Planning, Portland State University, Portland, OR 97207 (Email: chapmann@pdx.edu).

Teresia Hazen, MEd, HTR, QMHP, is Coordinator, Legacy Therapeutic Gardens. Legacy Health System, 1015 NW 22nd Avenue, Portland, OR 97210 (Email: thazen@lhs.org).

Eunice Noell-Waggoner, BS, Int Arch., LD, is President, Center of Design for an Aging Society, 9027 NW Bartholomew Drive, Portland, OR 97201 (Email: Eunice@centerofdesign.org).

This project was supported by grant # 2003-00705 from the Better Nursing Home Fund of the Oregon Community Foundation.

[Haworth co-indexing entry note]: "Gardens for People with Dementia: Increasing Access to the Natural Environment for Residents with Alzheimer's." Chapman, Nancy J., Teresia Hazen, and Eunice Noelle-Waggoner. Co-published simultaneously in *Journal of Housing for the Elderly* (The Haworth Press, Inc.) Vol. 21, No. 3/4, 2007, pp. 249-263; and: *Outdoor Environments for People with Dementia* (ed: Susan Rodiek and Benyamin Schwarz) The Haworth Press, Inc., 2007, pp. 249-263. Single or multiple copies of this article are available for a fee from The Haworth Document Delivery Service [1-800-HAWORTH, 9:00 a.m. - 5:00 p.m. (EST). E-mail address: docdelivery@haworthpress.com].

program was developed and tested to increase the knowledge of activity staff about horticulture and how to involve their residents in the outdoor environment. Staff members were able to introduce changes both to their activity programs and to the outdoor environments in their facilities as a result. doi:10.1300/J081v21n03_13 *[Article copies available for a fee from The Haworth Document Delivery Service: 1-800-HAWORTH. E-mail address: <docdelivery@haworthpress.com> Website: <http://www.HaworthPress.com>* © *2007 by The Haworth Press, Inc. All rights reserved.]*

KEYWORDS. Therapeutic horticulture training, long-term care, elderly, outdoor environment, older adults, dementia

INTRODUCTION

In 1998, the American Society of Landscape Architects committed to donating members' design services to create 100 new gardens nationwide to celebrate their centennial year. In partnership with the Alzheimer's Association, eight of these were developed as "Memory Gardens," designed specifically to fit the needs of people with memory disorders and their caregivers (Brawley 2004). One of these, the Portland Memory Garden, was developed in a public park through the volunteer efforts of a team of professionals from the Oregon chapter of ASLA, the Center of Design for an Aging Society, Legacy Health Systems, Portland State University's Institute on Aging, Portland Parks and Recreation, and the Alzheimer's Association (Chapman, Hazen & Noell-Waggoner, 2005). As the garden was completed, the team expanded its attention to developing and implementing a training program for activity staff caring for people with dementia. Despite a growing body of research on the healing power of nature, many elders living in congregate facilities have limited access to the natural world (Chapman & Carder, 2003). Many of these facilities lack adequate outdoor environments and easy access to the outdoors for residents (Cutler & Kane, 2005). In addition, limited knowledge, time, and funding, may prevent nursing facilities from incorporating the use of plants and natural settings into their daily activities. It became clear to the team that simply building gardens does not guarantee that they will be used, or that staff members have the knowledge they need to take full advantage of what the outdoor environment can offer to their residents.

The Importance of the Natural Environment

Access to the natural environment and health. Following Ulrich's (1984) discovery of the relationship between views of nature and reduced use of pain medications and quicker recovery among surgery patients, theory and research have explored the healing qualities of the natural environment. Ulrich posits that exposure to the natural environment promotes recovery from stress (Ulrich et al., 1991; Ulrich, 1999). Kaplan (1995), in a somewhat different formulation, argues that natural environments are restorative because they allow relief from the fatigue created by the directed attention needed to complete complex tasks. In his view, the natural environment has characteristics that attract involuntary attention (or fascination) and allow the organism to rebuild depleted reserves of energy. Although the lower demands of viewing the natural environment may provide relief from complex tasks, architects, environmental psychologists and horticultural therapists (Cohen & Weisman, 1991; Haas, Simson, & Stevenson, 2003) propose that they may offer needed stimulation to residents of long term care facilities.

The natural environment and dementia. Researchers have studied access to the natural environment for people with dementia as a means of providing stimulation and reducing agitation. Access to well-designed gardens may encourage walking (Joseph, Zimring, Harris-Kojetin & Kiefer, 2005; Mooney & Nicell, 1992), and decrease pacing, wandering, and agitation (Cohen-Mansfield & Werner, 1998; Namazi & Johnson, 1992). Gardens and outdoor areas are often also preferred locales for visits between residents with dementia and their families and friends (Chapman & Carder, 2003). They offer a focus for attention and "props" to spark conversation (even if one-sided) with people who may have a limited ability to communicate.

Exposure to natural light is another potential benefit of access to gardens for this population. It has long been known that light exposure synchronizes the circadian rhythms that control our sleep-wake cycles with the solar day. Disturbance of circadian rhythms may play a role in the agitation and sleep disturbances that are common among people with dementia. A specialized cell in the retina of the human eye has been identified as the human pacemaker (e.g., Klerman et al., 2002). This cell's peak sensitivity is in the blue range (Berson, 2003; Klerman et al., 2002; Lockley, Brainard, & Czeisler, 2003), similar to light from the blue sky. So the exposure to daylight associated with the outdoor environment may also be an important factor in the well-being of people with dementia.

Gardening is a very common hobby in America–according to Butterfield (2006), 40% of Americans identify themselves as "gardeners," 38% as nongardeners, and 23 % as lacking a space to garden. A Canadian survey (Craig, Russell, Cameron & Beaulieu, 1998) found that the most popular physical activities were walking and gardening for age groups 25-44, 45-64 and 65 + . Thus, horticultural activities provide an opportunity for many individuals to draw on past experience and skills. The natural environment offers the potential to include features and activities that are familiar to people with dementia, which they remember from earlier in their life even if their memory for recent happenings is very limited. Thus, designers of dementia gardens have included familiar plants and flowers rather than the newest trend in garden design (Cooper Marcus, 2005). Gardens may also incorporate clothes lines, mailboxes, and vintage cars that can spark well-remembered daily activities.

The Purpose of the Training Project

Lovering et al. (2002) offered four components as central to the success of gardens in dementia facilities based on their three-year follow-up of the success of such a garden. These components are (1) support from the organization, integrating the garden into its mission and use of resources, (2) application of design principles specific to people with dementia, (3) staff "creativity, knowledge and skill to design and implement programs that maximize the garden's potential and the client's well-being," and (4) a good maintenance program. Our training program aimed particularly at developing organizational support within the facilities involved and in training staff to advocate for and use plants and gardens as part of their activity program.

The project provided therapeutic horticulture training to activity staff from long-term care facilities Therapeutic horticulture can be characterized as "the purposeful use of plants and plant-related activities to promote health and wellness for an individual or group" (Larson, Hancheck & Vollmaar, 2006, Introduction, ¶2). The sessions familiarized activity directors and recreational therapists with the importance of exposure to the natural world and increased their skills in working with the outside environment using techniques from the field of therapeutic horticulture (e.g., Wells, 1997).

Specific Objectives and Activities of the Training

The training program had the following objectives:

- To demonstrate the therapeutic benefits of plants, gardens and natural settings, including emphasis on the cognitive, psychosocial, sensory, and restorative benefits of gardening.
- To teach activity directors and recreational therapists basic horticultural skills (i.e. plant care techniques, plant identification) that they could easily implement in their own facilities.
- To teach participants to task-analyze horticultural activities, including grading techniques to make their activities appropriate for people with different levels of function.

- To teach participants two to three strategies for engaging both family members and residents in therapeutic horticulture activities.
- To emphasize the importance of incorporating gardening, nature, and horticulture activities throughout the year. To understand and be able to conduct sessions involving sensory stimulation during all four seasons.
- To provide training in various sensory stimulation activities that can be used both indoors and in the garden.
- To provide activity staff with information that allows them to assess and further develop their own in-facility gardens, thus making them more useful to the intended population. The main areas of assessment included plant safety, availability and location of seating areas, and plant collections for four seasons of sensory stimulation.
- To use the Portland Memory Garden and increase awareness about its potential as a therapeutic setting for people of all ages, with varying levels of ability.

TRAINING METHOD

Participants attended five training sessions between September of 2003 and May of 2004. The first session was six hours in length and the others four hours, for a total of 22 contact hours. The first four sessions were held at Legacy Good Samaritan Hospital in Portland, and made use of the therapeutic garden at that location for part of the instruction. One session included a field trip to a major local nursery, and the final session was held at the Portland Memory Garden.

Participants

Facilities in the Portland, OR metropolitan area with dementia care units were the original target of recruitment. Recruitment was expanded to facilities attending a statewide conference when the funding agency required that 20 participants from 10 facilities be recruited prior to releasing funding. In both cases, facility directors received letters describing the free training project and inviting their participation. Participants were accepted on a "first come, first served" basis; 20 facilities were admitted to the training and 12 were placed on a waiting list. In the end, 28 staff members from 20 facilities throughout Oregon were admitted to the training program with 25 staff members from 18 facilities participating in the first session. Of these, 72% were activity directors, 12% were activity assistants, and the remainder included a resident care manager, a discharge planner, and a social services coordinator. Ninety two percent were women. Forty-eight percent of the participants rated their gardening experience as "none" or "minimal," 38% cited gardening experience (two with at least one class) and 8% had training in horticultural therapy.

Attrition took two forms: absence from training sessions and changes in the personnel attending the sessions. Of the 20 facilities accepted into the training program, six attended all five sessions, four attended four sessions, one attended three sessions, five attended two sessions, two attended one session, and two attended none. Attrition was probably increased by the inadvertent scheduling of two of the five sessions on days that were holidays for some participants.

There was also some change in personnel attending the sessions. Although there were 25 participants in the first session, there were a total 33 different people represented across the five sessions. Many of the participant changes were a result of staff turnover. In addition, several participants left their facilities following the training but prior to the final evaluation visit.

Participating Facilities

The 18 participating facilities had the characteristics summarized in Table 1. Of these facilities, ten were located in the Portland Metropolitan area (within 30 miles of the training site), six were 45-100 miles from the training site, and two were 300 miles from the site.

Training Curriculum

The following paragraphs summarize the elements of the training curriculum most relevant to the outdoor environment, led by the second author, a horticultural therapist with the Legacy Health System, assisted by several students from her Horticultural Therapy Certificate Program. Guest speakers included Brain Bainnson, the landscape architect most closely associated with the design of the Portland Memory Garden; the third author, an interior architect and lighting specialist; and the first author, an environmental psychologist specializing in gerontology. Each participant was provided with a notebook and written information to help them recall all of the activities included in the training. The learning model used throughout was interactive, often modeling activities with participants that staff might take back to their facility to use with their residents. At each session, participants reported ideas they had developed and implemented at their facilities since the previous session.

Plant Identification in the Garden. Plant identification in the garden was a key part of the training day. Participants gathered in the therapeutic garden at the hospital where the instructor identified by common and Latin name at least

TABLE 1. Characteristics of Participating Facilities

Levels of Care	No. of Facilities Beginning Training	No. Completing Training
AD only	2	2 (100%)
AD, ALF	4	3 (75%)
AD, NURS	5	2 (40%)
NURS	3	1 (33%)
MLF	4	2 (50%)
Total	18	10

Note: AD=dementia special care unit; ALF=assisted living facility; NURS=nursing facility (ICF, SNF, RCF), MLF=continuing care retirement community or multi-level facility including independent living.

10 different types of plants in the garden, focusing on those with interest during that month. For example, cherry trees might be mentioned during their bloom season in March or April. Participants learned the value of being able to identify plants in order to use resource materials to assist them in choosing and maintaining them. Discussion included:

• Cultural information for each plant, such as the type of light or soil the plant needed and its mature size;
• The therapeutic values of each plant. Plant features that provided stimulation for the senses (touch, taste, sight, audition, smell) throughout the four seasons were considered therapeutic. For example, the Cornelian Cherry is a small tree with edible fruit, good fall color, and yellow blossoms in the spring.
• How to incorporate the plants into garden group activities, indoors or outdoors.

Container Gardening. The participants from each facility received a large container and a variety of plants to go into it. The container provided an easy way to increase the outdoor gardening amenities available at each facility. Participants learned basic guidelines for container gardening and how to maintain them to ensure quality throughout the year. Basic pruning, fertilizer, watering, and planting instructions were demonstrated. Planting plans suitable for each of the four seasons were presented at each session and participants were given three different sets of plant material over the course of the training to renew their containers or begin new ones. The participants were encouraged to involve residents in planting and maintaining their container gardens. They also learned adaptive strategies for container gardening such as using a teepee trellis for vines and how to make container gardens accessible for people using wheelchairs and walkers. In the final session, they received a low container, a tomato trellis, and vegetables to create a salad garden.

Resources. At each session participants learned about new resources that could be used to help plan a therapeutic horticulture program, such as books on gardening and membership in the American Horticultural Therapy Association. A central resource, particularly in those facilities with residents prone to eating plants, is a source on toxic plants, such as *Common Poisonous Plants and Mushrooms of North America* (Turner & Szczawinski 1995). At the final session, each facility attending received a copy of the *Sunset Western Garden Book,* a source of information about plants, plant care, and gardening that is tailored to specific climate regions of the west. They also shared their own resources with the rest of the group, including useful internet sites and relevant classes in their community.

Activity Planning. During each session, participants were shown how to plan at least one, one-hour garden session for each week of the month. They learned how to organize the activity step by step through preparation, therapist steps, client steps, and then how to evaluate the session. Participants learned how to grade a horticulture activity to adjust it to the variety of residents and their individual needs.

Site Visit to a Local Nursery. A site visit to a retail garden center taught participants how to use the nursery as a learning tool and as a resource for resident outings. The participants explored plants of seasonal interest, adaptive gardening tools and container options as well as the variety of plants offered by the center.

Improving the Outdoor Environment at their Facility. The course included an introduction to how to develop a therapeutic garden design for nursing and dementia facilities, with presentations by a landscape architect and a gerontologist. Topics included developing a garden team planning committee and the characteristics of a therapeutic garden for this population. This part of the curriculum drew from the literature on planning gardens for people with dementia (e.g., Beckwith & Gilster, 1997; Cohen-Mansfield & Werner, 1999; Lovering et al, 2002; Lovering, 1990; Zeisel & Tyson, 1999), as well as from our own experience in creating the Portland Memory Garden. Important considerations included both the structure of the setting and the plantings. Structural features included the security of the setting, places to sit, accessible pathways and plantings, shade and absence of glare, and interesting things to observe in the garden. Planting features included the use of planters and raised beds, plantings with year-round interest, and plantings that offer stimulation for all of the senses.

EVALUATION

Goal

The evaluation was designed to gauge the success of the training by assessing (1) the extent to which the information provided was put into practice, and (2) the barriers encountered by participants in applying their knowledge.

Method

The evaluation included the following steps:

- A pre-training interview with the participant(s) was conducted with responses recorded in writing and, where feasible, a visit was made to the facility with a photo and written record. Respondents were asked about their indoor and outdoor plantings and nature-related items, garden supplies, current nature-related activities, level of horticulture experience, and expectations regarding the training.
- Activity calendars and questionnaire responses for the six months prior to the training were compared to activity calendars and interview responses following training to assess change in activities and garden development.
- Written evaluations of the content and presentation of each training session were gathered at the end of each session.
- During each training session participants responded to a brief questionnaire asking them to describe any activities they were able to carry out since the last meeting that involved plants, gardens, or the natural environment, to assess the success of those activities, and to report any barriers they encountered.
- One of the authors visited each of the facilities completing the training three months following the final training session to interview the participants about their experience and see any changes they had implemented as a result. They were asked about changes in staff, any physical changes made in the interior or exterior of the facility or in the activity program as a consequence of the training, and their future plans. They were also asked about any barriers or issues that had arisen in their attempts to implement change. Responses were recorded in writing and with a photo record.

Training Outcomes

A major barrier to successfully implementing change through training activity personnel was the turnover in staff members at the facilities, and thus in those attending the trainings. Staff turnover or change in position was one reason facilities dropped out of the training process. Only ten of the eighteen facilities beginning training attended at least four of the five sessions. The evaluation that follows is focused on the ten facilities that completed the training, and relies most heavily on the post-training visits and interviews.

Overall, the facilities and staff participating accomplished the following:

Knowledge. The staff members reported increased knowledge, enthusiasm, and confidence for working with plants and nature-related activities. Participants reported during the first training session that the main thing the participants wanted and needed was more knowledge about plants and gardening. Several noted this as critical in helping them develop and continue such activities with the residents. One said that she was more willing to accept plants donated by families because she now knows whether or not they will survive and be appropriate for the residents. Others noted that their enthusiasm generated enthusiasm among residents, families, and other staff members, who became involved in a variety of ways.

Activities. Based on analysis of the activity calendars and questionnaires collected before and after training, there was an increase in the number and variety of nature-related activities. Participants reported learning from each other as well via sharing of experiences during the training. Since the training extended from September to May, many activities during the winter months were indoors. As the weather improved, visits to nurseries and gardens in the vicinity became more common, as well as activities in the gardens at their facilities. Examples included encouraging residents to become involved in choosing plants, planting, watering and deadheading, and often eating the produce from their gardens. In one case, the family of a man who had been a farmer brought in seed potatoes of varieties he recommended, and they were planted and later harvested for a stew shared by residents of the unit.

Physical changes to gardens. Major new structural changes, plantings and/or numerous containers that exemplified the principles of therapeutic horticulture were present in at least five of the ten gardens in the follow-up evaluation. Examples include adding accessible pathways, a large new raised bed (Fig. 1), new beds with appropriate plantings (Fig. 2), large containers with seasonal plantings outside each resident room, a gazebo and renovating outdoor patios. Most facilities had more changes in the planning stage. A sixth facility, working with a landscape architect, developed plans and raised funds to completely re-landscape their extensive outdoor areas using these principles.

FIGURE 1. New Raised Bed

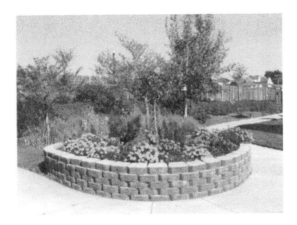

The other four facilities had made use of the container and plant materials we provided but other changes were minor.

Barriers to Engaging Residents in Garden–And Nature-Related Activities

There were a number of barriers to change that were identified by participants throughout the training, some of which had moved toward solutions by the end of the training. The most commonly mentioned were:

Garden design. Issues included existing plantings that were limited and did not offer different kinds of sensory stimulation; patios that were too hot, lacked in shade, or experienced glare from concrete pathways and surrounding buildings; a lack of covered areas; a lack of raised beds accessible to wheelchairs; background noise that interfered with working with groups; and unavailability of water (on large balconies). Staff were more able to intervene in changing plantings than in dealing with issues such as shade and glare, but a few had been able to make or get commitments for change in these areas as well.

Accessibility. In some cases it was difficult for residents to access outdoor areas due to lack of visibility from the windows, sloping sites, being located on a different floor, lack of secure fencing, and not being wheelchair accessible. Doors to the garden were sometimes too heavy for residents to open, locked or alarmed, discouraging residents from using the garden on their own initiative.

FIGURE 2. New Outdoor Planting

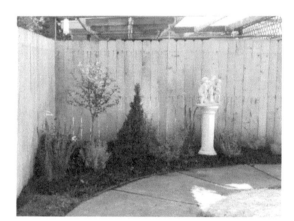

Money and time to develop ideas. In the end, most seemed able to find the resources to do more than they (and we) had expected despite the fact that activity staff rather than administrators were the target of the training.

Staff turnover. Turnover in activity staff and/or key administrators hindered continuity at times. This is a difficult issue to overcome for both a one-time training program and a long-term care facility. This type of training could best be integrated into general training for activity directors and into training for administrators. Some who participated were already passing what they learned on to other activity directors in their community through their local organization for activity staff, suggesting that such organizations might be good sites for ongoing training on this topic.

Resistance to change. A few said that "new ideas are not accepted" in their facility. This was particularly problematic in a large continuing care retirement community that gave priority to the more independent elderly in prioritizing use of outdoor areas.

Maintenance. Outdoor landscaping was often cared for by a contracted provider who was not able/willing to provide more than very basic care. This made it more difficult for staff to bring in diverse new plantings and to see that they were adequately maintained. Activity staff tried to take responsibility for maintaining plantings, but it was difficult to work into their schedules. A few were looking for new contracted providers or renegotiating with their existing provider to provide more care.

Resident issues. Some staff experienced problems with residents who attempted to eat plants or soil, who pulled up new seed starts or plants, who over-watered plants, or who didn't want to get their hands dirty. Solutions here included planting larger plants less likely to be pulled up, and instituting "plant hospitals" to nurse sick plants back to health. Staff also reported that some residents lacked interest or motivation to engage with the outdoor environment.

CONCLUSION

The project was able to demonstrate that long term care facilities can be attracted to training programs related to access to the natural environment. The funding source for the project originally required recruitment of 20 participants from 10 facilities prior to releasing the funding, indicating their doubts about the potential for recruiting participants. It is possible that offering the program without charge on a 'first come, first served' basis reduced commitment to the training and increased the drop-out rate. Although it is challenging to retain participants across a nine month schedule, we consider it an important component of the training process.

Although most of the facilities were still far from providing the ideal outdoor setting for a memory care garden at the completion of training, the attendees of the training program understood the principles and were applying them as they could. Most had taken steps to alter the indoor and outdoor environments as well as the nature-related activities that occurred in those settings. Unfortunately, we were not able to track the frequency with which residents were involved in outdoor activities. Increasing use of outdoor environments by long term care facilities will hinge on having activity staff that are comfortable with gardens and garden activities and understand their importance. In the long run, it will be important to convince facility administrators of the importance of nature and garden activities so that they can become a higher priority in the planning process. One attendee noted that she wished her administrator could experience a well-designed therapeutic garden to understand what could be accomplished.

REFERENCES

Beckwith, M. E., & Gilster, S.D. (1997). The Paradise Garden: A model garden design for those with Alzheimer's Disease. *Activities, Adaptation & Aging, 22,* 3-16.
Berson, D. M. (2003). Strange vision: ganglion cells as circadian photoreceptors. *Trends in Neurosciences, 26,* 314-20.

Brawley, E. C. (2004). Gardens of memories. *Alzheimer's Care Quarterly, 5*, 154-64.

Butterfield, B. (2006). *2005 a banner year for the gardening industry.* Paper presented at the 2006 Garden Writers Association virtual conference. Retrieved October 9, 2006, from http://www.gardenwriters.org/Meetings/benefits_of_gardening.pdf

Chapman, N. J. & Carder, P.A. (2003). Privacy needs when visiting a person with Alzheimer's disease: Family and staff expectations. *Journal of Applied Gerontology, 22*, 506-522.

Chapman, N. J., Hazen, T. & Noell-Waggoner, E. (2005). Encouraging development and use of gardens by caregivers of people with dementia. *Alzheimer's Care Quarterly, 6*, 349-356.

Cohen-Mansfield, J., &Werner, P. (1998). Visits to an outdoor garden: Impact on behavior and mood of nursing home residents who pace. In B. Vellas, J. Fitten, & G. Frisoni (Eds.), *Research and Practice in Alzheimer's Disease 1998* (pp. 419-436). New York: Springer.

Cohen-Mansfield, J. & Werner, P. (1999). Outdoor wandering parks for persons with dementia: A survey of characteristics and use. *Alzheimer Disease and Associated Disorders, 13*, 109-17.

Cohen, U. & Weisman, G. (1991). *Holding on to home: Designing environments for people with dementia.* Baltimore: Johns Hopkins University Press.

Cooper Marcus, C. (2005). No ordinary garden. *Landscape Architecture, 5*(3), 26, 28-30, 32, 34-39.

Craig, C. L., Russell, S. J., Cameron, C. & Beaulieu, A. (1998). *1997 Physical Activity Monitor: Foundation for joint action: Reducing physical inactivity.*. Retrieved October 9, 2006 from Canadian Fitness and Lifestyle Research Institute Web site: http://www.cflri.ca/pdf/e/97pam.pdf.

Cutler, L & Kane, R. (2005). As great as all outdoors: A study of outdoor spaces as a neglected resource for nursing home residents. *Journal of Housing for the Elderly, 19*(3), 29-48. doi: 10.1300/J081v19n03_03

Haas, K., Simson, S.P. & Stevenson, N. C. (2003). Older persons and horticultural therapy practice. In S. P. Simson & M.C. Straus (Eds.), *Horticulture as therapy: Principles and practice* (pp. 231-255). New York: Food Products Press.

Joseph, A., Zimring, C., Harris-Kojetin, L., & Kiefer, K. (2005). Presence and visibility of outdoor and indoor physical activity features and participation in physical activity among older adults in retirement communities. *Journal of Housing for the Elderly, 19*(3), 141-165. doi: 10.1300/J081v19n03_08

Kaplan, S. (1995). The restorative benefits of nature: Toward an integrative framework. *Journal of Environmental Psychology, 15*, 169-82.

Klerman, E. B., Shanahan, T. L., Brotman, D. J., Rimmer, D., Emens, J. S., Rozzo, J. F., III, et al. (2002). Photic resetting of the human circadian pacemaker in the absence of conscious vision. *Journal of Biological Rhythms, 17*, 248-555.

Larson, J., Hancheck, A. & Vollmaar, P. (2006). *Accessible gardening for therapeutic horticulture.* Retrieved October 9, 2006 from University of Minnesota Extension Service Web site: http://www.extension.umn.edu/distribution/horticulture/DG6757.html

Lockley, S. W., Brainard, G. C. & Czeisler, C.A.. (2003). High sensitivity of the human circadian melatonin rhythm to resetting by short wavelength light. *The Journal of Clinical Endocrinology & Metabolism, 88,* 4502-5.

Lovering, M. J. (1990). Alzheimer's disease and outdoor space: Issues in environmental design. *American Journal of Alzheimer's Care and Related Disorders & Research, 5,* 33-40.

Lovering, M. J., Cott, C. A., Wells, D. L., Schleifer Taylor, J., & Wells, L. M. (2002). A study of a secure garden in the care of people with Alzheimer's disease. *Canadian Journal on Aging, 21,* 417-27.

Mooney, P. & Nicell, P. L. (1992). The importance of exterior environment for Alzheimer residents: Effective care and risk management. *Healthcare Management Forum, 5*(2), 23-29.

Namazi, K. H. & Johnson, B.D. (1992). Pertinent autonomy of residents with dementias: Modification of the physical environment to enhance independence. *American Journal of Alzheimer Care Research, 7,* 16-21.

Turner, N. J. & Szczawinski A. (1995). *Common poisonous plants and mushrooms of North America.* Portland, OR: Timber Press.

Ulrich, R. S. (1984). View through a window may influence recovery from surgery. *Science, 224,* 420-421.

Ulrich, R. S. (1999). Effects of gardens on health outcomes: Theory and research. In C. Cooper Marcus & M. Barnes (Eds.), *Healing gardens: Therapeutic benefits and design recommendations* (pp. 27-86). New York: John Wiley & Sons.

Ulrich, R. S., Simons, R. F., Losito, B. D., Fiorito, E., Miles, M. A. & Zelson, M. (1991). Stress recovery during exposure to natural and urban environments. *Journal of Environmental Psychology, 11,* 201-30.

Wells, S. E. (Ed.) (1997). *Horticultural therapy and the older adult population.* Binghamton, NY: Haworth.

Zeisel, J. & Tyson, M. M. (1999). Alzheimer's treatment gardens. In C. Cooper Marcus & M. Barnes (Eds.), *Healing gardens: Therapeutic benefits and design recommendations* (pp. 437-504). New York: John Wiley.

doi:10.1300/J081v21n03_13

Designing Successful Gardens and Outdoor Spaces for Individuals with Alzheimer's Disease

Elizabeth C. Brawley

SUMMARY. There are many benefits derived from exposure to the outdoors for older adults with Alzheimer's disease, which include exposure to fresh air, sunlight and opportunities for walking and other forms of exercise. There are also opportunities for socialization that can minimize feelings of isolation and vulnerability, improve depression, enhance self-esteem, and simply experience the joys and surprises of nature.

While there seems to be universal agreement of the health and quality of life benefits in getting institutionalized persons into appropriate outdoor settings, in many ways gardens and outside spaces have failed. Time after time visitors stroll through the gardens admiring the landscaped grounds, the abundance of beautiful and fragrant flowers and other features, while noting the absence of residents.

Creditable research studies support the health benefits of exposure to the outdoors and nature. This discussion of design issues, barriers to use, the role of activity, the necessity of staff involvement, and design recommendations supports the urgent need for empirical research to inform the development of effective gardens and outdoor spaces to benefit older adults with Alzheimer's disease. doi:10.1300/J081v21n03_14

Elizabeth C. Brawley, AAHID, IIDA, CID, is President, Design Concepts Unlimited, Box 454, Sausalito, CA 94966 (E-mail: betsybrawley@attglobal.net).

[Haworth co-indexing entry note]: "Designing Successful Gardens and Outdoor Spaces for Individuals with Alzheimer's Disease." Brawley, Elizabeth C. Co-published simultaneously in *Journal of Housing for the Elderly* (The Haworth Press, Inc.) Vol. 21, No. 3/4, 2007, pp. 265-283; and: *Outdoor Environments for People with Dementia* (ed: Susan Rodiek and Benyamin Schwarz) The Haworth Press, Inc., 2007, pp. 265-283. Single or multiple copies of this article are available for a fee from The Haworth Document Delivery Service [1-800-HAWORTH, 9:00 a.m. - 5:00 p.m. (EST). E-mail address: docdelivery@haworthpress.com].

Available online at http://jhe.haworthpress.com

doi:10.1300/J081v21n03_14

KEYWORDS. Alzheimer's, outdoor environment, benefits, safety, activity

INTRODUCTION

The aging population is increasing dramatically in developed countries throughout the world. During the 20th century the U.S. population aged 65 and older increased tenfold, from 3 million to almost 35 million–a change from 4 to 13 percent of the population. This same group is expected to grow to 39.7 million by 2010 as nearly 77 million baby boomers begin to turn age 65 by 2008. That's more than double the current population of seniors (U.S. Department of Health and Human Resources, 2002). By 2050 more than 60 percent of people with Alzheimer's will be 85+, and of these, a high number will live alone (Alzheimer's Association, 2001). These compelling statistics underscore the need to change America's culture of long-term care.

As we age our ability to adapt to less than optimal conditions becomes more difficult, making the role of the environment increasingly important, particularly for those who are experiencing cognitive difficulties and diminishing physical dexterity (Lawton, 1989). Most people with Alzheimer's disease still have energy and the desire to remain active and involved in the world around them, which makes social life a high priority among family caregivers who instinctively seem to know that those who are allowed to freely socialize will form friendships and associations.

Throughout their lives, most people develop activities and interests–hobbies, likes and dislikes, skills and talents–that give their life structure and meaning and provide a sense of worth. These activities whether recreational or activities related to ordinary household tasks establish a routine, provide opportunities for socialization, and help define who we are. While cognitive decline tends to reduce participation, more often than not many individuals are limited in their ability to engage in community life because the daily program has not been adapted to their social and emotional needs. Integrating informal "everyday" activities into staff-led activities programs encourages many residents to participate and realize a satisfying social life.

Appropriate Alzheimer's care is focused on the psychosocial needs of the individual. Ideally, specialized Alzheimer's care settings provide environments customized to enhance individualized care, as well as to support behavioral approaches for care of residents with dementia. Activities are emphasized as a way to provide stimulation for residents' physical, cognitive and social skills (Ohta, and Ohta,1988); (Berg, Buckwalter, Chafez, Gwyther, Holmes, Koepke, Lawton, Lindeman, Magaziner, Maslow, Morley, Ory, Rabins, Sloane, and Teresi, 1991; Gold, Sloane, Matthews, Bledsoe and Konanc, 1991).These special care settings provide specific therapeutic activities designed to maximize remaining cognitive and physical abilities and diminish confusion, disruptive and agitated behaviors often associated with the disease.

Outdoor environments offer healthy exposure to fresh air and sunlight for residents and staff alike. Many older adults still enjoy gardening and other familiar activities and well designed gardens provide opportunities for raising vegetables and flowers, filling bird feeders and birdbaths, cutting flowers for table arrangements and sweeping the walk–activities that support movement and a sense of purpose. Until recently designing the outside environment has been an overlooked opportunity to create meaningful and accommodating spaces rich in association and responsive to the seasons.

Gardens provide a variety of opportunities for exercise. They encourage mobility and help older adults, especially those with cognitive impairment, to remain connected to nature and the world around them. Exposure to sunlight and healthy socialization in these outdoor settings can help to minimize feelings of isolation and vulnerability, improve depression, and enhance self-esteem (Van Someren, Hagebeuk, Lijzenga, Scheltens, DeRooji, Jonker, Pot, Mirmiran, and Swaab, 1996; Chen, Sloane, and Dalton, 2003).

Research specific to the value, benefits, design and use of outdoor environments for individuals with Alzheimer's disease is sparse at best. Until recently care settings for those with Alzheimer's have not focused on the outside environment and the need to encourage older adults to spend time outside in fresh air and sunlight (Brawley, 2002).

Carefully planned gardens and outdoor environments are a practical intervention that may well prove to be one of the safest and least expensive ways to encourage a healthy lifestyle, both in community and facility based settings. Too few care settings look beyond the obvious aesthetic concerns to skillfully address the more complex needs of physically and cognitively challenged seniors. In the design of residential Alzheimer's settings, gardens are particularly useful because they can be easily infused with cultural tradition, fond memories and compelling images that often stand in stark contrast to the prevailing clinical feel of many long-term care settings (Brawley, 1997). Well-executed outside spaces compensate for increasing frailty and sensory loss in cognitively impaired individuals, helping to reduce challenging behaviors, while poorly designed environments, unfortunately, often precipitate agitation and contribute to disorientation, and confusion.

RESEARCH

In the last fifteen years informational findings from the National Institutes on Aging collaborative studies have provided a wealth of information to help design more caring environments that support better quality of care outcomes. Additional studies have shown that care environments directly affect many resident behaviors and that Alzheimer's special care settings can affect agitation (Sloane, Zimmerman, Suchindran, Reed, Lily Wang, Boustani, and Sudha, 2002). Though studies evaluating the success of healthcare housing environments are increasing, there have been far fewer studies of healthcare facility gardens and outdoor environments (Cooper Marcus, and Barnes, 1995). Today, gardens and outdoor environments have taken on new significance and there is renewed interest in research exploring the numerous benefits of exposure to fresh air, sunlight and exercise.

There is general agreement that fresh air, sunlight, and natural settings are generally beneficial for good health, but only a few studies correlate nature scenes and stress reduction. A study on stress reduction was conducted in a laboratory setting where subjects evaluated pictures of scenes of nature and were then tested for emotional and psychological recovery, indicating the presence of natural greenery in a scene has a high correlation with stress reduction (Ulrich, 1979; Ulrich, 1984; Ulrich, 1986; Honeyman, 1987; Hartig, et al., 1990). Roger Ulrich's landmark study monitored hospital patients' recovery when looking out at vegetation as opposed to buildings, and found those with a view of nature recovered more quickly (Ulrich, 1984). Other studies indicated that participants in gardening activities reported positive mood shifts–sensory joy, peacefulness and tranquility (Ulrich, 1979; Kaplan, and Talbot, 1983). These studies, to be clear, did not evaluate particular gardens and outdoor spaces or the effects on participants.

The need for more documented, empirical research on gardens in healthcare settings is clearly evidenced. Evaluations of existing outdoor sites, the therapeutic goals and outcomes related specifically to Alzheimer's disease and dementia would be valuable in encouraging appropriate design and further development for gardens and outdoor spaces. Despite this lack of evidence-based research specifically related to people with dementia, there are a number of therapeutic benefits of outdoor spaces that can be reasonably theorized to have an impact on this population.

BENEFITS OF THE OUTDOORS

Light

Sleep disorders, depression and reduced calcium absorption are common problems in older adults who are light deprived (Chen, Sloane, and Dalton, 2003; Von Someren, Hagebeuk, Lijzenga, Scheltens, DeRooji, Jonker, Pot, Mirmiran, and Swaab, 1996). The benefits of sunlight are yet to be fully appreciated, particularly in relationship to synchronizing circadian rhythm, sleep disorders, and the synthesizing of vitamin D, which directly affects osteoporosis and vulnerability to falls. While exposure to high light levels during the day provides a strong natural regulator to synchronize the wake/sleep cycle with the day/night cycle, (Mishima, Okawa, Hishikawa, Hozumi, Hori, Takahashi, 1994) light deprived individuals do not experience the full effect of the light/dark cycles, causing the circadian rhythm or the internal body clock to malfunction. It can take as little as 15-20 minutes exposure to natural sunlight a day to reset and maintain these body rhythms, (Rea, Figueiro, and Bullough, 2002; Roberts, 2002) but unfortunately as mobility decreases, so does the exposure to the outdoors, the full intensity of daylight and the necessary high light levels.

Sixty five percent of those over age 65 experience some problems sleeping (Clapin-French,1986). According to the 1993 National Commission on Sleep Disorders Research, the annual cost for sleep disorders was reported to be $15.4 billion (National Commission on Sleep Disorders Research). Providing easy access to the outdoors is an effective, low cost, energy efficient intervention that every healthcare setting can use to maintain and increase resident health and wellness, allowing the use of natural daylight or sunlight to provide the essential high levels of light necessary for good health, as well as increased opportunities for exercise and mobility.

Adequate light exposure is also required for vital vitamin D synthesis and calcium metabolism (Holick, 2002). Vitamin D synthesis declines dramatically as mobility decreases, resulting in decreased bone mass, a contributing factor to falls and fractures (Hollick, 1994). Since nursing home residents are the elderly group found to be most deficient in the essential vitamin D (Clapin-French, 1986), it shouldn't be surprising that falls are even more common in nursing homes than for the same age group living elsewhere in the community (Ancoli-Israel, Jones, Hanger, Parker, Klauber, and Kripke, 1991). This would seem to be a strong indicator that exposure to the higher natural light levels found outside may be even more important than we had previously believed, for the health of nursing home residents.

Many residents in long-term care settings suffer from debilitating depression, making it one of the most serious chronic problems. The variety of an interesting garden is a powerful strategy to entice residents outside into warm sunlight, which can fight both depression and the boredom related to a chronically under stimulating environment (Cooper Marcus, and Barnes, 1999). Physical exercise, often attributed with improved results in psychological well-being, is now being shown to be especially beneficial in reducing depression. A 1994 study found that higher levels of physical activity were associated with lower rates of depression among the elderly in nursing homes (Ruuskanen, and Parketti, 1994). Getting older adults outside for exercise and exposure to high light levels offers a healthy, low cost intervention to fight depression, sleep disorders, mobility loss and other chronic problems of aging.

Exercise and Physical Activity

A growing body of research in the past decade has shown that exercise is one of the best medicines for older people who have or hope to forestall disabilities, even for people 85 and older. The concern with exercise has repeatedly caused The Centers for Disease Controls and Prevention to urge older adults to increase exercise and mobility (Centers for Disease Control and Prevention National Center for Injury Prevention and Control, 1999). Exercise is associated with a broad range of significant physical health benefits. Older adults with disabilities including chronic conditions such as arthritis, diabetes, heart disease, osteoporosis, sleep disorders and depression can greatly reduce their risk for secondary conditions by remaining–or becoming physically active (Rimmer, 2004). James Rimmer, director of the National Center on Physical Activity and Disability funded by the Centers for Disease Control and Prevention is particularly concerned with the correlation between physical fitness and physical health and well-being. He suggests making exercise a priority for all those involved in dementia care. Increased physical strength and emotional well-being are added benefits of physical activity (Rimmer, J., 2004).

Older adults especially value stimulation and the social experiences that bring an improved quality of life for individuals with dementia and caregivers alike. Exercise, for example, offers important opportunities for socialization and accepted physical touch. In the process of assisted walking, walking arm in arm is vitally necessary and socially accepted touching happens naturally (Brawley, 2002).

Current research studies are exploring mobility and sleep cycles to determine whether more exercise in the daytime helps residents sleep better at night and/or results in less roaming about in the middle of the night. It's encouraging and empowering to know that something as basic as physical activity and exercise can produce fundamental health benefits activity (Rimmer, 2004).

The design of outdoor spaces should be included in overall design plans to encourage exercise, support better health, maximize remaining abilities and possibly reduce the use of costly prescription drugs in our older adult population. This is therapeutic intervention and preventative medicine at its best.

DESIGNING FOR SAFETY AND SECURITY

Access to safe and secure outdoor spaces can provide opportunities for exercise, socialization, and a wide range of activities that stimulate long-term memories of previous home life, such as mowing the lawn with a push mower, raking leaves, and gardening. These outdoor spaces help to maintain a connection with the natural environment and can also provide places for privacy that may be difficult to find inside.

In addition to being physically safe and secure, it is essential that the garden be perceived as safe by staff, family and residents. Designs for outdoor space will vary according to location, availability of space and existing features, but the single greatest barrier to the use of accessible outdoor space may be staff concern that a resident may wander away or be injured (Brawley, 2005).

Outdoor spaces must be secure. With the exception of interior courtyards, gardens must be safely enclosed by a fence or a wall. The challenge is to create an enclosed space without the feeling of confinement. The skills of landscape architects and knowledgeable consultants in design and activity programming for older adults in outside environments can be invaluable in planning successful gardens and outdoor spaces for people with Alzheimer's disease. The goal is to provide secured spaces that encourage a variety of activities without causing a sense of feeling "fenced in." Good design techniques can successfully disguise or even hide fencing, making more interesting garden spaces that focus attention on a variety of activities in the garden rather than focusing on how to get out.

Many residential gardens provide good inspiration. The imagination and beautiful design of many small residential gardens in the center of Charleston, South Carolina provide excellent examples of how even small, awkward spaces can be adapted into very positive garden spaces for dementia. These small spaces are so well planned and skillfully executed with beautiful colors, fragrant blossoms and wisteria covered arbors that it prevents one from noticing the ten foot high brick walls that enclose the small garden spaces, sheltering them from the noise and distraction of traffic. The imagination, abundant creativity and skill of landscape architects and designers can transform a small space enclosed by high walls from an imprisoning enclosure into a beautiful and secure dementia garden for even the most vulnerable users. The security of this active and happy space invites residents, staff and families to enjoy the pleasures of the outdoors.

HOW DO RESIDENTS PERCEIVE SAFE ENVIRONMENTS?

Older persons express strong preferences for physical features that compensate for physical impairments and support safe passage. Those features include handrails and wide, glare-free, non-slip walkways that accommodate two-way traffic without physical contact (Brawley, 1997). Safety is a crucial aspect of design in relationship to physical mobility. Because of the progressive lack of coordination in Alzheimer's disease some individuals tend to shuffle rather than walk, making balance a problematic challenge (Gill, Williams and Tinetti, 2000). This reinforces the premise that gardens for older adults, especially those with Alzheimer's must be level.

Level, slip-resistant, glare-free walking surfaces help to minimize falls due to the high incidence of osteoporosis in the elderly. Surface materials should provide uniform texture in a medium color value and good contrast between the walking surface itself and the immediate surroundings. Wide, glare-free pathways with easily distinguishable borders encourage walking (Brawley, 2005).

Good design incorporates just enough slope of the surface to avoid puddles in wet weather and to insure that walking surfaces remain "non-slip" in wet or dry conditions. Properly maintaining walkways to remain free of irregularities such as cracks, potholes or uneven spots will help to support good balance and coordination. Falls in the outdoor environment are also often caused by glare reflected from bright white paving into the eyes of elderly walkers. It adversely affects balance and is particularly problematic for older eyes that no longer adjust easily to strong changes in light levels. Sufficiently tinting concrete and other surface materials enhances safety by eliminate hazardous glare.

Outdoor spaces that fail to accommodate for special needs by incorporating solutions designed to better support diminished physical capacity, as well as changes in awareness, orientation, interaction, privacy and independence will not be successful, actively used gardens.

MOBILITY AND FALL PREVENTION

It is important for staff to keep residents in view and the use of larger windows provides greater visibility to the outside and helps alleviate staff stress. It is important to develop policies of shared risk. In an elderly population in the most safely designed settings falls may occur even with the most caring staff. Normal aging changes common to older persons, particularly in those 85 and older, make them more prone to falls and at increased risk of hip fracture (Gill, Williams and Tinetti, 2000). The fear of falling itself can drastically limit mobility.

A recent study from Yale University indicates that poor vision and lack of exercise are factors most associated with falls in the elderly population. As Alzheimer's disease progresses, lack of coordination and balance can add to problems in walking causing some individuals to shuffle rather than walk. This reinforces both the need for level, glare-free pathways and the need for increased exercise. Exercise, including walking, offers protection against falls, through improved strength and balance (Gill, Williams and Tinetti, 2000).

KEY CONCEPTS FOR BUILDING BETTER GARDENS

There are concepts in the previous paragraphs that are key to understanding essential ingredients for successful gardens and why so many outdoor spaces are under used or altogether unused.

- Secured space should not scream confinement;
- Staff concern for resident safety;
- Fall Prevention: poor visual acuity and lack of exercise are top two causes of falls;
- Shared risk policies; and
- Activity. Fun, interesting gardens provide meaningful activity choices, somewhere to go and something to do while encouraging socialization and inclusion.

Culture Change in Long-Term Care

Culture change is the new "buzz word" in long-term care. In the world of aging, culture change embodies an emerging, progressive view of aging that means systems change throughout a facility from both the individual and the organizational perspective. "Residents first!" (Brawley, 2005).

Before culture change in long-term care do you remember how residents gathered around the nurses station? They drew up a chair at the nurses station because it's where the action was. It was the activity center–often the only activity going on and their presence allowed them to be part of the group. They were close enough to see and be seen and experience an abbreviated version of socialization.

While there is no single approach to culture change in long-term care, it must start at the top with an organizational structure that embraces total support and participation from all levels of management. This approach empowers staff, inspires creativity and puts more focus where it belongs, on direct care staff, who provide for residents' needs. *The goal is to redesign care settings as places for meaningful living, with good care supporting rather than dominating daily life* and to transform the environment from focusing first on the institutional need to meeting resident needs resulting in what is now known as "resident-centered" care (Fagan, 2002).

The three environments essential for culture change are the organizational environment, the psycho-social/spiritual environment, and the physical environment (Fagan, 2002). The culture change movement recognizes that many of the traditional methods of "doing things" don't achieve the results we hoped for. Culture change offers a more responsible approach to turning the process around to insure the outcomes we want. The very culture of the care setting changes, creating a sense of belonging where each individual's contributions are valued. A sense of community develops connecting residents, staff and families and promotes joy and aliveness. It is a *process based on inclusion*; everyone is actively involved and working together. To be successful it is essential that the whole organization be involved (Fagan, 2000).

WHY GO OUTDOORS IF THERE'S NOTHING GOING ON?

Outside environments must be better adapted to compensate for the physical and sensory changes related to aging and the special needs of those with Alzheimer's disease. Capacities of strength, endurance, balance and co-ordination, as well as decreased visual acuity must be addressed. However, *gardens fail primarily because they aren't designed for activity*. Fun, interesting activity means somewhere to go and something meaningful to do while encouraging socialization and inclusion. While many gardens are beautiful they aren't designed to support a meaningful, varied and well-planned activity program that focuses on the needs or desires of older adults.

GARDENS MADE FOR REMEMBERING

Experience has made it very clear that the "build it and they will come" theory (i.e., assuming that people will use gardens if they are built), is not borne out by reality. There are an abundance of pretty gardens that often improve marketing attempts but rarely seem to interest or engage residents.

Activity is the heart of residents' experience and it is just as inextricably tied to the success of the Alzheimer's care garden as it is to the success of the care setting. Gardens expected to be utilized as part of the overall therapeutic program must be woven into the care plans developed by the clinical staff (Brawley, 2002). This is a critical piece of the plan that rarely seems to be communicated with the design team or is not communicated in such a way that designers understand its significance.

Developing a strong outdoor activity program before–not after the garden is designed and built is the foundation that determines how the design can best support activities and ultimately, the residents. A successful garden is one that becomes a part of residents' lives and is constantly used.

As in designing interior environments, it is important to envision a clear and detailed picture of the experiences you want to create and the activities you want to accommodate before putting pen to paper to begin designing the garden. The most successful gardens are designed and built to accommodate robust activity programs. Too often the challenge of operating programs in spaces not designed for that purpose becomes overwhelming and rarely fulfills the needs of residents, especially those with dementia. This results in outdoor spaces going unused.

Professional landscape architects and designers can be invaluable in determining the location, orientation, and functional aspects of the garden. They are, for example, able to turn boring "wandering loops" into lovely walking paths that meander through the garden, and they can provide valuable assistance in the selection of paving surfaces that curtail glare and are smooth enough to accommodate unsure feet.

Gardens can be a symphony of color, fragrances, sights and sounds. Birds and small animals are a wonderful source of sensory stimulation, while delightful whimsical spaces are proven welcome additions to many gardens. Fragrance gardens, butterfly gardens, bird houses and bird feeders, garden ornaments, weather vanes, and flag poles are interesting focal points and opportunities for interaction and activity. Raised vegetable beds, even an occasional visiting Clydesdale provide interesting diversions that motivate people to go outdoors and offer relief from the interior environment.

Most people in the early and middle stages of dementia–even beyond still love getting outside. Those in middle to late-stages of dementia often respond to more peaceful, calm environments while many less severely impaired residents delight in an active and stimulating environment. This brings us again to the interesting dilemma of why we don't we find more older adults enjoying the garden?

Identifying potential pitfalls and developing appropriate outdoor activities and programs before initiating design development for outdoor spaces are strategies designed to insure positive outdoor environments and enjoyable experiences for residents with Alzheimer's disease.

DESIGN ISSUES

- The *layout* of the garden must be easily understood. To minimize confusion for cognitively impaired individuals the layout must be simplified. Larger garden spaces can be divided into areas of varying size and level of privacy. Some spaces are designed for socializing and a higher activity level, while other parts of the garden are designed for privacy. Various spaces can accommodate walking, exercise, gardening, visiting with other residents, family and visitors or places to sit comfortably in privacy.
- *Safety and security* are important. If the garden is not secure and designed to support safe, independent mobility staff won't feel comfortable letting residents outside on their own. Doors remain locked–an obvious impediment to using outdoor environments. To encourage the use of outdoor spaces the design must adequately address safety concerns and accommodate for diminished physical capacity. Decreased strength, endurance, balance and co-ordination, as well as diminished visual acuity are all factors associated with falls in the elderly.
- Visibility of garden spaces from inside by both staff and residents is critical to its use. Highly visible outdoor spaces help to maximize staff comfort levels about residents being outside. Providing several easily accessible, unlocked doors increases access to the outside. Locked doors increase frustration for individuals who resent being confined, and they may express their resentment in aggressive behavior.
- Visible connection to destinations is important. Some residents can become easily disoriented and need recognizable clues to lead them back to a more familiar area.
- *Walking.* Walking benefits residents and caregivers alike and provides a high degree of self managed healthy exercise. There is no question that for elders walking can be accompanied by risks however, the benefits of improved muscle tone, increased appetite and enhanced social opportu-

nities are significant. The environment should support walking in both interior and exterior settings.

- *Walking paths* are opportunities for innovation. Places for socialization and activity, for example, can be woven into the path as destinations making the walk significantly more interesting. Seating areas along the walking path give walkers and watchers an opportunity for greeting and conversing with others. These and other creative strategies encourage mobility and exercise.
- *Places to sit*–The more opportunities there are to sit and rest the more likely it is that older adults will get out and walk. It pays to provide plenty of comfortable seating along walking paths, allowing places to rest, places to enjoy watching birds at the feeder, rabbits, squirrels, cats, dogs and other visiting pets and animals, as well as to engage in nearby activities.
- *Proper size seating*–Size and design are important. Much of the furniture designed today for outdoor use is inappropriate and unsafe for frail older adults. The selection of garden furniture is often inappropriately based on personal preference rather than the special needs of older adults. Poorly balanced or poorly constructed furniture is unsafe and oversized seating is uncomfortable for sitting too and difficult to get up and out of the chair safely. Many finishes are too rough for fragile skin. Whether selection is at the discretion of the landscape designer or someone else, there is an obligation to insure the seating is comfortable and safe for the primary users.
- *Activities* such as raking leaves, sweeping the walkways, filling bird feeders, watering flowers, various types of gardening or even hanging clothes on a clothes line can stimulate long term memory of home life or professional tasks.
- *Gardening* is a familiar activity for many residents and provides an opportunity to plant and raise vegetables for meals. This gives individuals an opportunity to contribute to their community and a way to positively affect self-esteem. Raised planters allow residents to sit or stand while gardening rather than having to get down on hands and knees.
- *Outdoor activities that include staff* enhance staff comfort levels by allowing them to keep an eye out for those who might need help. A generous size pavilion to accommodates tables, chairs and storage for supplies is a wonderful sheltered space for activities such as arts and crafts, painting classes, gardening, flower arranging, even outdoor concerts. The pavilion can be screened and include lighting and a fan for ventilation. If you're stumped for activity ideas check with the experts–adult day care programs.

- *Exercise* Early morning walks provide essential light exposure, exercise and an opportunity to spend time outdoors. Create new opportunities for active participation in exercise programs such as Tai Chi, which helps to develops good balance. If there is no activity, nothing going on–no action, it is more difficult to get residents outside.
- *Opportunities for social engagement* are enhanced by careful design planning and the arrangement of spaces. Older adults prefer shaded places when the sun is bright. Seating areas under the trees can filter sunlight and give the illusion of privacy while tables with adjustable umbrellas provide shaded areas for protection from the sun and shelter from showers. Interestingly, accommodating the need for privacy may actually encourage socialization.
- *Transition spaces*–Porches are transition spaces that provide an invitation and a way of beginning to ease residents to the outdoors. Rocking chairs often entice reluctant residents outdoors to rock and watch the activities in the garden. A cup of coffee or tea, snacks or food on the porch can be incentives or first steps to the walking path and other activities. Transition spaces are vitally important in linking older adults to the outdoor environment. It is important to recognize in the progressive course of dementia individuals are likely to become less capable of initiating behavior–even walking through the door to reach the porch. Many other elders don't see or hear well and added to diminished strength and stamina, walking itself can be difficult.

CREATING A BEAUTIFUL GARDEN IS NOT ENOUGH!

Only recently have care settings for those with Alzheimer's disease begun to focus on the potential therapeutic value of the outside environment and encouraging older adults to spend time outdoors in fresh air and sunlight. Simply being outdoors is therapeutic in the most basic sense but the ability to go outside takes on added significance for those who have lost much of what they were once able to do.

For example, walking outdoors can help to reduce agitation while allowing persons with dementia to experience the benefits of fresh air and sunlight, vital to good health, better quality sleep patterns, and increased well-being (Brawley, 2005). Additionally, by accommodating activities in carefully designed outdoor environments there is enormous potential for increasing the variety and flexibility of activity spaces that are always in short supply.

A garden will never be successful if it is not used, which often has as much to do with policies and staff concerns as it does with the design of the garden space. While many factors that contribute to poor results can be identified, the basic flaw is the process itself. Talented landscape designers are often commissioned to create beautiful gardens that are a pleasure to behold and a watershed for the marketing group, but don't seem to attract residents. After all their planning and hard work, these designers often seem as mystified as many others as to why the gardens go unused. Delivering a beautiful garden is not enough!

The traditional process is one that involves the selection of a design firm, identifying priorities, designating tasks, and periodic meetings for progress reports and review. Everyone is very busy as each group operates in its own vacuum, completing individual assigned tasks. They come together, report on results and move on to another project. Too many contributors work independently. Tasks are completed but the process is not one that inspires an abundance of interchange, creativity or excitement.

Post occupancy evaluation is rarely used to evaluate results, in fact it is rarely used at all. Questions such as what were the project goals? Did the outdoor space meet the project goals? Is it being used the way it was intended? Do residents spend more time outside? Has the garden helped to increase mobility and exercise? Is it being properly maintained? These are all important questions designed to determine what works, what doesn't and what changes might improve results. These questions should be asked and the responses used to evaluate results, to learn from the experience, to share valuable information and to inspire better design for gardens and outdoor spaces for persons with Alzheimer's disease and other frail, vulnerable older adults.

Care settings involved in culture change have turned this process up side down. The decision to create a garden is fully supported by the administration, from the top down, insuring that everyone is actively involved with total support and participation from all levels of management. Culture change recognizes that staff participation in planning and design is *essential* and encourages direct care-staff involvement throughout the process rather than just a 15 minute meeting for input and a final meeting to announce the opening of the garden. Ultimately staff reactions will influence the success of the project. For example, their comfort level for safety and security determines if the doors are locked or unlocked. Their level of enthusiasm for the potential of the garden creates excitement about the prospects, planning activities and creating way to encourage residents to go outdoors. Are they finding ways to be outdoors themselves? This is an approach that empowers staff, inspires creativity and dedication and is proving highly successful.

Simply creating a beautiful garden is guaranteed to create far less enthusiasm and excitement with staff than a garden they have actively contributed to and been involved with developing from its inception. Selecting one or two staff representatives to be committee members during design development fosters a sense of inclusion. Continuing participation and active involvement throughout are hallmarks of the process. It creates the kind of excitement that is contagious, a positive investment in the outcome and a very real sense of ownership. The garden becomes *their* garden long before it is ever completed. They are able to solicit valuable feedback from other staff members and often prove to be a source of excellent ideas.

The activity program, so essential to a successful Alzheimer care setting, will positively benefit from creative care-staff input. A successful, well organized activity program insures that current activities are working for residents and allows opportunities to adapt and expand these programs with some assurance of success.

Too often various activities are identified and placed on a list for the landscape designer to accommodate in the garden rather than incorporating current successful activity programs. Without understanding how the abilities of younger adults differ from the special needs of frail older adults, for example, a space designed for T'ai Chi, may go unused. A more productive strategy would have staff and activity program specialists working together to develop and agree on an effective program for the outdoors. The environment can then be designed to better accommodate and support specific activities and functions that help to insure the overall success of the garden.

Landscape designers who are willing to "jump in" and participate *with* residents in many of these programs will better understand how the design must adapt to special needs. Understanding expectations makes it easier to provide for more activities and this is the best on the job training available for designers. Their willingness to participate is invaluable in building comfortable relationships with staff, who contribute so many valuable ideas, teach so much and ultimately strongly influence the success of the garden.

GARDENS ARE ABOUT QUALITY OF LIFE

Gardens are more than just another amenity or form of therapy. They are ultimately about quality of life. We miss an enormous opportunity to enrich lives, contribute to better quality care and a better quality of life if we think of design only as decoration. Improving the aesthetics would be a positive benefit for many long-term care settings, but using design strategies to create imaginative, safe, secure gardens and outdoor environments that concentrate on meeting the special needs of vulnerable residents can be a special gift!

Gardens should be considered as preventative medicine. They nurture and support residents with dementia and provide quality spaces for rest and renewal for families and staff. Perhaps the greatest strength of the garden is to bring a healthier sense of calm and well being, as individuals are buffeted by forces around them, With more persuasive information on the behavioral, medical and social benefits of outdoor environments, it is hoped that more gardens and outdoor spaces will be implemented early when they have the greatest impact for aging residents. Our challenge is to encourage research.

BIBLIOGRAPHY

Alzheimer's Association. Alzheimer's disease and the U.S. Population. 2001. Chicago, IL.

Ancoli-Israel, S., Jones, D.W., Hanger, M.A., Parker, L., Klauber, M.R., Kripke, D.F. 1991. Sleep in the nursing home. In S. T. Kuna, et al., eds. *Sleep and Respiration in Aging Adults.* Elsevier Science Publishing Co.

Berg, L., K.C., Buckwalter, P.K., Chafez, L.P., Gwyther, D., Holmes, K., Koepke, Lawton, M. P., Lindeman, Magaziner, J., Maslow, K., Morley, J., Ory, M., Rabins, P., Sloan, P. D., and Teresi, 1991. Special Care Units for Persons with Dementia. *Journal of American Geriatrics Society.* Vol. 30, No. 12(December, 1991): 1229-1236.

Brawley, E. 2005. *Design Innovations for Aging and Alzheimer's: Creating Caring Environments.* New York: John Wiley & Sons, Inc.

Brawley, E. 2002. Therapeutic Gardens for individuals with Alzheimer's Disease. *Alzheimer's Care Quarterly,* vol. 3 (Winter 2002): 7-11.

Brawley, E. 1997. *Designing for Alzheimer's Disease: Strategies for Creating Better Care Environments.* New York: John Wiley & Sons.

Centers for Disease Control and Prevention National Center for Injury Prevention and Control. 1999. *Falls in Nursing Homes.*

Chen, C., Sloane, P. D., and Dalton, T. 2003. Lighting and Circadian Rhythms and Sleep in Older Adults. *Electric Power Research.*

Clapin-French, E. 1986. Sleep patterns of aged persons in long-term care facilities. *Journal of Advanced Nursing.* 11:57-66.

Cooper Marcus, C., and Barnes, M. 1995. *Gardens in Healthcare Facilities: Uses, Therapeutic Benefits, and Design Recommendations.* Martinez, CA: The Center for Health Design.

Cooper Marcus, C., and Barnes, M. 1999. *Healing Gardens: Therapeutic Benefits and Design Recommendations.* New York: John Wiley & Sons, Inc.

Fagan, R. 2000. "Recreating Our Nursing Homes Through Culture Change." *Elders with Illness.* April, 2000: 21.

Fagan, R.M. "Pioneer Network: Changing the Culture of Aging in America." In A. Weiner, and J. Ronch, (eds.). 2002. *Culture Change in Long-Term Care,* (Vol. 2). New York: Haworth Social Work Practice Press.

Fagan, R.M. 2002. "Turning the Tables: who directs care at your community? Staff or Residents?" *Assisted Living Today.* October 2002: 36-38.

Gill, T., Williams, C., Tinetti, M. 2000. Environmental Hazards and the Risk of Nonsyncopal Falls in the Homes of Community-Living Older Persons. *Medical Care.* (38)12:1174-1183. Philadelphia: Lippincott Williams & Wilkins Inc.

Gold, D.T., Sloane, P. D., Matthews, L., Bledsoe, M., and Konanc, D. 1991. Special Care Units: A Typology of Care Settings for Memory-Impaired Older Adults. *Gerontologist.* Vol. 31, No.4 (August 1991): 467-475.

Hartig, T. et al. 1990. *Perspectives on Wilderness: Testing the Theory of Restorative Environments.* The Use of Wilderness for Personal Growth Therapy and Education. General Technical Report RM 193. Ft. Collins, CO: United States

Holick, M. 2002. "Vitamin D: A Required Supplement or a Sunshine Hormone." The Fifth International Lighting Research Office Lighting Research Symposium–Lighting and Human Health (November 3-5, 2002).

Holick, M. 1994. "Vitamin D–New Horizons for the 21st Century." McCollum Award Lecture. *American Journal of Clinical Nutrition.* 619-630.

Honeyman, M. 1987. Vegetation and Stress: A comparison study of varying amounts of vegetation in countryside and urban scenes. Manhattan, KS: Kansas State University, MLA Thesis.

Kaplan, S, Talbot, J. 1983. Psychological Benefits of a Wilderness Experience. In I. Altman, and J. F. Wohlwil (eds.). *Behavior and the Natural Environment.* New York: Plenum.

Lawton, M.P. 1989. Environmental Approaches to Research and Treatment of Alzheimer's Disease. In E. Light, and B.D. Lebowitz, (Eds.) *Alzheimer's Disease Treatment and Family Stress: Directions for Research.* Rockville, MD: National Institute of Mental Health, U.S. Department of Health and Human Services.

Mishima, K, Okawa, M., Hishikawa, Y., Hozumi, S., Hori, H., Takahashi, K. 1994. Morning bright light therapy for sleep and behavior disorders in elderly patients with dementia. *Acta Psychiatrica Scandinavica.* 1994: 89: 1-7.

National Commission on Sleep Disorders Research. 1993. Wake Up America: A National Sleep Alert. Submitted to the U.S. Congress and to the Secretary of the U.S. Department of Health and Human Services.

Ohta, R.J., and Ohta, B.M. 1988. Special Units for Alzheimer's Disease Patients: A Critical Look, *Gerontologist.* Vol. 28, No.6 :803-808.

Ory, M., Rabins, P., Sloane, P.D., and Teresi, J. 1991. Special Care Units for Persons with Dementia. *Journal of American Geriatrics Society.* Vol. 30, No. 12: 1229-1236.

Rea, M., Figueiro, M., and Bullough, J. 2002. "Circadian Photobiology: An Emerging Framework for Lighting Practice and Research." *Lighting Research Technology,* Vol. 34, No. 3: 177-190.

Rimmer, J., 2004. Exercise Can Ease Chronic Conditions. *Aging Today.* January- February, XXV: 7-9.

Roberts, J. 2002. "Light Interactions with the Human Eye as a Function of Age." Fifth International Lighting Research Symposium–Light and Human Health (November 3-5, 2002).

Ruuskanen, J., Parketti, T. 1994. Physical Activity and Related Factors among Nursing Home Residents. *Journal of the American Geriatric Society,* 42: 987-991.

Sloane, P., Zimmerman, S., Suchindran, C., Reed, P., Lily Wang, L., Boustani, M., and

Sudha, S. 2002. The Public Health Impact of Alzheimer's Disease, 2000-2050: Potential Implication of Treatment Advances. *Annals of Public Health Review,* 23: 213-231.

Ulrich, R. 1979. Visual Landscapes and Psychological Well-Being. *Landscape Research,* 4: 17-23.

Ulrich, R. 1984. View Through a Window May Influence Recovery from Surgery. *Science,* 224: 420-421.

Ulrich, R. 1986. Human Responses to Vegetation and Landscape. *Landscape and Planning, 13*: 29-44.

Van Someren, E., Hagebeuk, E., Lijzenga, C., Scheltens, P., DeRooji, S., Jonker, C., Pot, A., Mirmiran, M., and Swaab, D. 1996. "Circadian Rest-Activity Rhythm Disturbances in Alzheimer's Disease." *Biological Psychiatry.* Vol. 40 : 259-270.

U.S. Department of Health and Human Services. 2002. A Profile of Older Americans. Hyattsville, MD: U.S. Department of Health and Human Services.

doi:10.1300/J081v21n03_14

Garden of the Family Life Center, Grand Rapids, Michigan

Clare Cooper Marcus

SUMMARY. Landscape architects are often asked to design and install outdoor space for older adults with Alzheimer's disease and other dementias. This paper explores behavioral issues and the process of outdoor design for dementia, from the perspective of a landscape architect focused on therapeutic use of outdoor gardens. Specific design recommendations are followed by a case study of an exemplary garden, with experiential descriptions of usage by residents, staff and families. doi:10.1300/J081v21n03_15 *[Article copies available for a fee from The Haworth Document Delivery Service: 1-800-HAWORTH. E-mail address: <docdelivery@haworthpress.com> Website: <http://www.HaworthPress.com>*

KEYWORDS. Alzheimer's, garden, design elements, therapeutic, outdoor, landscape, plantings

Clare Cooper Marcus is Professor Emerita, Department of Landscape Architecture, University of California, Berkeley (E-mail: clare@mygarden.com).

She is the author/co-author/editor of several books including *Housing as if People Mattered, People Places, House as a Mirror of Self*, and *Healing Gardens*. She speaks internationally on the topic of outdoor space in healthcare facilities, and is the Principal of Healing Landscapes, Berkeley, CA

This article is republished with permission from *Landscape Architecture*, as a revised version of "No Ordinary Garden," published in March 2005, Volume 95, No. 3, 26-39.

[Haworth co-indexing entry note]: "Garden of the Family Life Center. Grand Rapids, Michigan." Cooper Marcus. Clare. Co-published simultaneously in *Journal of Housing for the Elderly* (The Haworth Press, Inc.) Vol. 21, No. 3/4, 2007, pp. 285-304; and: *Outdoor Environments for People with Dementia* (ed: Susan Rodiek and Benyamin Schwarz) The Haworth Press, Inc., 2007, pp. 285-304 Single or multiple copies of this article are available for a fee from The Haworth Document Delivery Service [1-800-HAWORTH. 9:00 a.m. - 5:00 p.m. (EST). E-mail address: docdelivery@haworthpress.com].

Available online at http://jhe.haworthpress.com
doi:10.1300/J081v21n03_15

INTRODUCTION

With the aging of the US population and larger numbers afflicted with dementias, restorative settings are expected to be more and more in demand. Today, approximately 10 percent of those over 65 have Alzheimer's disease, with the percentage nearly five times that (47.2 percent) among the group over 85. In 2050, the US will have 67.5 million people over the age of 65, over two and a half times the 25.5 million there were in 1990. If a cure or significant means of prevention is not found soon, the Alzheimer's Association estimated that 12 to 14 million Americans will be affected by the year 2040.

Landscape architects need to become familiar with, and advocates for, the particular needs of dementia patients and their care givers so that appropriate, supportive environments become an important component in the whole spectrum of care. Gardens for people with Alzheimer's disease present clients and designers with a very special set of opportunities and challenges, summarized thus by John Zeisel and Martha Tyson (Zeisel and Tyson, 1999, p. 501).

- "To provide a prosthetic environment that is also spiritual and uplifting.
- To create a safe place that supports independence while remaining interesting and challenging.
- To respond to a complex set of needs . . . while being easy to understand without instructions.
- To enliven gardens with events while promoting places for people to relax alone . . .

To provide healing opportunities for residents while participating in garden life or observing its use."

CREATING GARDENS FOR PEOPLE WITH DEMENTIA

From the perspective of landscape design, here, in brief, are some of the main issues a designer must consider when creating a successful garden for people with Alzheimer's disease and other forms of dementia. The case study garden at the Family Life Center in Grand Rapids illustrates many of these essential qualities.

Visibility and accessibility. Patients need to know that a garden or courtyard is available for use by seeing it from a well-used interior space (activity room, dining room, etc.). There must also be easy access from that space into the garden. A less clear or more circuitous access route may trigger frustration, even anger and aggression on the part of the patients. It is preferable that there only be one access door. Patients can easily become confused and need to know that the door they exited is the one they return to. To ease supervision, the whole garden should also be visible by staff who bring patients outside. If patients go out alone, the whole garden should ideally be visible from an interior nurses' station. In some situations where this is not the case, staff keep the exterior door locked, thus precluding patients from the benefits of spending time outdoors (Grant, 2003).

Provide a Covered Patio or Terrace

One of the features most often overlooked is a shaded patio or terrace right outside the access door (Cooper Marcus and Barnes, 1999; Grant, 2003; Mahan, 2004). Many patients like to sit and view the garden while remaining close to the building's amenities; some like to go out when it rains to smell the ozone; many programmed activities (barbecue, crafts, etc.) need a hard-surface area with tables, provisions for sitting in the sun or shade and enough space for a group activity, people in wheelchairs, etc.

A Simple Path System

Alzheimer's patients often engage in "wandering" behavior so places to walk are essential. Since many have cognitive problems with spatial orientation, it is imperative that the circulation consist of a simple returning path system (looped, circular, figure of eight, bisected loop) with a minimum of choice points which may cause confusion, and no dead ends. Where space is tight, a continuous loop can be created with an outdoor path and a parallel interior corridor.

Path Design

As we age, our eyes are less able to cope with the glare caused by light bouncing off light-colored materials (or by oncoming headlights). Hence outdoor spaces for all older adults should have paths of tinted concrete with strong edge delineation. Ideally, paths should be a minimum of six feet wide and of brushed concrete for good traction.

Destination Points

To encourage people to walk–which is healthy at every age–a garden for dementia patients needs visible and memorable destination points such as a seating arbor or gazebo at one or more places along the looped path system.

FIGURE 1. Easy transition from the inside to the outside through a marked threshold

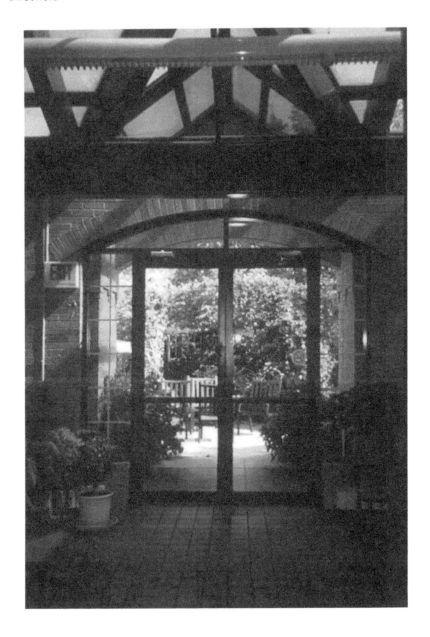

FIGURE 2. A brick-paved pathway the loops around permits garden users a choice of route without creating confusion.

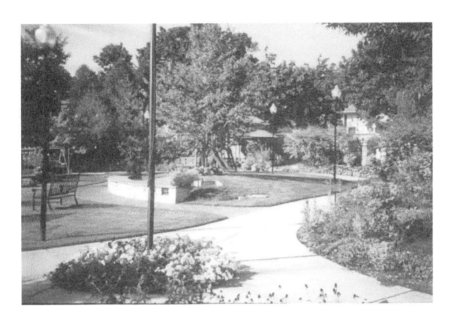

Ample Seating

Dementia patients are often restless and engage in pacing behavior along with a brief rest, then pacing again. It is important to provide plenty of seating of different types (fixed, movable, a glider or swing seat) in different locations, and with a choice of sun or shade. All seating should have sturdy arms projecting just beyond the seat edge to facilitate an older person pushing themselves up from a seated position.

Create an Outdoor Space That is Domestic in Scale and Appropriate to Local Culture

Research indicates that residents exhibit fewer dementia symptoms in more familiar homelike environments than in larger institutional settings. This finding should also apply to outdoor space, as the Family Life Center garden case study beautifully illustrates. Since many Alzheimer's patients recall details from their childhood, the design should incorporate plants and other elements which might trigger long-ago memories. For example, landscape architect Edward Stillinger, on discovering most of the residents of a new facility in Victoria, BC had grown up on the Canadian prairies, incorporated prairie grass, a typical back yard shed, and a large outdoor thermometer in his design.

A lawn provides an area for programmed events (movable chairs in a circle, barbecue, croquet, etc.) as well as being a reflection of the home settings of many patients.

Features to stimulate activities reminiscent of daily routines at home are often provided in Alzheimer's gardens, including washing lines for hanging clothes, cans for watering, brooms for sweeping paths. In one Canadian facility in Victoria, BC, an old red Buick is bolted down on a concrete slab; residents wash the car and "go for a drive."

Space for gardening activities. Simple gardening tasks provide an opportunity for people suffering from dementia to engage in familiar activities. A small working garden, a garden shed, raised beds, a potting table accessible by a person in a wheelchair, and outdoor faucets can support gardening, whether in a formal horticultural therapy program, or informal activities with family members.

FIGURE 3. Movable furniture facilitate the creation of conversational grouping on the lawn.

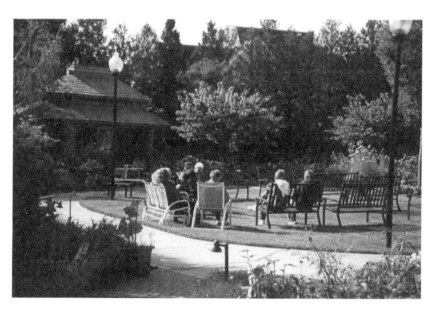

Provide ample shade. In recent post-occupancy evaluations of eight east coast Alzheimer's facilities, Catherine Mahan, FASLA, and colleagues noted that shade was often woefully inadequate (Mahan, 2004). Since one characteristic of Alzheimer's patients is that they have difficulty recognizing when they are too hot and would not think to put on a hat or sun block, adequate shade is essential. This can be provided by umbrellas, trees, canopies, solid-roofed arbors or gazebos. Slatted roofs should be avoided since the shadows of slats on paving can be perceived as depressions and thus be confusing, as also can the juxtaposition of dark and light paving. Shade provided by a canopy or vine-covered arbor is essential at all exit doors since the eyes of Alzheimer's patients–as is true for all elderly people–have difficulty adjusting from indoor light levels to bright sunlight.

Maximize Planting of a Wide Variety of Perennials

Funds for garden maintenance are often limited; the planting and re-planting of annuals can be costly. Perennials should be selected to reflect what might

FIGURE 4. An arbor marks the transition from a working garden with raised beds and a small orchard into a large area with lawns, paths, perennial beds and places to sit.

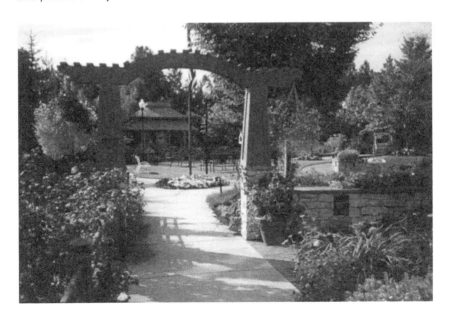

have been familiar flowers in the youth of the residents, to create color throughout the seasons, and to provide elements to be used in craft activities. In areas with snowy winters, select trees and shrubs with interesting and colorful branching systems.

Avoid Poisonous Plants

In late stage Alzheimer's disease, people tend to put everything into their mouth, whether suitable or not. To relieve staff of the responsibility of watching every patient at every moment, plants which have any toxic component should be avoided. Commonly used poisonous plants which could be quite appropriate in another situation include azalea, black-eyed susan, bleeding heart, chrysanthemum, daphne, daffodil (bulbs), English holly, English ivy, foxglove, hydrangea, lily of the valley, lupine, mistletoe, monkshood, oleander, poinsettia, St. John's wort, spider plant, wisteria, yew. (For additional information on toxic plants see www. ansci.cornell.edu.) If a facility has separate units and gardens for those in the early, moderate and late stages of Alzheimer's disease, it should be noted that plant toxicity is not an issue for those in the early stage.

A Sense of Enclosure

An outdoor space for dementia patients needs to be securely enclosed with a fence, walk or railings screened with vegetation so that patients seeking to "find their way home" are not tempted to leave. A gate to enable maintenance staff to enter, or residents to leave in an emergency, needs to be subtly located and/or designed to look like part of an opaque fence, not recognized by residents as "the way out."

Involve management and staff in the design of the garden. Research indicates that management policies and staff attitudes and training affect the success of outdoor space in a facility for dementia patients as much as–or more than–the actual garden design (Grant, 2003).

Case Study: Family Life Center, Grand Rapids, Michigan

Entering the Family Life Center garden on a sunny morning in early October, one is immediately entranced by the colors of autumn flowers, the sounds of falling water, the feel of a secure, restful refuge. And that is exactly what it is for the twenty-five or so people who live at home with their families but who come here, to the Sophia Louise Durbridge-Wege Living Gardens almost every day. Some were professional people, heads of corporations; others never worked anywhere outside the home. Now approximately half have Alzheimer's disease; the remainder have other forms of dementia, schizophrenia,

FIGURE 5. The garden offers places to sit in an enclosed space

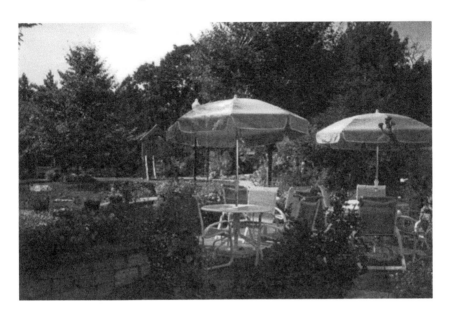

MS, Parkinson's or Huntington's Disease. The oldest patient is 90, the youngest 36.

Several aides bring patients out and a group of nine pull their chairs around in a semi-circle on the lawn to talk about the garden—the colors and sounds; ripe beans and tomatoes people can take home. A man comes outside and sits swinging in a glider, some distance away. Another man who is restless listens for a while and then paces impatiently back into the building and out again. The lone man on the glider gets up, walks past the grotto and starts eating ripe cherry tomatoes off the vine.

"What are the flowers you can see?" asks a staff member sitting with the group.

No one answers.

"What about the yellow ones you can see all over?"

"Marigolds?" someone answers.

"Yes, that's right! Mary, the gardener says we can pick straw flowers this afternoon . . ."

FIGURE 6. Site plan for the Family Life Center garden in Grand Rapids, Michigan

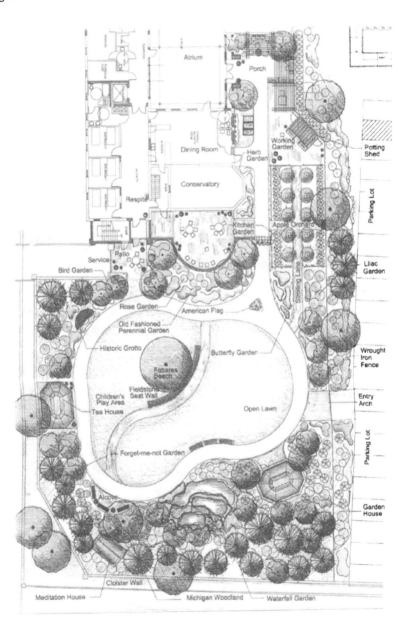

Another aide approaches the group. "Anyone want to help me pick some beans?" Two women get up and follow her to the vegetable garden on the east side of the building.

This garden was designed by Martha Tyson of Douglas Hills Associates for individuals with Alzheimer's and other forms of dementia; it was the first of its type in Michigan. There are two main components to the half-acre Living Gardens: the main strolling and viewing garden, and the working garden. The working garden is a rectangular area east of the building with raised beds and trellises for horticultural therapy; a potting area with shade and a sink; a garden shed; a small orchard; a butterfly garden; and an area for seating with umbrellas for shade near the atrium entry door. The larger component of the garden entered via an arbor from the working garden consists of lawns, paths, perennial beds, gazebos, a waterfall and pond, and various places to sit.

The garden was financed entirely by private donations resulting from a very successful fundraising campaign organized by Cindi Longchamps, former Director of the Center. Money was donated by many individuals and companies, the largest donation coming from Peter Wege, CEO of the Steelcase Company, which has its headquarters in Grand Rapids. The garden is named in honor of his mother.

The garden opened in 1999 and is maintained by a staff gardener who works three days a week, and a landscaping service which comes once a week. Maintenance is financed through endowments as well as by renting the outdoor space for weddings and receptions. (This practice has recently been discontinued due to vandalism of plants and clean-up costs.) In the first three years of the garden's operation, a grant covered the costs of a successful horticultural therapy program, but since change of ownership of the Family Life Center, this formal program has been discontinued.

The Family Life Center (founded in 1991) is housed in what was once a convent. One wing of the Center houses a six-bed residential facility for the elderly mentally ill. The day-center building consists of a large activity space (formerly the convent chapel), a kitchen and administrative offices. With views and access to the garden are a dining/activity room, and a large glass-roofed atrium with a fountain, tile floor and many plants. Overlooking the entire garden is a large conservatory, heavily used in colder weather for indoor horticulturally related activities–sorting seeds, sowing seeds, pressing flowers, turning gourds into bird feeders. (Raising plants under grow-lights in winter was enhanced when local police donated the lights seized in a marijuana-growing bust.)

In any healthcare facility garden, it is very important that potential users know it is there and have easy access into it. This is especially so where users are individuals with dementia, for whom graphic signage or a circuitous route

FIGURE 7. The garden includes a waterfall and a pool

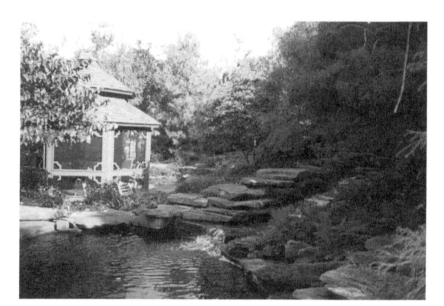

would be daunting. The Family Life Center has spacious views to the garden and entries into it primarily from the atrium, and secondarily from the dining room. The doors remain unlocked during the day.

Daily life at the Center revolves around programmed indoor activities (Social Hour, Tai Chi, Sing-along, Mood Music, etc.), and two visits each day (weather permitting) to the garden. Some of the Center's customers (this is the term preferred by the Center's staff), who do not need to be watched constantly, go freely back and forth from the building to the garden to walk, sit and smoke. But many–especially those with Alzheimer's–*do* need constant care. In late-stages of the disease, people regress to a state not unlike infancy. They have to take liquid food and will put anything they can into their mouths, including flowers or plants. Hence the necessity to use non-toxic plant material, which Tyson was careful to do in this garden.

People attending the day center are brought into the garden almost every day in good weather. The design of the garden works extraordinarily well for these programmed activities: chairs in a semi-circle on the lawn for conversation; the Garden House (which has electricity) for listening to music and singing; a flat lawn for croquet; the concrete path for wheelchair races; a number of

FIGURE 8. A resident paces the looped pathway around the garden.

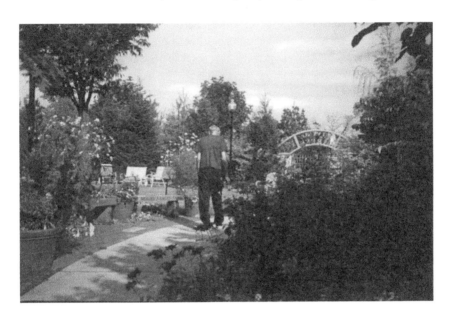

faucets for watering the flower beds; raised beds, tables and a potting shed for gardening.

"The garden also works very, very well for Physical Therapy staff working with people who have had a stroke or need help in walking," I am told by Sherry Gaines, the Program/Activity Manager as we rock gently in a glider. "It has a wonderfully calming effect on people who are agitated. We have two customers who are totally blind and two who are legally blind. They like to hear the waterfall, birds . . . We have a ratio of staff to customers of 5 to 1; when you factor in volunteers and interns, it is 2 to 1."

In a facility with such a high staff/patient ratio, it is essential that the designer bring staff into the design team. This is not a museum courtyard or a corporate plaza where the goals of the fee-paying client may dominate, or observation of a few similar settings may provide sufficient user-information. A garden such as this is an important component of daily therapy; for some, it may be just as important as a dose of medication. The design of the Living Gardens is successful because it included so many significant actors in the design process, in addition to the landscape architect. These included representatives of the families who were using the Center; the Center's staff; and horticultural therapists from the Meijer Botanical Garden, Grand Rapids.

Consulting advice was also sought from Gene Rothert, the Chicago Botanic Garden; landscape horticultural students from Michigan State; garden designers from a Grand Rapids nursery; and a local garden contractor. Input from such a range of experts has insured that the garden serves the needs of patients, families and staff; that the selection of plant materials is appropriate; and that built and movable features in the garden meet the needs for programmed activities.

Martha Tyson is uniquely qualified to design this type of garden. Courses in cultural geography during her BLA studies at the University of Minnesota alerted her to interactions between people and the physical environment. Nursing home visits to elderly relatives who had grown up on farms and yearned to be outdoors aroused Tyson's sensibilities. Not only was there a meager provision of outdoor space, doors to the outside were often kept locked. Her senior project was a nursing home garden.

Continuing her landscape architecture studies at the University of Illinois Urbana-Champaign, Tyson was inspired by the books of Carstens (1985) and Regnier (1985, 1995) and courses taught by Sue Weidemann, Katherine Anthony and Amita Sinha in a department long at the forefront of behavioral studies in landscape design. For her MLA thesis she studied an Alzheimer's garden in Urbana which was functioning poorly. Using behavior mapping techniques, she pinpointed the roadblocks, redesigned the space and led a team of students who installed new elements in the garden.

"Sometimes I had a hard time finding employers who wanted to follow this approach," Tyson told me. "One of them–in the mid-'80s–told me: 'Why bother to design for Alzheimer's people when they don't even know what's going on?'! But I also found good people willing to 'deal with me' and let me search out clients amenable to a behavioral and participatory emphasis."

Tyson has had her own business since 1989 and has designed approximately thirty gardens for nursing homes and Alzheimer's facilities in Minnesota, Michigan, Illinois, and Massachusetts. She keeps up with research by attending–and presenting at–at least one conference on aging each year and has herself published in the field (Tyson 1998, 1999). Her current projects include gardens for a hospice and a home for developmentally disabled men. She is also working on a line of outdoor furniture for people with disabilities.

Not only does Tyson provide for the known needs of *Alzheimer's patients* (a visually enclosed setting, no toxic plants, plants which were popular during the youth of current patients, for example), she also creatively draws upon the work of Kevin Lynch (1960) about how all of us tend to create cognitive maps of familiar places.

"Five elements by which people cognitively organize the city: paths, places, landmarks, nodes, and edges, are organizing cognitive principles that seem to hold for people with Alzheimer's as well" (Zeisel and Tyson, 1999). At the Family Life Center Garden, the *path* offers a walking route and a fundamental orienting element; specific *places* such as the working garden or the lawn provide gathering places encouraging physical and social interactions; the entry arbor, flagpole, a grotto with a statue of the Virgin Mary (50 percent of the Center's users are Roman Catholic), bird feeders hanging from trees provide *landmarks* or visible cues to aid orientation; the Tea House and Garden House create *nodes* or hubs of activity; the building, walls, fence and peripheral planting provide *edges* defining the space and offering a sense of security. Tyson is the only designer, to my knowledge, to employ Lynch's elements in garden design, particularly useful in this kind of setting since they relieve the user from having to organize a mental map, thus making it easier for those with Alzheimer's to navigate and use a garden.

A garden that meets the needs of Alzheimer's patients and their carers is no ordinary garden. Just sitting in this setting for a day, overhearing various conversations between staff, family members and patients, I began to appreciate how enormously important is the variety of flowers to look at and talk about; vegetables to touch and perhaps eat; sub-spaces where people alone or in a group can find a place to sit for a while. Such a space must allow for people to see the layout at a glance and offer a simple circular or figure-of-eight circulation system. The main garden, entered via a wooden arbor, has a clear perimeter path of tinted concrete, bisected by a curving brick pathway, thus allowing patients (who tend to pace) a number of alternatives for moving around the garden. Too many choices, however, can lead to confusion, agitation, even aggression. One trip around the six-foot wide loop path provides a 300-foot route with changing path-side details but no anxiety-provoking choices in way-finding.

Many people with Alzheimer's and other mental illnesses tend to be restless. During a one-hour period, I noticed Dwight (not his real name), a middle-aged man with schizophrenia in jeans and a check-shirt–enter and leave the garden five or six times. He walked, he sat for a while; walked some more; went back into the building; returned, joined a group that was talking, left, walked, sat, walked. Hence, a garden serving those with mental disabilities needs to provide multiple places to pause, sit, and view the garden (and be seen by the staff). The Family Life Center Garden does this in a superlative fashion. There are two wooden gazebos–or, as Tyson prefers to call them–Garden Houses. One of these has fixed perimeter seating; the other, with easily-movable, padded chairs and screened windows, looks out onto a waterfall and pond. There are three comfortable gliders alongside the perimeter path and

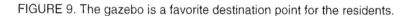

FIGURE 9. The gazebo is a favorite destination point for the residents.

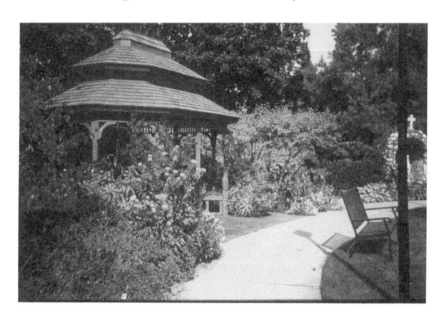

one near the potting shed; patio seating with tables and umbrellas outside the conservatory; a curved stone seating wall; and numerous movable chairs for one or two persons scattered throughout the garden.

The only unattractive seating consists of three marble slabs facing the waterfall, inscribed: "In Loving Memory. . ." This sometimes is a problem in the gardens of nursing homes, hospices, and Alzheimer's facilities: family members want to dedicate a tree, a flower border, an arbor, a bench in memory of someone who has died. One has to wonder–how is this for the living, reminded of death each time they walk in the garden? Sherry Gaines told me that several times a year, someone will ask her: "Is someone buried here?" "No, but people who loved our program so much donated money in memory of someone in their family." A better solution might have been one employed in the garden of the San Diego Hospice, where the names of donors are recorded in tiny letters on small ceramic leaves which together form an attractive *in-laid pattern* on a garden wall.

One of the characteristics of Alzheimer's patients is that they are frequently trying to "find their way home." Thus, an outdoor space or garden needs to be visually enclosed so that people are not exposed to tempting, often frustrating, views to "the outside world." Tyson's design of the Family Life Center garden fulfills this need in a functional and aesthetically pleasing manner. The garden is bounded on the north side by the building and conservatory; on the west and south sides by high walls of mellow, buff-colored brick; and on the east side (facing the parking area) by a steel fence. The walls and fence are virtually invisible, screened by a variety of trees–mostly evergreen–so that even in winter, the boundaries of the garden are blurred. One exception is a steel gate allowing entry from the parking lot for service personnel and people arriving for an event in the garden (fund raiser, memorial).

In early October, there were over twenty-five varieties of flowers in bloom at the Family Life Center Garden, including roses, zinnias, cosmos, begonia, salvias, petunias, alyssum, lobelia, nasturtium, pansies, African marigolds, cleome, clematis, sedum and pelargonium. Staff "use" these flowers to press blooms for use in arts and crafts activities, to collect seeds, to talk about the seasons and next year's garden, to stimulate conversation and memories of flowers from childhood–people with Alzheimer's may forget their name or whether they have eaten lunch, but have vivid memories of songs from their youth or of flowers from their grandmother's garden. Star jasmine and tobacco flowers stimulate a sense of smell; the feathery blooms of amaranthus, the seed-heads of cone flower tempt you to reach out and touch them. A garden needs to stimulate the senses, particularly for those who are beginning to lose their memory. Color and smell stimulate parts of the brain not reached by "intellectual" activities, and even those with little cognitive ability seem able to sense the tranquility and beauty of a garden on a precognitive, affective basis. A garden–in contrast to an unchanging building's interior–is also a cogent metaphor for observing and talking about growth, blossoming, maturity, decay, renewal.

While the boundaries of the garden are marked by moderately tall trees stepping down in height to shrubs (lilac, roses, rhododendrons, dogwood) and perennial borders, the center of the garden is open lawn which in turn is bounded by the circular concrete path and bisected by the curving brick path. The lawn towards the eastern side is flat and has movable chairs for casual seating. The slightly mounded western lawn is partially bounded by a stone seating wall (permitting transfer from a wheelchair onto the grass) and punctuated by a beech tree and a playhouse with steps and a slide. Though this might seem a surprising feature in a garden for (mostly) elderly clients, those who live in the residential wing of the facility have family visitors. For lively grandchildren such a visit may seem boring, or–if they remember their grandparent before the onset of the disease–troubling, even frightening. A play feature in the garden provides a welcome diversion.

In one corner of the garden, just outside the staff room is a sheltered corner with movable chairs, umbrella and a barbecue; this is a seating area for patients in the residential wing and for the staff. "How do you like our garden?" asks a staff member who comes outside for a smoke, a bunch of keys jangling at her belt. I am sitting nearby on the patio, writing. "It's our little bit of heaven." She gestures to the blooms of cosmos and cleome, moving in a light breeze. For the staff here, as in any healthcare facility, the garden provides an essential respite from the stress of work and the demands of patients. Though (in my observations) few leave this patio, they still have an expansive view of the garden, its colors and innumerable shades of green, the sound of birdsong and breezes moving through the trees. All of these have a remarkable effect on reducing stress, even, as researchers Roger Ulrich and Terry Hartig have discovered, in as short a time as five minutes (Ulrich, 1991; Hartig, 1993).

Not only does this garden work extraordinarily well and provide a beautiful, colorful refuge for those who use it daily, it also provides a soothing milieu for occasional users and important ceremonies. Hope Network which owns the Family Life Center also owns other facilities in the area. In one such facility, for example, the seriously mentally ill live in a locked facility where the only outdoor space is a parking lot. Sometimes residents in these facilities come to the Living Gardens for a picnic.

Other occasional users are family members in a support group which has its quarterly meeting at the Family Life Center. "We start out in the garden," Sherry Gaines informs me. "I tell them: 'Leave your stress at the door. Walk or sit; just be by yourself.' Later, we gather in the gazebo for pizza and lemonade, and talk about the care-giving journey. Many of these people are grieving for the loss of a companion, a husband or wife of fifty or sixty years who now doesn't recognize who they are. For some, it's the first time they've met someone else in the same situation."

I must confess I barely took note of a flagpole in the garden until Sherry Gaines took me on a tour and explained its significance for occasional ceremonies. "This is very important to us," she said. "We have several gentlemen patients who are veterans–several from World War Two. They feel they've been forgotten so every national or patriotic holiday, we come out here, one raises the flag, the others salute, and then we all hug them and thank them for what they did for our country."

Perhaps the only element in this garden that doesn't work so well is the Waterfall Garden. The sound of falling water adds a soothing touch, but to curb those patients who might try to get *into* the water, the pond and waterfall had to be largely screened from view by shrubs at the southern end of the garden.

To understand the importance of gardens such as this one, we need more post-occupancy evaluation studies such as that conducted by Charlotte Grant for her Ph.D. at Georgia Institute of Technology (see sidebar and map). Another recent study shows just how important a garden can be in the care of dementia patients.

Julie Galbraith and Joanne Westphal studied the Martin Luther Alzheimer Garden at a Third State Alzheimer's Dementia Unit in Holt, MI, and reported their findings at the recent ASLA conference in Salt Lake City. The garden was constructed in Fall, 1999. The following year, nursing records were examined for eight variables (aggressive and non-aggressive behavior; physician ordered and as needed medications; pulse rate; diastolic and systolic blood pressure; and weight change) during April and May (pre-garden use) and July and August (high garden use). When the variables were compared with the amount of time residents spent outside, residents showed significant improvements on virtually every parameter (one stayed the same; none deteriorated) with as little as 10-15 minutes of unprogrammed activity in the garden each day during the summer months.

A significant result like this can translate into substantial savings in staff stress, the cost of medications, and other important benefits. Landscape architects need to have this kind of information ready to quote to potential clients to convince them that investment in a garden for a dementia unit will not only create a restorative setting for patients and staff, but is likely to lead to long-term financial savings.

PROJECT CREDITS

Client: The Family Life Center, Grand Rapids, MI
Landscape Architect: Douglas Hills Associates, Evanston, IL
Project Landscape Architects: Martha Tyson, Elizabeth Dunn, Jeanne Senis.
Landscape Contractor: Everett Nursery, Grand Rapids, MI
Consultants: Gene Rothert, Chicago Botanic Garden; Horticultural Therapy Professional Group, Meijer Botanic Garden, Grand Rapids, MI; Landscape Horticulture students, Michigan State University, with Professor Ron McCollum, Storm Hill Nursery, Grand Rapids, MI
Fundraiser: Cindi Longchamps, Director, The Family Life Center

REFERENCES

Carstens, D.Y. (1985). *Site Planning and Design for the Elderly: Issues, Guidelines and Alternatives.* New York: Van Nostrand Reinhold.
Galbraith, J. and Westphal, J. (2004). "Therapeutic Garden Design: Martin Luther Alzheimer Garden," *Proceedings of ASLA Conference,* Salt Lake City.

Grant, C. (2003). *Factors influencing the use of outdoor space by residents with dementia in long-term care facilities.* Ph.D. thesis, Dept. of Architecture, Georgia Institute of Technology.

Hartig, T. (1993). *Testing Restorative Environments Theory.* Unpublished Doctoral Dissertation, Program in Social Ecology, University of California, Irvine.

Lynch, K. (1960). *The Image of the City.* Cambridge, MA: MIT Press.

Mahan, C. (2004). "Lessons Learned: Post Occupancy Evaluation of Eight Dementia Facilities," *Proceedings of ASLA Conference,* Salt Lake City.

Regnier, V. (1985). *Behavioral and Environmental Aspects of Outdoor Space Use in Housing for the Elderly.* Los Angeles: School of Architecture, Andrus Gerontology Center, University of Southern California .

Regnier, V. (1995). *Assisted Living for the Aged and Frail: Innovations in Design, Management and Financing.* New York: Columbia University Press.

Tyson, M. (1998). *The Healing Landscape.* New York: McGraw-Hill.

Ulrich, Roger, et al. (1991). "Stress recovery during exposure to natural and urban environments." *Journal of Environmental Psychology,* Vol. II. pp. 201-230.

Zeisel, J. & Tyson, M. (1999). Alzheimer's treatment gardens, in Clare Cooper Marcus and Marni Barnes (Eds.) *Healing Gardens: Therapeutic Benefits and Design Recommendations,* pp 437-504. New York: John Wiley and Sons, Inc.

doi:10.1300/J081v21n03_15

Index

Page numbers in *italics* designate figures; page numbers followed by "t" designate tables.

T - #0997 - 101024 - C332 - 212/152/18 - PB - 9780789038050 - Gloss Lamination